T0323225

TRANSITION TO PROFESSIONAL NURSING PRACTICE

Sara Miller McCune founded SAGE Publishing in 1965 to support the dissemination of usable knowledge and educate a global community. SAGE publishes more than 1000 journals and over 800 new books each year, spanning a wide range of subject areas. Our growing selection of library products includes archives, data, case studies and video. SAGE remains majority owned by our founder and after her lifetime will become owned by a charitable trust that secures the company's continued independence.

Los Angeles | London | New Delhi | Singapore | Washington DC | Melbourne

2ND EDITION

TRANSITION TO PROFESSIONAL NURSING PRACTICE

ROB BURTON
GRAHAM ORMROD

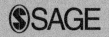

Los Angeles | London | New Delhi
Singapore | Washington DC | Melbourne

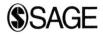

Los Angeles | London | New Delhi
Singapore | Washington DC | Melbourne

SAGE Publications Ltd
1 Oliver's Yard
55 City Road
London EC1Y 1SP

SAGE Publications Inc.
2455 Teller Road
Thousand Oaks, California 91320

SAGE Publications India Pvt Ltd
B 1/I 1 Mohan Cooperative Industrial Area
Mathura Road
New Delhi 110 044

SAGE Publications Asia-Pacific Pte Ltd
3 Church Street
#10-04 Samsung Hub
Singapore 049483

Editor: Alex Clabburn
Editorial assistant: Ozlem Merakli
Production editor: Tanya Szwarnowska
Copyeditor: Tom Bedford
Proofreader: Derek Markham
Indexer: Judith Lavender
Marketing manager: George Kimble
Cover design: Wendy Scott
Typeset by: Cenveo Publisher Services
Printed in the UK

Library of Congress Control Number: 2020932916

British Library Cataloguing in Publication data

A catalogue record for this book is available from the British Library

ISBN 978-1-5264-4465-3
ISBN 978-1-5264-4466-0 (pbk)

At SAGE we take sustainability seriously. Most of our products are printed in the UK using FSC papers and boards. When we print overseas we ensure sustainable papers are used as measured by the PREPS grading system. We undertake an annual audit to monitor our sustainability.

In memory of my mother, Gillian Burton and for
my grandchildren Isabelle and Jack, with love, Rob

Special thanks to Pat, Jake, and Polly, with love, Graham

CONTENTS

LIST OF TABLES

LIST OF FIGURES

ABOUT THE EDITORS

Associate Professor Dr **Rob Burton** is International Program Director in the School of Nursing and Midwifery, Griffith University, responsible for leading a post-registration transnational Bachelor of Nursing programme based in Singapore and leading the strategy for internationalization. He is a UK Registered Nurse (Learning Disability) and is a registered Lecturer/Practice Educator. He has been involved in Nurse Education since 1990, his previous educational career roles have encompassed contributions to teaching, delivery, development and leadership of courses at Undergraduate, Postgraduate and Doctoral levels as well as Transnational projects. His specialisms are Health Professional Education, Transition to Professional Practice, Leadership, Personal Development, Research, Internationalization and Transnational Education.

Dr **Graham Ormrod** recently retired from the University of Huddersfield where his latest role had been The Director of Health Partnerships. He has extensive experience in both teaching and management in academia and nursing practice. Previous roles have included being the Divisional Head for Acute Care at the university, and prior to joining the university he had a number of roles at the Leeds Teaching Hospitals NHS Trust, including Divisional Nurse and Associate Director of Professional Development. He has a particular interest in enhancing student nurses' experiences, exploring their shifting identities, ethical decision-making, and recognition of their accountability.

ABOUT THE CONTRIBUTORS

Dr **Angela Darvill** is a Senior Lecturer in Children's Nursing at the University of Huddersfield. Angela is also programme leader for the Postgraduate in Health Professional Education. Angela has over 20 years' experience in higher education and has been responsible for the education of nurses, mentors and lecturers. Angela engages in continuing professional development in teaching and learning pedagogy, incorporating research, scholarship and the evaluation of professional practices. Angela's PhD was a study of newly registered children's nurses' transition into children's community nursing teams. She is a Senior Fellow of the Higher Education Academy.

Dr **Nichola Barlow** qualified as a nurse in 1984 and has worked in mental health, acute medicine and acute medicine for the older person settings, before working in nurse education and undertaking a PhD in nursing ethics. Nichola now works both in education for The Open University and clinically within a palliative care setting.

Val Ely was a registered nurse for 40 years. Her career at the University of Huddersfield culminated in her becoming a principal lecturer and subject leader for continuing professional development (CPD) for all health professions other than medicine. Her early career was spent in surgery and operating departments, and she was one of the first leaders in day surgery. Since becoming an educationalist over 30 years ago, she has specialized in teaching legal and CPD issues to a mainly post registration audience. She has taught and published in non-medical prescribing and was involved in this policy initiative from its inception.

PREFACE

As you come towards the end of your nurse training, you will have developed the clinical skills needed to demonstrate your proficiency in your chosen field of practice. You will have also developed a greater awareness and appreciation of the complex roles and responsibilities of the registered nurse. In this book, you will find information and guidance that explores the issues that you will experience as you become a qualified nurse. You will need to make decisions concerning both your own practice and the practice of others. Your scope of practice will include the need to make decisions concerning those for whom you are caring, their relatives and carers, the team with which you are working, and the wider interdisciplinary team. All of these areas will generate issues with which you will be expected to deal. The main aim of the book is to provide you with reassurance about these challenges by exploring aspects of practice such as improving safety and quality of care, the legal and ethical context of clinical decision-making, accountability, leading, managing and working in teams and teaching and assessment in practice.

Related theories, influential policies and professional standards are critically discussed, explored and clarified to provide a fundamentally practical approach to the types of situation that you will face, no matter what your chosen field of practice. Although this book is primarily designed to assist you in the latter period of your pre-registration course, it will also be invaluable for your initial post-qualification experience, with chapters specifically devoted to areas such as the need for ongoing and continuing professional development and offering advice on helping you get the job that you want.

What this book covers

Chapter 1: Becoming a qualified nurse

This chapter introduces the concept of the transition from student to newly qualified nurse. There is an introduction to the NMC Standards of Proficiency for registered nurses and the seven platforms that the proficiencies are grouped under and which support the subsequent chapters in the book. It looks at the changing responsibilities, expectations, challenges and experiences of those facing this transition to becoming a fully professional qualified nurse working in a healthcare team. There is discussion highlighting the different fields of nursing: Adult, Children's, Learning Disability and Mental Health, including the main philosophies, responsibilities and environments where they practise. The chapter concludes with a summary of professional skills and responsibilities.

Chapter 2: Transition

This chapter will build upon some of the issues already highlighted above. The concept of transition will be explored generally and applied to the situation of a newly qualified nurse entering the profession. It must be remembered however that throughout a career of nursing you may often find yourself changing career path or direction which will bring with it further issues of transition. Stages of transition will be discussed and supported by personally reported experiences of transition. Potential strategies needed to navigate such a transition will be highlighted and there will be some discussion on the need for resilience and the support and strategies related to this as well as providing opportunity for reflection as you prepare to enter the profession as a qualified practitioner.

Chapter 3: Improving safety and quality of care

Improving safety and quality of care and maintaining and developing standards is an essential part of the responsibilities of a qualified nurse (NMC, 2018b). This chapter will cover the main areas that fall within improving safety, maintaining standards and ensuring quality of care. Your responsibilities as a nurse in providing 'good quality care' will be explained and relevant policies that influence quality of care will be explored to identify what they mean in genuine, practical terms. The various bodies and organizations set up to monitor standards in areas in which you might find yourself working as a qualified nurse will be critically discussed.

Chapter 4: Accountability and ethical decision-making

Nurses abide by *The Code* (NMC, 2018a). This chapter will focus on the various professional roles of the qualified nurse and how *The Code* impacts on them. It outlines the responsibilities of a nurse in maintaining safety and making ethically sound decisions. Issues relating to the concept of ethics will be explored including maintaining confidentiality, acting in a spirit of beneficence and non-maleficence, and making decisions while remaining non-judgemental. Consent, capacity, and safeguarding the interests of patients and service users will also be investigated.

Chapter 5: Accountability, decision-making and the law

The legal, professional, and ethical issues, and the decision-making approaches that need to be considered by a qualified nurse, will be discussed in this chapter. The nature of professional employment brings with it many obligations that a nurse must abide by, including aspects related to ensuring anti-discriminatory measures that form the basis of the nurse's practice. The concepts of nurses' responsibilities in relation to civil and criminal law will be discussed. Considerations related to personal and public liabilities will be explored in detail.

Chapter 6: Leading, managing and working in teams

This chapter will look at what it means and what it takes to make the transition from being a student one day to suddenly, the next day, finding out that you are the one who is supposed to be responsible not only for your own welfare, but also for the welfare of the patients/service users, staff, visitors, and anyone else who happens to access the service, whether it is in a hospital or community setting. Although as a newly qualified nurse expectations of leadership and management may not be in your immediate thoughts, it is imperative to understand the theory and practice of both, as you may find yourself leading care for a number of patients, managing small care teams or the whole care environment. Understanding the relationship of leadership and management and the application in practice is important.

This chapter will also look at the elements of a good functioning team, how teams differ from simply collections of individuals and what skills are needed in team members. It will also explore how to subsequently lead and manage a team. There will be some discussion related to the formation and structure of teams as well as some exploration of the necessity for interprofessional teamworking. Again, the established theories in this field will be explored, as will real-life management scenarios and experiences both in the NHS and in education.

Chapter 7: Learning, teaching and assessment in practice

A large part of the responsibilities of a qualified nurse are related to their own personal development and also the development of those around them. This chapter will focus on the personal and professional development issues faced by nurses every day. It will include discussions related to setting outcomes, identifying needs, and taking action to meet them. Theories of learning, managing learning environments and teaching strategies will be discussed, so you can understand your role in developing yourself and others more clearly. Learning opportunities present themselves in practice every day and it is up to you to seize those opportunities readily when they arise.

Chapter 8: Getting the job that you want

The chapter will begin by exploring what interviewing for a job is really about. The success criteria of an interview will be discussed and reframed from the most commonly held misconception that success means 'getting the job' to success means 'getting the *right* job', which might not be the one for which you have just been interviewed. The chapter will next focus on getting the right job, beginning with the filling in of application forms and creating a suitable CV, through to preparing for the interview, dealing with interview 'nerves', and performing well at the interview. We will give some hints and tips for how to answer those awkward questions around the themes of the book. It will also cover how to deal with the 'nightmare' questions.

Chapter 9: Preparation for personal and professional development

Returning to the issues of personal and professional development, this chapter will build from the earlier learning, teaching and assessing chapter with more of a focus on yourself. Issues related to your transition, continuing personal and professional development planning and NMC requirements for further education and training will be discussed, including the concept of preceptorship, supervision, and important aspects and requirements related to continuing professional development. We will also touch on coaching, regarding how you can use specific goal-setting techniques to enrich your personal and professional life, and how this could then assist you in helping others in your field of practice and work.

Chapter 10: Global and international nursing

You may be preparing for a job as a newly qualified nurse within your local area or region, however nursing is a worldwide profession and health issues such as ageing populations, chronic disease and socioeconomic influences on health are all affecting the way nursing develops all around the world. The world is becoming figuratively much smaller due to more accessible transport, access and communications between countries globally. The Coronavirus pandemic of 2020 confirmed the commonality of many of the challenges facing nurses throughout the world and emphasized the need to recognize many of the shared priorities of all nurses and the essential requirements of good practice, team working, communication and the sharing of research and best evidence in a rapidly changing environment. This chapter discusses the concept of global nursing and explores issues of nurse migration. You may have already planned – or at some point in the future should the opportunity arise you may wish – to pursue a nursing career overseas and these aspects are also discussed.

Chapter 11: Conclusion

This concluding chapter has exercises and examples, and will demonstrate how, although we have covered many separate themes, they all come together to form a holistic view of the roles and responsibilities of the newly qualified nurse.

EDITORS' ACKNOWLEDGEMENTS

Producing the book has involved many people and we would like to thank the following for their support and assistance at various stages in the process: Nichola Barlow, Val Ely and Angela Darvill for their essential contributions, and Sheena Hiller, Ruth Elliott, Karen Currell, Jackie Vasey and Victoria Kain for the scenarios and information that they provided to promote reflection and discussion.

Throughout the book there are resonances of those who have motivated us throughout our careers. Those we have valued as role models and mentors, and students and colleagues too numerous to mention who have inspired us by their compassion, caring and unwavering commitment to patient care and the nursing profession. We are forever grateful for their influence, guidance and positivity.

Lastly, we would like to thank our families for their patience and tolerance during the writing of this book.

Rob Burton and Graham Ormrod

PUBLISHER'S ACKNOWLEDGEMENTS

The editors and publisher would like to thank the following for permission to reproduce copyright material:

Angela Darvill for permission to use the figure 'stages of the transition process' (Figure 2.1). Darvill and Croughan (2018) *Transition to Nursing Practice: From Student to Registered Nurse*.

Belbin for permission to use Belbin's team roles (Table 6.2).

Cambridge University Press publishers for permission to use Figure 5.3, reprinted from Church and Watts' (2007) Assessment of mental capacity: A flow chart guide. *Psychiatrist*, 31: 304–307.

Cengage publishers for permission to use Figure 7.5, adapted from Hughes and Quinn's (2013) *Quinn's Principles and Practice of Nurse Education* (6th edn).

Elsevier publishers for permission to use Figure 6.4, reprinted from Gallo's (2007) The new nurse manager: A leadership development program paves the road to success. *Nurse Leader*, 5(4): 28–32.

Elsevier publishers for permission to reprint Figure 10.2 from Crisp and Watkins (2018) The triple impact of nursing. *International Journal of Nursing Studies*, 78: A3–A4.

John Wiley & Sons publishers for permission to use the 'balancing transition' figure (Figure 2.2) from Feltrin et al. (2019) How graduate nurses adapt to individual ward culture: A grounded theory study. *Journal of Advanced Nursing*, 75(3): 616–627.

Pearson Education Inc for permission to reprint Figure 7.7, adapted from Kolb, D.A. (1984) *Experiential Learning: Experience as the Source of Learning and Development* (2nd edn, © 2015).

The editors and publisher are grateful to the following academics for their work reviewing the first edition of this text and the revised material:

Amanda Smith, University of Southampton

Claire Peers, University of Plymouth

Dawn A. Morley, Bournemouth University

Debbie Casey, Leeds Beckett University

Peter Ellis, Independent Nursing Educational Consultant and Writer

Su McAnelly, Northumbria University

1

BECOMING A QUALIFIED NURSE

Rob Burton, Graham Ormrod and Angela Darvill

THE AIMS OF THIS CHAPTER ARE TO:

- Explore the expectations of a newly qualified nurse.
- Discuss the challenges involved in the transition from student to qualified nurse.
- Highlight the experiences of newly qualified nurses.
- Discuss the roles of the nurse in different fields of nursing.
- Provide an overview of the structure and rationale of the book.

Introduction: How this book can help you to become a qualified nurse

Becoming a qualified nurse is quite an achievement. After three or four years of education involving experiences both in practice and in the academic context, entering the nursing register of whichever field of nursing you qualify in is something to be proud of. The hard work pays off and you are able to become a professional in your own right. Undoubtedly this achievement brings with it challenges as well as rewards. You may now find that there are different expectations of you, and a set of roles and responsibilities that are different from those that you experienced as a student under supervision.

The aim of this book is for you to be able to explore and develop understanding of the varied important aspects of the roles and responsibilities of the qualified nurse in order to prepare you to successfully make the transition from student nurse to registered professional. It can also be used as a resource for those who may already be qualified and registered, but who are looking for helpful advice and are wishing to continue their professional development.

The roles, responsibilities and accountabilities of a qualified nurse include essential professional skills described as 'platforms' by the Nursing and Midwifery Council (NMC). The seven platforms are:

- Being an accountable professional.
- Promoting health and preventing ill health.
- Assessing needs and planning, providing, coordinating and evaluating care.
- Leading and managing nursing care and working in teams.
- Improving safety and quality of care.
- Making ethical and legal decisions.
- Teaching others.

(NMC, 2018b)

The focus of the book is not about clinical practice, or the theory of nursing interventions or clinical nursing skills, because in order to become a qualified nurse these aspects should be addressed satisfactorily within the nursing course undertaken to demonstrate proficiency in order to register with the Nursing and Midwifery Council (NMC, 2018b). Instead, the intention is to prepare you for the challenges that you will face on being a newly qualified nurse by providing the knowledge, skills and values required to become effective and accountable practitioners. Clinical decisions will still have to be made in relation to meeting the needs of the people within your care; however, becoming a qualified nurse brings with it wider responsibilities in making and taking decisions related to the nursing team, other staff, and the work environment as a whole. These changes require a large shift from the experience of being a student and a supervised learner, so it is essential that you are equipped with all of the skills required to successfully make the transition. There are countless texts available on providing clinical nursing care, but there are few designed specifically to help final-year student nurses to develop the transferable professional skills necessary for the role of the registered nurse, and so this text sets out to assist final-year students by clearly outlining these.

The professional skills that you require as a nurse must be developed in a contemporary context in which nursing careers are changing radically, with nurses now working in a wide array of new roles in a variety of healthcare settings. Today, you must be able to demonstrate these skills in job applications and interviews as well as develop employability skills for a career in which continuing professional development will be a key to success. Throughout your career, you may work in a variety of care settings and specialized nursing roles, but you will always require skills in teamworking, leadership, management, decision-making, and teaching.

The approach taken throughout the rest of this book will be to provide a discussion of the main theories, concepts, and issues related to the professional skills listed above. We will discuss the meaning of these concepts and their importance for nurses and provide some practical contextual examples. Throughout the book, you will find exercises designed for you to read and reflect on the material presented and to encourage you to recognize how to use these in your own field of practice. Examples from all fields of practice will be used to illustrate the theories, with the inclusion of scenarios to illustrate how to consider and apply these to nursing practice. We also recognize that a pertinent issue in the transition from student to qualified nurse is that of getting a job and building a career, so skills such as preparing for interviews, interview skills, and continuing professional development are also included.

Changing expectations: From student to qualified nurse

Many student nurses will tell you that their nurse education course passed quickly. Within that time, a student would have had a vast range of experiences and been exposed to many theoretical and practical aspects in their educational and practice settings. On qualifying, nurses are required to demonstrate a high level of knowledge, understanding, and application of high-order skills, not only with patients/service users, but also with other team members and those within, entering, and leaving the workplace. These are all skills that they should have developed in their journey to qualifying and are also highlighted as required standards of proficiency (NMC, 2018b).

The seven platforms within the standards of proficiency (NMC, 2018b) also include essential aspects of care, such as communication and relationship management skills; assessing needs; planning; provision and management of person-centred care; use of evidence-based practice in meeting the needs for care and support with rest, sleep, comfort and maintenance of dignity, hygiene and skin integrity, nutrition and hydration, bladder and bowel health, mobility and safety, respiratory care and support, prevention and management of infection, end of life care and medicines administration and optimization.

With registration comes a shift in professional accountability, together with wider clinical, leadership, management, and teaching responsibilities.

On becoming a qualified nurse, the expectations and dynamics of relationships change fundamentally. Suddenly, the newly qualified nurse is the one who must 'know the answer', whether it is a query from a patient, a carer, a work colleague or a student. As a newly qualified nurse you will encounter many challenging situations in which you must lead care delivery. This includes dealing with care management within the team, dealing with patients/service users, dealing with other professionals, and dealing with the needs of the whole workplace environment and those within it. The NMC requires a student nurse to demonstrate professional values in leading and coordinating evidence-based, compassionate person-centred care. They should be able to work autonomously within interdisciplinary teams, demonstrate emotional intelligence communication skills, decision-making, and show personal and professional development in order to join the register (NMC, 2018d).

The challenges of moving from a student to a newly qualified nurse

You may find that moving from being a student to a newly qualified nurse is an exciting but challenging time. As a newly qualified nurse you may need to adapt to working independently in a workplace environment that is rapidly changing, fast paced, may have staff shortages and an increased patient workload. A study by Halpin et al. (2017) found that workload was consistently the highest reported stressor for newly qualified nurses with inadequate staffing and managing multiple role demands. In addition, attrition is a consistent problem, with 18 percent of nurses leaving the profession within three years of qualification, and the highest figure being apparent within the first 12 months of registration (RCN, 2017a). According to the NMC, during 2016–17 more than 29,000 registered nurses allowed their registrations to lapse. Therefore, there is the real potential for newly registered nurses to leave the profession due to a lack of personal resilience and adequate coping strategies when their experiences in practice do not match their expectations (RCN, 2017a). According to the NHS Long Term Plan (NHS England, 2019a: 4.35) the leaver rate for nurses was eight percent in 2017 up from six point eight percent in 2013. Current insights into the experiences of newly registered nurses entering the world of work are founded on the concept of transition (Darvill et al., 2014). This concept will be developed further in Chapter 2.

The transition from student to newly registered nurse is acknowledged as having a significant social, physical, intellectual, and emotional response that is also influenced by the context of the individual's situation (Boychuk Duchscher and Windey, 2018). Overall, it is a complex process of evolving professional development, socialization and adaptation (Boychuk Duchscher and Windey, 2018). Therefore, to fully understand responses to transition and develop strategies to ameliorate adverse effects, it is important you understand the conditions that influence it, including the factors that facilitate and disrupt progress towards a positive outcome (Darvill et al., 2014).

The transition from student to newly registered nurse is a temporary phase which involves a period of adjustment and change. Transition begins with the first anticipation of the change and continues until stability occurs in the new status and within a defined time frame. Every newly registered nurse will experience this transition; however, each nurse will interpret the experience from their own subjective and unique perspective. You will have differing expectations, will require differing levels of support and yet undoubtedly require a certain amount of resilience in what is recognized as a crucial stage in your professional career.

Experiences of newly qualified nurses

With registration and a career as a qualified nurse comes a shift in professional responsibilities and, on becoming a qualified nurse, the expectations and dynamics of relationships change fundamentally. The NMC requires a registered nurse to demonstrate professional and ethical practice and provide, lead and coordinate care that is compassionate, evidence-based and person-centred. The nurse is accountable for their own actions and works autonomously and as an equal partner with other professionals in teams, and they must be emotionally intelligent and resilient and able to manage their own health and well-being. This is a large leap from the culture of being a student and a mentored, supervised practitioner, so it is essential that student nurses are equipped with all of the skills required to successfully make the transition. The different fields of nursing undeniably have differing roles and differing priorities of care, however there is also great similarity in the skills and knowledge required by all qualified nurses, and these broad, transferable skills that can be applied to all fields can certainly be developed.

All newly qualified nurses have been deemed fit for practice and have been robustly assessed as proficient to practice as a registered nurse. However, many newly registered nurses often identify significant concerns about their preparedness and frequently perceive themselves as not being ready for some aspects of their clinical practice. This can be attributed to anxiety and shock generated by a greater awareness of the increased responsibility and accountability, the expectation of extensive knowledge and skills and a subsequent confidence deficit, particularly at the start of the first stage of transition, and particularly if there is a perceived lack of sufficient support (Kumaran and Carney, 2014; Morrell and Ridgway, 2014; Whitehead et al., 2013).

There are a variety of strategies and interventions that are available to support you during your transition. Edwards et al. (2015) identified that these transition interventions and strategies can help to develop confidence and competence, job satisfaction and critical thinking, and reduce stress and anxiety in newly registered nurses.

Other studies have also identified that preparation for transition can ease some of the detrimental effects of reality and transition shock (Kaihlanen et al., 2018; Morrell and Ridgway, 2014). Identifying the strategies that might be helpful for managing your transition may enhance the process and outcome. These strategies will be further discussed in Chapter 2, but include mentorship/preceptorship type supervision for a period of time, formal induction/orientation/transition programmes and online or simulation courses as well as strategies for developing resilience.

In meeting the NMC (2018b) standards of proficiency for registered nurses, the nurse should have demonstrated the relevant knowledge and skills in order to practise in their relevant specialized fields. However, it is important to recognize that not every nurse knows everything about everything in their field, especially if they are practising in highly specialized fields. What they need is to be able to develop and adapt to changing situations. This is similar to the popular saying:

> Give someone a fish and you feed them for a day, teach them how to fish and they feed themselves for a lifetime!

Therefore, as a newly qualified nurse, it is impossible to know everything, but you should have developed the skills to find out relevant information, reflect on it, and apply this to your practice. In essence, you should have learned how to learn. There is a great deal to be learned once qualified – especially related to a nurse's 'new' area of work – and a good deal of the development needs to take place 'on the job'.

Issues and expectations for newly qualifying nurses

Currently, in the United Kingdom, nurses undertake a three- or four-year programme, which is split 50/50 between theory and practice.

In practice, student nurses are supervised throughout by approved practice supervisors, practice assessors, mentors, and registrants (NMC, 2018e) to support the application of the theory to practice and to assess the competency and skills of the nurse in clinical health and social care settings. The NMC (2018a) explicitly identifies that the qualifying nurse should be competent to practise safely. Therefore, the experiences that nurses are exposed to throughout their nursing course should be a vehicle for this. On qualifying, this competence is accepted as a given and highlights that the skills the nurse requires for professional practice incorporate not only the need for clinical skills and knowledge but also 'people' and environmental management abilities underpinned by finely tuned interpersonal skills.

In this way, positive outcomes for both service users and staff can be ensured. As a qualifying nurse you are given the remit to practice, yet the need to continually and consistently meet the standards of proficiency means that further and continuing professional development and training is also necessary to ensure that you remain a competent and developing practitioner.

Before going any further, it is appropriate to reflect on one of Rob's own experiences of becoming a newly qualified nurse (many years ago!).

I had studied and practised hard for three years. Each year I had revised and prepared for my exams and undergone practical examinations. These aimed to demonstrate that the potential qualified nurse was clinically competent, just as the NMC require for those qualifying today. There were some questions and assessments related to managing the clinical area and I'd had the opportunity to lead shifts in under supervision. All of these aspects had gone well. So, on commencing my first job as a qualified nurse, I felt very well prepared for the job with my main fears being related to perhaps being faced with clinical situations that I did not know the answer to.

In my early weeks, I tended to work with more senior nurses and was expected to carry out tasks relevant to the qualified nurse (such as administering and dispensing medications, writing reports, giving handovers and general unit tasks) that had been delegated to me. After a relatively short period of time, the first shift that I was to be solely in charge of came around (these days there is a much more structured approach for preceptorship and support for the newly qualified nurse). The handover was given to me, and the all-important and symbolic 'unit medication keys' also handed over.

As the previous senior nurse left the area, I was suddenly aware of the eyes of all the staff on duty being trained towards me. I was in charge and no longer was there any other person for me to turn to for advice, each of these staff were now awaiting instructions in an expectant manner. This was a daunting experience.

I realized that my every move was now being scrutinized and assessed by every member of the team. I had to delegate duties to staff for the coming shift, some of which were less popular than others. This required me having to answer certain questioning staff (many that were much older than I) as to why I had asked them to carry out these tasks (after all, it had been they that had done the same task yesterday!). My answers needed to be good! Over the coming weeks, I realized that it was not to be my clinical knowledge and skills that were put to the test as had been my initial fears; rather it was the tasks related to dealing with staff and aspects such as having to make difficult phone calls to distraught relatives or to other services and professionals where their input was urgently demanded.

I had to quickly develop assertiveness skills. I had to deal with situations such as staff squabbling amongst themselves, staff refusing to carry out tasks, emergency situations, running out of resources (such basics as there not being enough dinners available for the patients) and much more. I had to account to other professionals and staff why certain things had been carried out in a particular way or not and defend decisions to others that I had perhaps not even made. I had to defend patients and staff as well as give bad news to patients/clients/service users.

Overall, the first year as a qualified nurse was one of adjustment and was very different from our previous expectations. Therefore, it might be useful at this juncture for you to reflect on your own expectations on becoming a qualified nurse.

--------------------------------- **ACTIVITY 1.1** ---------------------------------

What are your expectations, concerns, and anxieties regarding becoming a qualified nurse? Identify both positive and any negative aspects.

A great deal of the literature and policy in place today highlight the fact that the context of health and social care is changing. According to *Leading Change, Adding Value: A Framework for Nursing, Midwifery and Care Staff*, for example:

the pace of change is sometimes so great it is hard to imagine what the future looks like. (NHS England, 2016: 6)

The NHS Long Term Plan (NHS, 2019a: 6) speaks of the need to 'accelerate the redesign of patient care to future proof the NHS'.

This is going to require a significant change in values, attitudes, philosophies, and roles of nurses and other health and social care professionals. Nurses are one of the important groups of professionals who will have to respond to these changing roles as flexible and creative working practices are the expectation in current nursing roles. This includes dealing with the complexity of an increasingly ageing population, the increase of chronic health conditions such as obesity, increasing mental health issues in young adults, potential future pandemics and other health and social factors that affect people's ability to live independent lives. The changes are not just related to societal, demographic, and health/illness issues, but also to positive changes such as advances in medical, health, social and pharmacological interventions, and the rapidly expanding integration of digitally enabled care, specialized technologies and communication systems and approaches, and many other innovations.

The necessity for nurses to work flexibly to meet the changing needs of patients and service users is not necessarily a new trend, however, as changes in roles, boundaries and services have been gathering pace since the 1980s with earlier initiatives from the forerunner of the NMC, the former United Kingdom Central Council (UKCC), and the Department of Health (DH) such as *Project 2000* (UKCC, 1986), *Making a Difference* (DH, 1999) and *Modernising Nursing Careers* (DH, 2006). In 2004 The Royal College of Nursing (RCN, 2004) had argued that nurses were crucial for the changing emphasis in health and social care services, which were becoming increasingly person-centred and focused, in order to remove barriers to support for individuals and their families.

Presently the NMC (2018a: 25) suggest that exhibiting leadership potential – an ability to guide, support and motivate individuals and interact confidently with others – is essential for addressing the complexities of these changes in society generally and the health and social care systems within it.

Despite some of the concerns about the NHS, including funding, staffing, increasing inequalities and so on (King's Fund, 2019c), there remains optimism about the possibilities it can deliver and the potential for improved quality outcomes of care (NHS England, 2019a). Nurses have an important role to play in ensuring that health services are fair, personalized, effective and safe, not least as they are often seen by the public as the main point of support while receiving care in their own homes or community or during hospital stays. It is therefore important that nurses fulfil their responsibilities and are confident in their roles. The main goal of nurses is to provide holistic healthcare for their patients/service users and their families while maintaining all aspects of the healthcare environment.

This means communicating with, and at times managing, others around them, including other professionals as part of a multidisciplinary team. The nursing profession is unique because of these characteristics, the interventions that nurses use, their knowledge domains, focus, value base, and commitment to working with others in partnerships (NHS England, 2016).

Roles of qualified nurses in differing fields

There are currently four fields of nursing in the UK – adult (RNA); children's (RNC); mental health (RNMH); and learning disability (RNLD) – serving the different patient/client groups (NMC, 2018b). These fields are all bound by *The Code* (NMC, 2018a) and registered with the NMC. They have some very similar underpinning philosophies and some similar knowledge and skills. However, while sharing common nursing goals, each field is also very different, not least because of the client groups they serve, in identity, environments, and in specific philosophies, attitudes, missions, knowledge and skills. Just as the armed forces in the main comprise the army, navy, air force, and marines, which have their own strongly defined identities; each with a common purpose (to protect the public and defend the nation); some shared aspects (uniforms, discipline and ranking etc.); but each having an entirely different set of values, approaches and contexts within which they operate and in how they achieve their aims (namely, sea, air and land), the fields of nursing each have similar but different dimensions too. Therefore, although there is some overlap in the roles, responsibilities and accountabilities of qualified nurses in the respective fields, there will also be some very specific differences. The NMC (2018b: 5) highlight:

> All nursing students across all fields of nursing must have the necessary learning supervision and assessment in preparation for professional practice as a registered nurse. The adult nursing field must also include the content and competencies specified in relevant EU legislation.

Below, we provide a brief description of the roles of qualified nurses in each field of nursing. Further information can be found at the National Health Service (NHS) Health Education England health careers website (www.healthcareers.nhs.uk/explore-roles/nursing/roles-nursing).

Adult nurses

Adult nursing could arguably be seen as the most recognizable field of nursing, particularly to the general public. It is the field of nursing, in acute and other hospital settings and a range of primary care and community settings, with which most of the population has some contact in their experiences with the health services and also forms the largest numbers of registered nurses. In fact adult nurses are the largest NHS workforce with over 176,000 currently working in acute settings alone.

This field of nursing is concerned with the care of adults over the age of 18, including working with older persons in a variety of settings for patients with wide-ranging levels of dependency. They work in varied settings such as hospital wards, outpatient units and specialist areas; community settings, GP clinics, walk-in centres and nursing homes, the prison service, the police; and the voluntary or private sector. Nurses engage in and develop therapeutic relationships that involve patients and their carers in ongoing decision-making that informs nursing care.

Adult nurses have skills to meet the physical, psychological, spiritual, and social needs of patients suffering from short- or long-term physical conditions, supporting them through care pathways and working with other health and social care professionals to maximize opportunities for recovery, rehabilitation, adaptation to ongoing disease and disability, health education, and health promotion.

Once qualified there are a range of specialities to enter such as working in operating theatres, caring for older persons, intensive care, accident and emergency (A&E), public health, community or moving into management, research or education (HEE, 2020).

Adult nurses are expected to have understanding of all of the other fields as they will come into contact with people of all ages with physical illnesses and/or mental health issues or a learning disability whilst working in some adult nursing areas such as A&E, amongst others (Davenport et al., 2015). The role is continually changing due to adaptations in dynamic health environments, people living longer and the increase in multiple and complex needs associated with this and therefore all adult nurses will continually be required to learn new skills and take on differing responsibilities (Davenport et al., 2015).

Children's nurses

The philosophy of children's nursing is based on the principle of family-centred care and the belief that children should be cared for by people they know and, wherever possible, within their home environment. Children's nursing involves work with newborn babies that may be sick to adolescents. Children's nurses work in a variety of settings, such as hospitals, day care centres, child health clinics and the child's home setting. They work across and beyond traditional boundaries, and within a multidisciplinary and multi-agency team. In particular, they contribute to child protection, in collaboration with other key professionals, respecting and promoting the rights of the child (HEE, 2020). Once qualified they can specialize in areas such as health visiting or school nursing, management, research or education.

This field of nursing tends to span the age group of children from birth to 19 years old. Changes in the way services for children are configured means that a children's nurse will need to be equipped to work across settings and agencies. As technology advances more children are surviving with complex health issues that need advanced nursing support. This also requires skills in working closely with families in partnership (Davenport et al., 2015).

Learning disability nurses

This field is probably the least well-known of all of the specialisms in nursing. The population of people with learning disabilities are increasing, and they face a range of physical, mental health, and social issues. There are many health inequalities faced by them compared to their non-disabled peers as their learning disability often creates barriers for them in accessing effective healthcare, therefore there is a demand for specialist learning disability services and learning disability nurses (Davenport et al., 2015).

The focus of learning disability nursing is influencing behaviours and lifestyles to enable a vulnerable client group to achieve optimum health, and to live in an inclusive society as equal citizens, where their rights are respected. This includes helping to improve the physical and mental health of persons of all ages with a learning disability; reducing barriers to them living independent lives and supporting them in leading a fulfilling life. Learning disability nurses work in a variety of settings such as people's homes; educational settings; workplaces; residential and community services; specialist hospital settings; mental health settings; and prisons. They adapt the level of support that they provide according to the complex needs of the individuals, families, and carers with whom they are dealing, and the settings that they are in. Risk assessment and risk management are key components of their work and enable individuals to exercise their individual rights and choices. On qualifying nurses can specialize in community settings, working with people with autism, management, research or education (HEE, 2020).

Mental health nurses

Mental health nurses care for people experiencing mental health issues, which may have a variety of causative factors, such as stressful life events, substance misuse and physical issues. The focus of mental health nursing is the establishment of effective working relationships with service users and carers to help to bring about an understanding of how they might cope with their experience, thus maximizing their potential for recovery. Users may be cared for in a variety of settings, including the community and their own homes. They may require care for an acute episode or ongoing support for an enduring illness. Mental health nurses work as part of multidisciplinary and multi-agency teams.

Mental health nurses work in a range of settings such as hospital or in the community. In hospital settings they may work in psychiatric intensive care, or longer-term care and rehabilitation, outpatient units, specialist units (e.g. for people with eating disorders) or secure settings. In community they may work in GP surgeries, prisons, community centres, residential centres and patients' own homes. They may specialize in children and adolescents, primary mental health, transcultural psychiatry, management, research or education (HEE, 2020).

In the past, mental health nursing (and to an extent learning disability nursing) has been associated with custodial care in institutions. However, the focus now is on working with people, their families, and other professionals and services in order to demystify these outdated views and assist individuals to maximize their independence over their conditions which can restrict and create barriers in their approach to living an ordinary life (Davenport et al., 2015).

What can be seen in all fields of nursing is that the registered nurse specializing within each field works in a variety of settings, with a variety of different specialist professionals, whilst working with families in partnership, to produce values-based person-centred care to the individuals they serve. Therefore, that is why the NMC standards of proficiency (NMC, 2018b) highlight the platforms that apply to each field and outline the requirements needed to become a professional nurse in whichever field is chosen.

ACTIVITY 1.2

At this point, take some time to reflect on the roles and responsibilities of the qualified nurse in the different fields. Whichever field you belong to, you may have had experience from placements during your training or by coming into contact with nurses from other fields in your work.

1   Describe the types of patient/service user, the settings/environments in which they worked, and the roles they were undertaking.
2   Identify the similarities and differences between the fields and compare them with your own.

As can be seen above, each field of nursing is a unique speciality. However, within each one there are sub-specialities in which the qualified nurse could choose to work, and they can follow specific or broad career paths via their choice of specialization. These specialities recognize that the needs of each client group can be diverse. They can be acute or chronic, health or social-related, involve family members and other members of the multidisciplinary team or a multitude of agencies, and be community or hospital-based. The fundamental transferable skills that all newly qualified nurses require are a high level of communication skills as well as a highly developed awareness of the approaches that can meet the clinical health or social care related needs of their patients.

—————————————————— ACTIVITY 1.3 ——————————————————

Some key words to consider up to this point which can be found or implied in the standards, challenges and specialist descriptions of the fields are: dynamic; unique; measured risk-taking; creativity; relationship-centred care; interpersonal sensitivity and intimacy; positive outcomes; person-centred; community; hospital; safe; effective; multi-professional; ethical principles; clinically competent; flexible; different contexts; rights; values; and specialized.

What do these words mean to you in relation to the role of the nurse?

As a newly qualified nurse you may not yet have decided which aspect of nursing you wish to go into, but you would have obviously chosen your field. During your career you may work in a number of specialisms within your field or even decide to go for further training to qualify in a different field. You need to remember that your first job is important but that a whole career in nursing is ahead of you and there may be many opportunities for you to access a variety of specialisms and services in which to find yourself a niche where you are most comfortable, or areas for you to further develop into specialist roles.

—————————————————— ACTIVITY 1.4 ——————————————————

Think of a member of qualified staff with whom you have worked. Describe their qualities in dealing with everyday issues, their clinical knowledge, skills, and abilities to manage people and communicate well with patients/service users and families.

What were their attributes, and what were the main aspects of the role that you learned about from working with and observing them?

As already mentioned above, it is apparent that nurses work within different disciplines and fields, specialities, and contexts, and play an important role in health and social services. Change has been a constant in the health and social care services for many years and continues to rapidly develop in response to changing trends in health and societal situations, and the economic and political responses to them. Despite these differences, there are some roles and responsibilities underpinned with relevant theory that are applicable to all nurses and which will always be deemed so, regardless of how services and nursing are reconstructed.

A newly qualified nurse will face challenges in whatever situation they are employed. In analysing the situation in which nurses from all fields find themselves at the current time, one thing that is clear is that nursing roles and responsibilities are constantly in a state of flux, having to respond to changing societal and healthcare issues. The newly qualified nurse of the future may not necessarily be entering employment into traditional roles. They need to develop skills that transcend the detailed knowledge and skills required to demonstrate that they are fit to enter the NMC register and therefore be eligible to practise as a qualified nurse.

This requires understanding and developing the professional skills discussed above so that they can be utilized effectively at work by nurses from all fields in a variety of contexts. The following chapters of this book will focus on these aspects in detail, with discussion of the main theoretical underpinnings and practical application.

Professional responsibilities and skills: Overview of this book

The focus in this book is related to the issues faced by a newly qualified nurse and some of the professional responsibilities and skills they will face. This includes:

- Transition.
- Improving safety and quality of care.
- Accountability and ethical decision-making.
- Accountability, decision-making and the law.
- Leading, managing and working in teams.
- Learning.
- Teaching and assessment in practice.

- Getting the job that you want.
- Preparation for personal and professional development.
- Global and international nursing.
- Putting it all together.

It is recognized that there is a certain amount of overlap in these professional responsibilities and skills and that some concepts are applicable across all of them, in that there are no clear lines drawn where one skill ends and another starts; however, there is still scope for scrutinizing the particular elements of each. Decisions are made and actions taken by nurses in light of the environmental situations that occur in day-to-day practice. You would not usually consider each of the skills or concepts in isolation in relation to particular incidents and environmental situations but would make a decision based on the factors contributing to the situation.

However, when analysing any situation, the decisions made, and the actions taken, some of the individual conceptual principles may be recognized and highlighted. For example, asking a member of staff to complete a task on your behalf is delegating. This fits neatly into leadership theory and also relates to aspects of accountability. Such an approach is something that you may find yourself doing quite often. Completing a health and safety audit in the work environment might relate to management theory. This may be another responsibility you have to take on. Completing a review of an individual's care and setting goals for them in multidisciplinary meetings might relate to teamworking theory. Reporting of poor practices or environments might relate to aspects of accountability and improving safety and quality of care. Demonstrating skills related to care needs to junior (or sometimes senior) staff might be considered teaching and assessing.

However, all of the above aspects could arise from analysing one situation in which the nurse has to make decisions about a certain aspect of care management, consider the human and environmental resources, and report these aspects to their seniors or employers. Therefore, all of these aspects are roles and responsibilities of the qualified nurse. The rest of this book will explore each of these theoretical and practical aspects in more detail.

—————————————————— **ACTIVITY 1.5** ——————————————————

Think back to some of the qualified nurses with whom you have worked.

1   Apart from their clinical duties and tasks, in what other aspects have you seen them often involved? Make a list of these other duties and tasks.
2   With regard to the concepts introduced above, which duties and which tasks more readily align with each concept?

Starting the journey to becoming a qualified nurse

Successfully completing the nurse preparation course and becoming registered with the NMC may appear to be an end point. However, in reality, it is just the beginning of what could be a long career. An analogy would be that this is the point similar to that at which someone passes their driving test and can take sole control of a car without supervision. In your role as a newly qualified nurse, there may still be some provision of further supervision and support, but in the main, many decisions have to be made by you and you alone. Therefore, this book aims to inform you of the considerations needed to make the transition to the role of a newly qualified nurse as smooth as possible. You will, of course, be supported in your transition, but it is not beyond the realms of possibility that you may be called on to demonstrate some of the shift leader and person management aspects within the clinical area in which you begin your career as a qualified nurse sooner rather than later!

The book can be used as a whole to read from beginning to end, or to look at particular sections in which you might be more interested, or you may wish to use it as a reference source. The accompanying exercises are designed to help you to reflect on the information provided and create some dynamic insights for you. Within the book, you will find advice, considerations, or theoretical direction to solve issues that you will come across in your qualified nursing career. As with any book the material is relevant at the date of publication. However, policies, procedures and regulations do change regularly over time so be aware to check on any of the issues and approaches discussed to ensure you access the most up-to-date information to help you in your nursing career. Enjoy the journey you are soon to undertake!

Summary

In this chapter we have looked at the expectations of a newly qualified nurse and what they may face on entering the profession. We have discussed the challenges involved in the transition from student to qualified nurse and highlighted the experiences of newly qualified nurses. There has been some focus on discussing the roles of the nurse in different fields of nursing and we have provided an overview of the structure and rationale of the book. Although aimed at final year nurses or newly qualifying nurses we believe the material will also help those already established in looking at some of the pertinent issues in relation to applying theory to more advanced practice.

2

TRANSITION

Rob Burton, Angela Darvill and Graham Ormrod

THE AIMS OF THIS CHAPTER ARE TO:

- Explore the concept of transition to professional practice.
- Outline the stages of transition.
- Examine experiences of transition.
- Analyse the concept of resilience and strategies to improve the adverse effects of transition.
- Examine the need for support during the transition period.
- Reflect on how you can prepare for the process as a final year nursing student.

Transition

Transition in nursing is a very important consideration. It occurs on a number of levels from becoming a student nurse to eventually joining the profession as a fully registered and licensed nurse, to becoming specialized and perhaps changing career direction. Benner's (1984) work 'from novice to expert' highlighted the process that nurses take in relation to their transitions and is well recognized within nursing literature. It outlines how nurses move through the stages of being a novice, to becoming an advanced beginner, and developing competence and expertise following exposure and immersion in settings where they gain technical, communication, moral, skills, knowledge and agency. It should also be recognized that transition occurs at all levels. This is because every time there is a change in position, such as from student nurse to qualified nurse or registered nurse to nurse manager or nurse educator, the process starts again, albeit in differing environmental conditions. The authors of this chapter and book have experienced this many times in their careers as they have changed jobs, positions, roles and areas of practice. Therefore, even though the newly qualified nurse may be knowledgeable and competent upon qualifying, the wider role of being a qualified professional encompasses new factors, within different settings and cultural systems in which the nurse once again finds themselves as a beginner.

Meleis (2009: 11) suggests that a common way of defining transitions is that of a passage from one life phase, condition or status to another, or from a

> fairly stable state to another fairly stable state triggered by change. Transitions are characterized by dynamic stages, milestones and turning points and can be defined through processes and/or terminal outcomes.

According to Chang and Daly (2016) there is a vast amount of literature that shows that the process of transition from student to graduate to professional registered practising nurse is multifaceted and complex. This is characterized by periods of intense socialization into the new culture and world of work. Nurses learn what others will expect of them in a specific contextual new role and they will need to learn how to exert control within these environments.

As well as roles and responsibilities in new environments that need to be quickly grasped and demonstrated, there are other factors that impact on transition. According to Meleis (2009), transitions can lead to losses of social networks and supports, and also meaningful and familiar objects. There can be periods of uncertainty as different skills and competencies might be required in new settings. This can lead to potential marginalization and vulnerability for nurses who had always been well-supervised and supported throughout their nurse training. She suggests that roles play an important part in transition as a person's roles are discovered, created, modified and defined. Such role transition needs to be considered within the context of a system. These roles are usually consolidated in relation to significant others within the context, who 'reinforce' or 'punish' the individual based on their performance in these new roles.

Transition is a process which can be short or longer term. A person in transition may often experience a sense of disconnectedness or social isolation due to loss of previous familiar reference points. Perception plays an important role as certain events influence reactions and responses making them less predictable. The process of transition comprises three main phases: entry, passage and exit. Within these processes there are aspects of adjustment by the individual in relation to becoming used to the working and professional environment, and role expectations (Meleis, 2009).

Brennan and McSherry (2009) support the concept that transition, such as when a student nurse becomes a qualified nurse, is a move from one state to another which brings with it issues in socialization. They outline that the process involves socialization (adapting knowledge, skills and values pertinent to the professional group) role identity and role confusion, reality shock, and formal and informal exposure. Their study found that those in transition from one role to another experienced 'culture shock', their 'comfort zones' were affected, and they had to consider clinical issues differently from the perspective of their new role than how they had done as students. These are all factors that can be applied in the transition from student to professional nurse. Orupabo (2018) also highlights that this process of socialization into the new role can be affected by cultural stereotypes such as race, ethnicity and gender. Orupabo (2018) suggests that in nursing, although in terms of numbers it is a predominantly female profession, there may still be some stereotypical 'cultural masculination' of competence and expectation. However, she suggests that the actual competences required and deployed in the education of nurses transcend this. All nursing students can position themselves as competent and demonstrate belonging within their professional community.

Phillips et al. (2015) argue that successful transition, therefore, requires support in the socialization of those individuals moving from being a student nurse into the role of a qualified nurse. This socialization occurs through a process of organizational approaches and influences leading to adjustments (clarifying of role, knowledge, and acceptance of organizational cultures) and finally into desired outcomes related to satisfaction, commitment and performance. Ankers et al. (2018) highlight that part of this process of transition is the necessity of dealing with 'reality shock'. They suggest this might occur due to the compartmentalization of the university aspect of nurse education to the physical, social and emotional aspects found in new responsibilities within the real-world practice of nursing. Reality shock for nurses was first discussed by Kramer (1974). Reality shock is also sometimes considered to be 'transition shock' (Blevins, 2018). Therefore, it is important to recognize this as a natural part of your journey to becoming a professional, registered practising nurse. Hodge (2018) suggests that this reality shock can occur because of discrepancies between your undergraduate education and the real-life situations faced in clinical practice. This may be due to having to deal with prioritizing tasks at the expense of meaningful interactions, therefore causing some inner conflict and a loss of an idealized view of what a nurse's role should actually be. Donnelly (2017), reflecting on her career transitions, identifies the journey through reality shock as adjusting to become 'professionally grounded', 'understanding and respecting cultures', and 'navigating chaos'. She points out that cataclysmic events impact on your career where these factors may be revisited, in order to readjust to the reality of a new situation. An example of this can be seen in a study by Halpin et al. (2017) which showed that newly qualified nurses faced stress within their first year of qualifying which appeared to be mainly associated with the 'shock' of the amount of work they were faced with.

This reality shock stage of transition is dominated by an increased awareness of accountability and a perception of being unprepared for the added responsibility of becoming qualified in clinical practice and not being fully prepared for some aspects of their clinical practice.

Negative experiences include feelings of being unprepared, fear of making mistakes, increased workload, lack of confidence and changes in responsibility and accountability (Darvill, 2013). The above-mentioned factors may become apparent to you during this journey and can also be identified within certain stages. The stages of transition will now be investigated more closely.

Stages of transition

As suggested above the period of transition is normally experienced in a series of stages. One suggested model of such stages developed by van Gennep in 1960 is identified as 'separation', 'transition' and 'incorporation' (Darvill and Croughan, 2018). Kramer et al. (2013) outline that this could also be considered as 'Knowing' (academic or education phase), 'Becoming' (developing professional skills, perhaps in an internship phase) and 'Integration' (developing accountability, professional identity and specialization skills perhaps following a residency phase).

Separation

Within nursing, separation is characterized by the movement from being a student nurse to becoming a newly registered nurse. This movement is inevitable as student nurses transfer from the comparative safety of being a student supported by the university environment to the unknown position of a newly registered nurse in a paid healthcare service environment, with further individual accountability related to your roles and responsibilities. This marks the end of your initial educational preparation and the beginning of your professional journey as a registered nurse. Blevins (2018) highlights the importance of this phase and the support required to assist the newly qualified nurse to not only become acculturated to the profession but also to the specific healthcare and professional environment they find themselves employed and deployed in. This is a crucial stage as these first experiences may influence decisions such as whether to stay or leave the profession. Slate et al. (2018) point out that support in this stage is very important as the onboarding of newly qualified nurses into the workforce is instrumental in the success or failure of retaining them, and therefore in the fiscal situation of healthcare services. There are many financial implications of constantly having to recruit more nurses if they are unable to be retained. Hence recognizing and providing very structured support is a worthwhile investment.

Transition

The next stage is the actual transition. There is some general agreement that the first phase of transition occupies the time between the first month and the third to fourth month after qualification. This stage is also identified as the most difficult period of transition for newly registered nurses. Nurses are often lost to the profession within the first year of practice as they come to terms with feelings of being overwhelmed, working in an increasingly ageing workforce, job dissatisfaction and workload issues (Schroyer et al., 2016). Silvestre et al. (2017) acknowledge that up to 18 percent of nurses may leave the profession in their first year and up to 33 percent by the end of their second year. However, they note that structured programmes including mentorship/preceptorship and formal orientation/transition programmes can help to reduce this amount of turnover.

Following this period, the individual normally begins to socialize and adapt to their new environment and there is a gradual increase in knowledge, skills and confidence as they develop professionally and through gaining experience.

Incorporation

Incorporation is characterized by the individual taking up their new status and identity, and them being accepted by the group. This stage is characterized as a relatively stable level of comfort and confidence with roles, responsibilities, and routines. The time period for this is usually 12 to 18 months. In this stage the individual can perform professionally, independently and demonstrate accountability. They may pick up other peripheral nursing skills such as teaching, management or research, as well as becoming active members of professional committees and advisory boards (Kramer et al., 2013).

Boychuk Duchscher and Windey (2018) suggest that in this stage the individual, although now belonging to the professional team with a professional identity, will also be able to distinguish themselves from other practitioners around them. They become able to provide guidance to others and can manage increasingly complex clinical and relational situations. See Figure 2.1, which depicts a summary of the stages regarding the transition process (Darvill and Croughan, 2018).

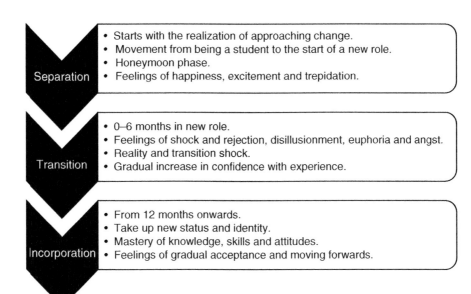

Separation
- Starts with the realization of approaching change.
- Movement from being a student to the start of a new role.
- Honeymoon phase.
- Feelings of happiness, excitement and trepidation.

Transition
- 0–6 months in new role.
- Feelings of shock and rejection, disillusionment, euphoria and angst.
- Reality and transition shock.
- Gradual increase in confidence with experience.

Incorporation
- From 12 months onwards.
- Take up new status and identity.
- Mastery of knowledge, skills and attitudes.
- Feelings of gradual acceptance and moving forwards.

Figure 2.1   Stages of the transition process (Boychuk Duchscher and Windey, 2018; Kramer et al., 2013)

Darvill and Croughan (2018) *Transition to Nursing Practice: From Student to Registered Nurse.* Adapted with kind permission of Angela Darvill

----------------------------------- **ACTIVITY 2.1** -----------------------------------

Sarah is a final year student preparing for her final placement. Throughout the three years of the undergraduate programme she has experienced a variety of clinical placements in both hospital and community settings. She feels she has made good progress with her academic work, having submitted and passed all requirements. She can demonstrate the ability to evaluate the knowledge that underpins practice. Sarah has been assessed in all her placements and successfully completed all her practice competencies required to date. Her assessors and practice supervisors have commented that she communicates well, demonstrates professional behaviour and works well as part of a team. She has also been able to demonstrate excellent leadership and management skills.

However, Sarah has asked to see her personal academic tutor at university because she feels anxious and concerned about the required expectations on her final placement.

Reflect on your own experiences and situation and consider the factors that might have contributed to Sarah seeking this advice at this stage.

1   How do these factors in Sarah's situation compare to your own?
2   What advice should the academic supervisor provide to Sarah?
3   What would you want to hear?

This is a situation often experienced by final placement students. You may perceive that you have knowledge and skills deficits, and this may be a cause for concern when approaching your transition into professional practice.

Final-year student nurses may have the ability to assess, plan, implement and evaluate care and have excellent communication skills, demonstrate the ability to work in a team and have a high level of ethical awareness. However, they may have concerns about being accountable for their actions.

You will see from Figure 2.1 that the student in the case study is experiencing entering into the separation stage of the transition process. There is a realization that change is approaching and although they may be looking forward to some aspects of being a registered nurse, they may also be experiencing feelings of stress and anxiety at this daunting prospect. It is now appropriate to focus on the experiences of transition.

Experiences of transition

Rob recalls his first experiences as a newly qualified staff nurse.

I was nervous about whether I knew enough clinically (even having passed the course in all academic and practical aspects successfully), however, this did not appear to be the major challenge. There was no shortage of people around to support and advise in clinical matters and people to learn from (especially working in a true interdisciplinary area); the issue was actually developing relationships with experienced qualified and non-qualified staff working within the clinical area. This included having to delegate tasks to people who (at that time) were much older than myself. The issues were not about remembering clinical procedures or drug side effects and dosages, it was how am I going to convince a nursing auxiliary or other nurse to perform a task they might not be willing to do. Taking responsibility and accountability for patients was obviously a big requirement, but it was learning the rules of the cultural environment and the navigating of the social relationships within it that created the bigger stress.

According to a systematic review conducted by Arrowsmith et al. (2016) it was found that transition occurs through pathways for novice nurses in pre-registration and newly qualified stages and for experienced nurses at times of clinical role change, moving to specialization and moving through nursing registration levels. They found the transitions were related to the striving for a new professional self, including emotional upheaval and identity, and know-how related to competence and role boundary changes. Adams and Gillman (2016) found in their review that transitioning nurses found the process stressful, as they were overwhelmed by expectations of the role, and faced difficulties with time management. Other factors identified included lack of confidence with clinical skills and decision-making. They recommended support in the socialization of new graduate nurses, and facilitated learning opportunities preferably via formal, structured approaches.

Suresh et al. (2012) looked at stressors of final year students and newly qualified nurses. They investigated factors such as workload, dealing with death and dying, inadequate preparation, lack of staff support, uncertainty concerning treatment, conflict with physicians and conflict with other nurses. They suggested that excessive workload, difficult working relationships, unmet clinical learning needs, and combining academic demands with clinical placement were factors that raised stress amongst these groups. Due to these perceived deficits, preparation for transition for final year nursing students is an important factor and one that can ameliorate against the negative effects of transition. Meleis (2009) identified that anticipatory preparation can aid transition whereas lack of preparation can inhibit the process and outcome. Numerous studies have identified that preparation for transition can ease some of the detrimental effects of poor graduate transition (Broad et al., 2011; Doody et al., 2011; Kaihlanen et al., 2018; Morrell and Ridgway, 2014; Ong, 2013).

Labrague and McEnroe-Petitte (2018) identified from an integrative review that nurses in their transition period experience low- to moderate-level stress. This is often related to heavy workloads and lack of clinical competence. They suggested that cultural differences also affect the responses to these stressors highlighting that coping depends on the cultural norms individuals are exposed to in dealing with such situations and expectations. It could be argued that as student nurses, you are exposed to the reality of the clinical area whilst being protected within it and not fully integrating as part of a team or culture. Labrague and McEnroe-Petitte (2018) also argue the case for structured transition programmes and continuing professional development courses focusing on clinical skills and scenarios to assist in this cultural and professional integration.

Feltrin et al. (2019) found in their study that newly graduated nurses had to balance three main aspects:

- Self-embodiment and self-consciousness.
- Navigating the social constructs.
- Raising consciousness.

In self-embodiment and self-consciousness, newly graduated nurses had learned that they had to present themselves and demonstrate their competence within the workforce. They were often self-conscious of this as it would go a long way to showing whether or not they would be able to fit in with the social culture of the workplace. This did actually help with their adaptation into the workplace and profession as they had gained confidence through demonstrating their abilities.

In navigating the social constructs, newly graduated nurses first had to learn the culture of the workplace as well as the broader culture of the profession. At first this may have been challenging and some individuals felt out of place until they realized the commonalities and approaches used within practice. Therefore, they had to find their way through these social nuances until they became used to them, Race (2015), building on the 'unconscious incompetence' to 'unconscious competence' model, suggests that learning takes place through a process of what he terms 'uncompetence' (not yet competent) through to full competence. This goes through the stages of:

1 'Unconscious uncompetence' (not knowing what you don't know).
2 'Conscious uncompetence' (knowing what you don't know).
3 'Conscious competence' (knowing the skill/knowledge).
4 'Unconscious competence' (being able to automatically understand or conduct a competency without thinking).

This could be happening during this stage for newly qualified nurses navigating the social situation in the workplace. Navigating the social constructs relates to fitting in in the workplace and then fitting in in the profession.

In raising consciousness, the newly graduated nurses were involved in the adaptation process by reflecting on their experiences. In this

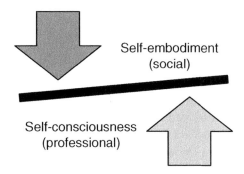

Figure 2.2   Balancing transition (Feltrin et al., 2019: 623)

Adapted with kind permission of © 2018 John Wiley & Sons Ltd

stage the newly graduated nurses were able to know whether they were fitting in (or not). They were able to understand that they had developed the skills needed to become a welcome part of the work-force and profession and could be more confident in their own abilities. They were able to tell the attributes or behaviours presented by others that would not be so popular in the workplace.

Balancing these aspects can be seen in Figure 2.2.

As well as newly qualified nurses entering practice as professionals for the first time, overseas qualified nurses (who may be very well experienced in their own countries) often join the healthcare workforce due to migration and opportunities to work globally. Going back to Benner (1984) and the concept of moving from novice to expert, such nurses may now find themselves moving back to a lower level of the stages, for example, moving back to be a novice due to the new situation they find themselves in. The challenges they face may not necessarily be related to their nursing qualification or ability but to issues related to culture, language and differing clinical approaches. They will follow the stages of transition identified above and have to deal with the issues of reality/culture shock and adjustment to these factors. A study by Iheduru-Anderson and Wahi (2018) found that Nigerian nurses moving to practice in the United States of America went through stages of fear and disappointment (some of this arising from racism and actual harassment), overcoming challenges (which was aided through gradual acculturation and resilience) to moving forward (occurring through professional development and becoming proficient as role models within their positions).

Ohr et al. (2016) note that even though experienced, such nurses will also need to undergo some kind of formal structured transition programme and support mechanism. This requires tailored support approaches not only for those entering the organization but for those that will be developing the programmes and those working with the overseas/international qualified nurses.

Bagley et al. (2018) also highlight similar transition experiences and barriers for nurses wishing to become academic faculty members. Again, similar factors relating to adapting to new cultural ways and confidence in abilities were major barriers for staff entering these roles. The author has experienced this shift in moving from practice to nurse education as well as more recently also moving to a role in an overseas institution. The lack of confidence experienced due to accessing new environments and cultural organizational practices can lead to what is known as 'imposter syndrome', i.e. believing that you do not belong in that area due to a lack of confidence, expertise or qualification in some factors. Therefore, even experienced nurses and nurse academics also need support in adjustment.

The ideal experience of transition

The notion of an ideal experience of transition which accommodates individual differences during the transition offers a solution to ease the experience of newly registered nurses. Darvill (2013) suggests that there may be some key components within organizational support, allocated time and personal and professional development that can lead to an ideal experience of transition. This is something you might want to consider when you start your first post. This ideal experience of transition should include the following components:

- A period of lengthy and consistent support.
- The allocation of contrived workloads.
- The physical presence of a supporting individual.
- Ability to spend time with different practitioners to observe different styles of practice.
- Having the confidence and competence to choose to commence working independently.

- Being allocated patients based on previous experience and capability level.
- Being provided with opportunities to develop your knowledge, skills and experiences.
- Being given the autonomy to work independently to gain confidence through experience.
- Being able to face challenges with the support of the organization and colleagues.
- Feeling valued and having your undergraduate learning experience recognized.
- Identifying learning needs, undertaking self-assessment, personal development planning and goal setting.
- Gaining consistent and continuous feedback on performance.
- Being given guidance, time and support.
- Facilitation of stress reduction.
- Networking with other newly qualified practitioners.
- Not being allocated complex patient cases requiring skills and knowledge beyond your competence level.

The factor of resilience will now be focused upon.

Demonstrating resilience

New nurses are required to develop resilience during transition and deal with adversity through taking control of their learning and development and gaining organizational support to enhance their transition experiences. Nursing involves complex caring work, and newly registered nurses need to prepare and develop strategies to avoid workplace adversity, stress, workplace incivility, burnout and neglectful care. According to McAllister and Lowe (2011) resilience is of vital importance and an essential skill that enables nurses to make sense of their experience and manage the stress of the workplace. Resilience is viewed as a critical graduate capability for new nurses entering professional practice. Grant and Kinman (2013) refer to resilience as the ability of an individual to adjust to workplace adversity, maintain equilibrium, retain some sense of control over their environment and continue to move on in a positive manner. This definition is similar to that provided by DuBois and

Zedreck Gonzalez (2018), who also add that it is the ability to adjust to stressful events such as those recognized in the stages of transition. It involves characteristics of self-efficacy, humour, competence and positivity. They highlight that resilience education should be part of any transition. This should include interventions focusing on the individual healthcare worker, such as mindfulness, improving communication and relationships, managing difficult situations and conflict, goal setting, and decision making. Kulka et al. (2016) found that mindfulness interventions helped nurses in transition to reduce their stress levels.

Currently, researchers have identified that resilience can be developed or enhanced (Stephens, 2013). Individuals can strengthen personal resilience by developing strategies for reducing the impact of workplace adversity. Strategies to enhance resilience include seeking and gaining supportive relationships, achieving a positive work–life balance, self-awareness, self-care and reflection.

Transition resilience is defined as the ability to cope with the stresses of the experiences of transition by demonstrating mental toughness, adjusting to adversity, maintaining equilibrium, retaining some sense of control over the environment and continuing to move on in a positive manner. Nurse graduate development programmes can assist new nurses to develop transition resilience through preparing and implementing transition focused personal and professional learning and development strategies. Further strategies to enhance resilience include seeking and gaining supportive relationships, achieving a positive work–life balance, self-awareness, self-care and reflection (McDonald et al., 2016). Meyer and Shatto (2018) found that resilience is necessary for nurses in transition and that it can be developed through a sense of community and communication throughout the transition period. Lekan et al. (2018) highlight that resilience should be cultivated through a student's nurse education experience to reduce the risk of anxiety, depression and post-traumatic stress experiences when it comes to entering the profession. This is crucial as Concilio et al. (2019) point out that ultimately reduced resilience in new graduate nurses can negatively affect patient safety outcomes, so it must be consciously tackled in nurse education programmes and in the period of transition into the nursing career. We will now look at the types of support for the transition process.

Support during the transition period

Accessing support

In the current environment, there is an expectation that nurses have a preceptor on qualifying to aid in their transition – in dealing with the conversion from supervised student to autonomous practitioner. There is strong evidence that newly registered nurses benefit from a period of supported and structured preceptorship, which translates to improved recruitment and retention for employing organizations (Whitehead et al., 2013). The perception of support by the organization is crucial to successful outcomes for newly qualified nurses.

Support from senior colleagues is highly valued and perceived as having a significant impact on new nurses' ability to cope with the demands of the job, gives an increase in confidence levels, and could lead to perceived stress reduction. Conversely, a perceived lack of support in the period of transition increases anxiety and feelings of disillusionment and inadequacy. Ankers et al. (2018) suggest that transitioning nurses found positive benefits in having dedicated staff assigned to assisting them through their transition experience. Baldwin et al. (2016) outline the benefits of integrating volunteer retired nurses as part of a structured programme to specifically mentor newly qualified nurses during their transition, particularly from an economic cost perspective.

The benefits of support during the transition period are expressed in terms of skills development, increased confidence, knowledge, critical thinking, communication, collaborative working and personal and professional development. There is also an indication that crucially recruitment and retention are improved through simple measures put in place for staff in posts at fixed points.

--------------------------------- **ACTIVITY 2.2** ---------------------------------

Research the areas where you might be applying for your first post, or your next post, and find out what strategies and interventions they have in place to support newly registered or transitioning nurses.

1   What kinds of programmes are there?
2   Is there any supervision?
3   Is there a period of probation?

(Continued)

(Continued)

These factors might influence your choice in your career progression and also provide you with valid questions to ask at interview.

There are lots of examples in the literature of the importance of structured, formal, orientation/transition/residency programmes that help in the transition of newly qualified nurses. Tyndall et al. (2018) found in their integrative review that newly graduated nurse transition programmes did show some contribution to improving patient safety. However, they point out that this was not wholly conclusive, and much more research is needed into understanding the nature of such courses and how they can contribute. It was clear in their study that there is a lack of consistency amongst the types of transition programmes offered.

According to van Camp and Chappy (2017) nurse residency programmes are designed to expand and develop the clinical and professional competencies of those joining the organization's workforce. As mentioned earlier, there are issues in retaining newly qualified staff early in their tenure. Nurse residency programmes are also costly but are an economically preferred approach compared to replacing staff. The study by van Camp and Chappy (2017) suggested that nurse residency programmes have positive outcomes and benefits for newly graduated nurses on the education, support and guidance received. According to this study such programmes foster positive transitions into practice and produce competent, confident nurses and staffing retention into the workplace. Another option for conducting a new nurse residency programme for organizations with limited budgets and resources is to provide an online programme.

A study by Wilson et al. (2018) found a gradual reduction of stress over time and had similar positive results to other formal and structured face-to-face programmes. An extended orientation programme is suggested by Baumann et al. (2018) in order to ensure that newly qualified nurses are specifically integrated when being deployed to work in specialist care environments. The use of simulation-based education is suggested by Rossler et al. (2018) who found some benefits in the approach in transition programmes. Newly qualified nurses were able to gain comfort in professional relationships by having the opportunity to develop working associations, and the approach gave them chances to thoroughly talk through clinical incidents and professionally develop via close communication and discussion with others.

A study by van Rooyen et al. (2018) investigated the best practice guidelines for supporting nurses in transition and found three main aspects were required. This included, first, formal and structured support for students in their final year as student nurses, followed by a structured programme in their first year post-qualifying. Second, providing opportunities for socialization and creating a sense of belonging within clinical teams by full integration into teams with less rotation. And finally having a positive clinical learning environment which values educators and learners in a welcoming and structured programme helps with transition by assisting in reducing the reality/culture shock and providing supervised clinical experiences to promote confidence.

Another approach suggested by Verret and Lin (2016) is 'Peer Mentoring'. This is a structured approach and programme where new graduate nurses are assigned a mentor. Usually this could be a 'veteran' nurse and a younger peer nurse. This helps as the veteran may demonstrate wisdom via their experience and the younger peer through technological understanding and social similarities. The results from their evaluation showed improvements in teamwork, increased satisfaction amongst new graduate nurses and on their retention rates. Retention is key to improving patient outcomes and safety in healthcare provision. A study by Williams et al. (2018) supported the notion that mentorship is important in the transition for new graduate nurses, their professional development and their stress management.

Reflection on preparing for transition

To assist you in the preparation for transition you can undertake a professional and academic self-assessment of your current knowledge skills and values. This will enable identification of any learning deficits that can be remedied on the final placements. Self-assessment for a final year nursing student entails a critical reflection on where you are now in relation to the expected professional standards of knowledge, skills and attitudinal values that you must acquire, and achieve competence in performing, by the end of your registration.

The NMC (2018a) considers that newly registered nurses should take responsibility for continuous self-reflection, seeking and responding to support and feedback to develop their professional knowledge and skills. The ability to reflect and make use of your experience in order to learn and enhance your knowledge and skills will be an important strategy for you to prepare for your transition to professional practice (Keeling and Major, 2018).

ACTIVITY 2.3

If you are still a student nurse and coming up to preparing for your transition to becoming a qualified nurse, reflect upon and list the factors that you believe may be the most stressful, or that you are most anxious about.

1   How might you go about addressing these concerns?

If you are already qualified, reflect upon the factors that caused you most stress during this period and how you addressed them.

2   What helped to reduce stress and improve transition?
3   What issues do you believe would need to be addressed in further role changes?
4   Consider which tools you might use to undertake this self-assessment of your current knowledge, skills and values.

You might have considered referring to your feedback from academic work or from your practice assessors. You could review your portfolio and practice assessment documents and clinical skills documents. After reviewing your progress to date, you could then formulate a SNOB analysis (Strengths, Needs, Opportunities and Barriers) as in Figure 2.3.

ACTIVITY 2.4

Use communication skills as an example and complete a SNOB analysis.

You might have identified your strengths as communicating with clients and their families, however you may have identified breaking bad news, communicating in challenging situations and delivery handover competently and confidently as your needs. Opportunities

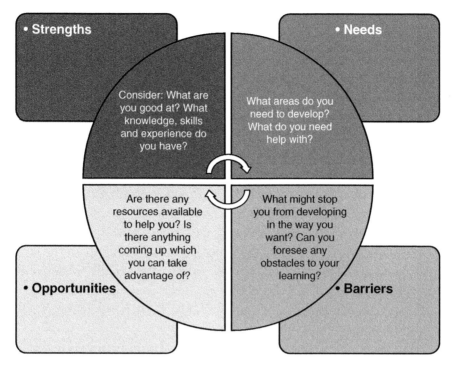

Figure 2.3 SNOB analysis

might include feedback from your assessor on your next practice placement or reading literature around certain specific topics; barriers could include being assertive enough to highlight your learning needs.

Through undertaking a range of self-assessments, you can clearly identify your personal transition development needs, and this may help you to be assertive and take control of your own learning both in the academic and practice settings.

There have been a variety of strategies and interventions put in place to support newly registered nurses during their transition. Recently, Edwards et al. (2015) identified that transition interventions and strategies do lead to improvements in confidence and competence, job satisfaction, critical thinking and reductions in stress and anxiety for new nurses.

Summary

This chapter has focused on the concept of transition. It has highlighted that this is a recognized factor for newly qualified nurses affecting their knowledge, skills, attitudes and behaviours as they move into the profession. This period is one of great importance as it is also the time when nurses make the decision to either stay or leave the profession. The outcome of such decisions affects nurse retention, which besides having an economic impact on the healthcare providing organization can also have a major impact on patient safety.

Transition is recognized in stages. The newly qualified nurse moves from the relative safety and protection of the nurse education environment to one of entering the 'real world' of healthcare provision. Here they are more exposed and vulnerable to the outcomes of their own decision-making and are accountable for them. Issues such as heavy workloads, conflict, dealing with death and dying and increasing exposure to wider sets of clinical skills can all add to the stresses of transition. This leads to nurses experiencing reality shock, culture shock or transition shock. As they go through a period of adjustment, they eventually are able to stabilize into their new positions as they develop competence and confidence.

It is recognized therefore that such transitioning nurses need a great deal of support, and communication with and support from nursing colleagues are crucial in assisting the nurse to navigate this period. It may not just be this initial phase either. Transition can occur at many points throughout a nurse's career as they develop in their roles and perhaps take up other positions in specialized areas of clinical care, management, research or nurse education.

Having experienced and encouraging preceptors or identified support staff assigned to newly qualified nurses can help. Formal structured courses such as transition/orientation/residency programmes can help in settling the newly qualified nurse into their careers. This should perhaps be factored into pre-registration nursing programmes as well as within the organizations where they commence their initial employment within the profession. Nurses need to be resilient to navigate through this period of transition, and such programmes should include some focus on resilience training and development, including mindfulness, communication and self-efficacy development.

In the UK and other countries, reflection plays an important role in the development, continuing professional development and revalidation/registration process. It is a useful tool to use in order to identify impacting factors in transition, resilience and supportive approaches required to address adversity and stress in the process.

Finally, transition does not only occur at the newly qualified stage but in all aspects of changing roles, responsibilities and career directions. Nurses migrating to other countries to practise nursing will also find transition a challenging process, and will need support in adapting to the new cultural environment and approaches.

With the correct support the challenges related to transition can be addressed and you can find yourself in a career that is very rewarding on a number of levels.

3

IMPROVING SAFETY AND QUALITY OF CARE

Graham Ormrod and Rob Burton

THE AIMS OF THIS CHAPTER ARE TO:

- Explore your role as a student nurse in improving safety, maintaining standards and ensuring quality of care.
- Explore your subsequent role as a registered nurse in improving safety, maintaining standards and ensuring quality of care.
- Critically review health policy and explore its impact on quality in clinical practice.
- Investigate what is meant by 'good quality care'.

Whilst reading this chapter, you will have the opportunity to discover how the experience gained on your placements can help you to contribute to improving safety and quality of care. It will help you to develop competence in improving care delivery and management and explore the mechanisms available to help to develop your authority to improve safety and deliver and maintain high standards of care confidently.

Improving safety and quality of care and the nurse's responsibilities

Improving and maintaining safety and developing quality standards of care is an essential responsibility for all registered nurses. Indeed, the Nursing and Midwifery Council (2018b) reiterate that public safety and safe and effective practice are central to the NMC Standards as nurses are often those who make the key contribution to quality of care and treatment and thereby enhance outcomes (NMC, 2018b). Improving safety and quality of care is 'Platform 6' in the *Standards of Proficiency for Registered Nurses* (NMC, 2018b: 21) where it emphasizes how registered nurses make a major and unique contribution to the continuous monitoring and quality improvement of care and treatment. Therefore, the care and safety of patients must always be nurses' main concern and it is essential that nurses lead and support good quality care, implement change as necessary and promote professionalism and trust by putting care and safety first (NMC, 2018b). Nurses should always put the needs of those receiving care or services first by identifying priorities, managing time, staff and resources effectively and dealing with risk to make sure that the quality of care or service delivered is maintained and improved (NMC, 2018a: 25.1).

The *Standards of Proficiency for Registered Nurses* insist that at the point of registration the registered nurse will be able to:

work with people, their families, carers and colleagues to develop effective improvement strategies for quality and safety, sharing feedback and learning from positive outcomes and experiences, mistakes and adverse outcomes and experiences. (Platform 6.9)

This principle is confirmed in *The Code* (NMC, 2018a: 25.1) where nurses are challenged to always:

> identify priorities, manage time, staff and resources effectively and deal with risk to make sure that the quality of care or service you deliver is maintained and improved, putting the needs of those receiving care or services first.

The Coronavirus pandemic of 2020 highlighted the profound difficulties inherent in always achieving these aspirations. Difficulty in the provision of certain *resources*, most particularly personal protective equipment (PPE), led the Royal College of Nursing (RCN) to suggest that if all measures to reduce risk have been exhausted and appropriate PPE was still not provided then, as a last resort, nurses were entitled to refuse to work (RCN, 2020). Whilst recognizing the 'enormously difficult decision' the RCN assured their members that they would be provided with legal representation and other support in any proceedings that might ensue. The circumstances nurses found themselves in during the pandemic had led to guidance that the RCN recognized would go against every instinct of nurses, and confirms the unprecedented nature of the circumstances confronting some nurses at that time.

So, what is high-quality nursing care?

What does it mean to say that a nurse or team of nurses delivered a high standard of care? Interestingly, nurses and other health professionals have historically struggled with articulating the concept of 'good care' and it appears that good care was not something talked about very much with colleagues (Dewar and MacBride, 2017; Goodrich and Cornwell, 2008). According to Maben and Griffiths (2008), there are six core elements to good-quality nursing care:

1 A holistic approach to physical, mental and emotional needs, patient-centred and continuous care.
2 Efficiency and effectiveness combined with humanity and compassion.
3 Professional, high-quality, evidence-based practice.
4 Safe, effective and prompt nursing interventions.

5   Patient empowerment, support and advocacy.
6   Seamless care through effective teamwork with other professions. (How this might be achieved will be discussed further in Chapter 6).

Maben and Griffiths (2008) also highlighted that nurses want many of the same things as patients and the public, the five main aspects being:

1   Making a difference to patients' lives.
2   Close contact with patients.
3   Delivering excellent care.
4   Working in a team and being a role model.
5   Continuous development with ongoing learning and improvement.

ACTIVITY 3.1

It has been said that some of the enduring qualities of nursing, such as care and compassion, have been lost and are now not demonstrated adequately by nurses. The implication seems to be that the humanity of caring and the more advanced technical tasks and roles that nurses are now undertaking are at polar opposites.
  Do you agree with this?
  Consider and write down why you answered as you did.

A brief history of quality in the UK health service – the political context

Your experience as a student will probably have helped you to form a perspective and opinion on what makes good-quality nursing care. However, to fully recognize where we currently are and where we might want to be in the future often requires looking back and reflecting on the journey. Think about this as we explore the history of 'the quality agenda' in healthcare.

It was initially assumed that the UK's National Health Service (NHS), as set up in 1948, with its fundamental welfare principles and aspirations of improving social justice, would inevitably result in quality standards of care being delivered. The NHS essentially worked with an implicit notion of quality – an assumption that if staff were well trained and good facilities and equipment were provided, then high standards of care would inevitably be achieved (Gottwald and Lansdown, 2014). However, as time progressed, it became clear that this was not necessarily so. This realization came due to a number of reasons, not least the changing attitudes and priorities in society. For example, by the 1970s, some of the original aspirations of the welfare state in general and the NHS in particular were being seriously questioned for the first time (Crinson, 2009). This questioning coincided with a steep economic decline in the British economy in that period, leading to shortages and subsequent debates about whether valuable, but limited, resources were being used in the best ways. There was also a dawning realization that the NHS had become far more extensive and complex than originally envisaged and therefore could no longer meet the demands placed on it. The original intention to provide services that met a range of basic human needs had changed into a service that was required to cater for the far more complex personalized requirements of the population (Bradshaw and Bradshaw, 2004). Comparable economic pressures in other countries led to similar debates concerning social welfare generally and 'universal' healthcare in particular.

The election of the Conservative government in the UK under Margaret Thatcher in 1979 indicated a belief that public services had become paternalistic and now had an unhelpful and inappropriate involvement in virtually all aspects of people's personal lives. The 'political' argument was that this created a culture of dependency, resulted in lack of choice in the services that were available, and, fundamentally, constrained individual liberty. Health was seen more as an individual's possession and therefore ill health was seen to a large extent to be the fault of the afflicted, thereby obscuring the impact of any socio-economic considerations and the potential impact of the broader context on an individual's health (Baggott, 2015).

Public expectations were also starting to challenge the power of the professionals – in particular, doctors – and this challenge, and what is often called the rise of consumerism, resulted in demands for greater choice, more information in any decisions concerning healthcare, and also a greater accountability of those delivering the service.

Some of these principles – greater choice, greater information, partnerships, transparency and accountability for example – might resonate with your previous and current experience. We shall see later in the chapter that some of these key ideas have been retained and remain central to the philosophies of current health policy.

Later in 1992 the Conservative government introduced *The Patient's Charter* (DH, 1992) which for the very first time set out in a very clear way the rights that patients had in relation to NHS services and the standards that they could expect in relation to waiting times for operations, ambulance response times, the timely handling of complaints, and so on.

For example:

> You have the right to have any complaint about NHS services (whoever provides them) investigated and to get a quick, full written reply from the relevant chief executive or general manager. The new complaints procedure means this will be within four weeks. (DH, 1992)

Also, for the first time, each patient in a hospital was required to have an identified nurse – *a named nurse* – to deliver and coordinate their care for the duration of their hospital stay or engagement with health services. Although some criticized many of the rights articulated in *The Patient's Charter* as being too easily achievable (Williamson et al., 2008), if nothing else, it represented a shift in thinking both for the public and also for professionals. The historical management of resources and demands by a combination of waiting lists, 'gatekeeping' by general practitioners (GPs) and clinical autonomy of physicians was beginning to break down (Harrison and McDonald, 2008). High-quality healthcare was viewed much more as a *right* and an entitlement rather than a system in which patients were simply passive recipients of care. Not only were such standards introduced, but they were also published, showing how well various organizations were doing in comparison with others. These were presented in the form of 'league tables', highlighting the increasing aspect of 'comparison and competition' in healthcare and also hinting at the future of patient choice and greater patient and public involvement in healthcare (Bradshaw and Bradshaw, 2004).

Supporters of greater patient and public involvement presented the ideal as a shared decision-making model (Crinson, 2009) and highlighted certain key characteristics, including that both the patient and the doctor or health professional are involved and share information to build a consensus about the preferred treatment. However, many studies indicate that there is little evidence that this participation in the consultation process occurred (Cave and Reinach, 2019; Rogers et al., 2005). Indeed, at best in many cases, patient self-management essentially constituted nothing more than compliance with medical instructions. Similarly, Smith (2001) questioned any developments that might challenge medical autonomy as this inevitably implies distrust of doctors and attempts to replace this trust in the individual with a supposedly more objective trust and confidence in systems: for example, guidelines and performance indicators. This, according to Smith (2001), fractures the therapeutic moral content of the client–practitioner relationship. In relation to this potential challenge it is interesting to consider the development in contemporary politics that appears to have cast doubt on the status of expertise and led to the claim that the public 'have had enough of experts' not least in what has recently been called a 'post-truth world' of fake news and misinformation. However, this rather bleak commentary has been challenged, suggesting that what evidence there is suggests a broadly positive public attitude toward experts (Dommett and Pearce, 2019).

In theory, such initiatives highlighted that not only could patients now appropriately expect universal or consistent standards irrespective of where they came in contact with healthcare, but they could also expect that all healthcare practice be supported by sound, current, and robust evidence.

However, some highlighted the possibility of tension between such consumerism and choice on the one hand, and evidence-based practice on the other. Simply put, the first suggests that people should have the services that they desire, while the second suggests that they should receive the services that, according to the evidence, are good for them (Harrison and McDonald, 2008: 150).

More and more during this period, healthcare began to adopt a philosophy that mirrored the world of business (Baggott, 2015), resulting in heated discussion of how healthcare could be run more efficiently, have greater financial accountability, and meet rising expectations. This subsequently led to profound changes in ideas of quality management. The effects of chronic underfunding had led to long waiting times and dilapidated premises, and despite the continued hard work and excellent care being delivered by many, this inevitably resulted in a great deal of hostile commentary in the British media. The shortcomings of the NHS at this time were undeniable, and yet the level of public support for the NHS remained constant (Welch, 2018).

Following the election of New Labour in 1997, it quickly became clear that one of the new government's priorities would be to attempt to address the concerns that the public had about the quality and standards of healthcare provision. *The New NHS: Modern and Dependable* (DH, 1997: 3.2), for example, promised that the service 'will have quality at its heart' and NHS organizations would have a statutory duty to ensure the quality of their services. Therefore, NHS trust chief executives were now made legally accountable for clinical standards, and each trust had to identify a designated senior clinician to ensure that systems of quality were functioning properly. Similarly, primary care trusts (PCT) – the new administrative bodies set up with the responsibility for commissioning primary, community and secondary health services from providers – had to nominate a senior health professional to lead on clinical standards and professional development. These 'systems of quality' are often encapsulated under the umbrella term 'clinical governance'.

The NHS Plan (DH, 2000) was the landmark document produced by the New Labour government highlighting its vision of this direction of change. The document highlighted a massive ten-year reform of the NHS, with setting and monitoring standards as a central theme. The plan attempted to set in place structures to improve efficiency, effectiveness, access and quality of services. As Bradshaw and Bradshaw (2004) explained, the strategies chosen by the government concentrated on the formulation of national standards, performance indicators, audit and inspection. Part of this was to create new structures, bodies, and guidelines to enable the plan to work. These included the setting up of the Commission for Health Improvement (CHI), the National Institute for Health and Clinical Excellence (NICE), the Modernisation Agency, and the introduction of national service frameworks (NSFs) to set minimum standards and expectations for key areas of health. Many of these initiatives were designed to address the apparent disparities in care and treatment throughout the country – a phenomenon often called 'care by postcode'.

By 2010, whilst the quality agenda remained as a pledge for the Conservative Party when they fought the general election of that year, the international financial crisis and economic recession in the UK meant that their election manifesto emphasized a belief in the need to substantially reduce the UKs public financial deficit, not least by a significant reduction in public expenditure which would have major implications for much social and health policy in the UK (Bochel and Powell, 2016).

Following the election result in 2010 the Conservative Party were 19 seats short of a majority government and therefore they formed a coalition with the Liberal Democrats, with David Cameron as Prime Minister and Nick Clegg as Deputy Prime Minister. The adverse economic climate, rising demands for healthcare, ageing population, costs of new technology and the comparison of the relatively generous increases in NHS funding under New Labour created considerable problems for the new Coalition Government (Baggott, 2016).

It is important to remember that most UK health policy is now devolved to the governments of Scotland, Wales and Northern Ireland – the key initiatives highlighted in this short section are undoubtedly more precisely focused on the impact of policy on England.

The Coalition's reform plan for England was said to be so big 'you could probably see it from space' (Greer et al., 2014). The Health and Social Care Act (2012) overseen by Health Secretary Andrew Lansley abolished Primary Care Trusts, established a national commissioning board (later named NHS England) to oversee the planning and commissioning of healthcare; and local clinical commissioning groups (CCGs) were set up to commission secondary care services, such as most hospital, mental health, and urgent and emergency services. A statutory body called Healthwatch England was also set up. The Healthwatch network is a network of patient and public involvement made up of 152 local Healthwatches across each of the local authority areas and the national body Healthwatch England. The purpose of this network is to understand the needs, experiences and concerns of people who use health and care services and speak out on their behalf (Healthwatch, 2019).

────────────────── ACTIVITY 3.2 ──────────────────

Access the Healthwatch website and explore the latest news and current work of Healthwatch. Healthwatch considers itself to be the champion for people who use health and social care services (www.healthwatch.co.uk).

Do the priorities expressed on the website match your experience of healthcare?

Greater choice remained a priority of the policy and this was evidenced by extending patients' rights to choose a named consultant, specific GPs and particular service providers. However, possibly due to the massive nature of the proposed changes, by 2014 then Health Secretary Jeremy Hunt – who had taken over in 2012 – declared that patient choice was now *not* seen as the main key to improving performance in the NHS (West, 2014).

Many of the performance management targets introduced by New Labour were pledged to be abolished if they were perceived as 'getting in the way' of achieving better clinical outcomes (Davis et al., 2015). The espoused principle was that measuring outcomes – mortality rates from cancer for example – should be the priority rather than the measurement of processes or systems such as waiting times for diagnosis and treatment. The belief was that such performance management would thereby focus on improving health and care rather than simply meeting targets. Targets that some now viewed as fundamentally bureaucratic and less related to tangible results in healthcare, outcomes or patient experience. Interestingly, in relation to quality and the patient experience, certain targets such as accident and emergency waiting times remained.

The Mid Staffordshire Inquiry (2013)

The Mid Staffordshire Inquiry (Francis, 2013) led by Sir Robert Francis, reaffirmed the Coalition's need to revisit *the quality agenda* as it highlighted that the poor quality and shocking neglect exposed at the Mid Staffordshire Hospital had to some extent been due to the encouragement of a culture focused on financial and management issues rather than patients' needs or experiences.

The impact, ramifications and implications of the Francis Report (Francis, 2013) on the whole of the NHS should not be underestimated. The seismic effect of the Report and the reflection, self-examination and self-analysis that it generated within the Health Service in the UK, the various health professions – not least nursing – and in the mainstream media and wider society in general was immense.

The Francis Report felt the need to explicitly reaffirm nurses' need to commit to compassionate and considerate patient care and emphasize practical hands-on training and experience as a pre-requisite to entry into the nursing profession (Francis, 2013). Moreover, the Report also confirmed that recruits to the nursing profession needed 'possession of the appropriate values, attitudes and behaviours' – and the 'ability and motivation to enable them to put the welfare of others above their own interests' (Recommendation 185). This was to be in some way assessed, prior to taking up nursing, by an aptitude test created by the NMC and universities together.

The Francis Report did **not** advise that the education of nurses should return to an educational level below a degree, however it did, by implication at least, suggest that the more recent registrants to nursing had in some way differing values than nurses who had qualified previously and perhaps that the 'old ways', as evidenced by these 'old timers', was in some way better or more appropriate to the needs of patients and service users. The Francis Report undoubtedly had a chastening message for nursing care provision, patient care, professional regulation, nurse education and particularly recruitment of students and the structure of nursing registration programmes (Hayter, 2013).

Much of the debate within the nursing profession post-Francis Report revolved around how apparently caring, compassionate and empathetic staff – including most specifically nurses – had 'allowed' this situation to come about and how and why had nurses apparently remained silent in the face of such lapses of care. In part resultant from these challenging revelations the NMC and General Medical Council (GMC) published guidance that reiterated the professional duty of candour and the important responsibility for nurses and other healthcare staff to be honest with patients when things go wrong (NMC and GMC, 2014). The Francis Report was also insistent that nurses who raise concerns about poor care – or 'whistle blow' – should be protected and supported in this endeavour (Francis, 2013: 188).

Other challenges highlighted by the Francis Report included a recommendation to move away from a culture driven by achievement of objectively measured targets – albeit set centrally by the Department of Health – that were essentially paper-based indicators of 'quality care' and 'success' (Hayter, 2013: 184).

Similarly, Berwick and the National Advisory Group on the Safety of Patients in England (DH, 2013a), in their report written in response to events at Mid Staffordshire Hospital, also challenged the NHS to change and embrace an ethic of learning. Berwick claims that the most powerful foundation for advancing patient safety and improving quality within the NHS is the potential for being a 'learning organization' rather than a culture of the 'mechanistic imposition of rules, incentives or regulations' (DH, 2013a: 45).

The renewed focus on quality and safety made essential by the Mid Staffordshire enquiry led to interventions in other healthcare providers as it was widely acknowledged that Mid Staffordshire was not an isolated 'bad apple'. The then NHS Medical Director Bruce Keogh's review of the care and treatment provided by 14 NHS trusts in England that had relatively high mortality led to 11 trusts being placed in 'special measures' and amongst other concerns showed that inadequate nurse staffing was an important factor in poor care and even persistently high mortality rates (Keogh, 2013).

Interestingly, students' and qualified nurses' assessments of a negative work environment and subsequent job dissatisfaction generally concur with those made independently by service users or patients, with job dissatisfaction among nurses contributing to incidents of quality of care deficits and subsequent increased risk to patients (Aiken et al., 2012; McHugh et al., 2011). A negative work environment may be the result of many variables – not least nurse staffing levels. For example, evidence indicates that an increase in a nurses' workload by one patient alone increases the likelihood of inpatient deaths (Aiken et al., 2014). Conversely hospitals with more positive work environments, as evidenced by considerations such as appropriate nurse staffing levels and managerial support for nursing care, good doctor–nurse relations, nurse participation in decision-making and quality of care being seen as an organizational priority, appear to result in improved outcomes for patients, nurses and student nurses alike. This claim of general improvement in patient care and greater staff and student satisfaction should such positive work environments pertain is supported by the research undertaken by Aiken and Sloane (2020) and Blackman et al. (2014).

It was clear that this period was one of great challenge for the NHS with real-term increases in funding much lower than in the previous decade. For example, 40 percent of NHS trusts and 51 percent of foundation trusts reported a deficit for the financial year 2014/15. Foundation trusts are trusts that are still within the NHS but have greater autonomy of decision-making, prioritization and strategy-making from central government in an attempt to more readily meet the needs of the local population.

Public satisfaction with the NHS fell between 2010 and 2011 from 70 percent to 58 percent but rose again to 65 percent in 2014. This offers a complex picture, with reductions in hospital-acquired infections and mixed-sex wards being positive influences on the patient experience, whereas the increased waiting times of over four hours from less than two percent in April 2010 to over eight percent by April 2015 and missed key cancer targets from 2014 onwards inevitably negatively impacted on patient and public perception of the NHS (Baggott, 2016).

Five Year Forward View (2014) and Next Steps on the NHS Five Year Forward View (2017)

In 2014 the new Conservative Government issued the *Five Year Forward View* (NHS England, 2014) and pronounced that although the NHS had improved and continued to lead the world in quality of the care it still had to be admitted and accepted that care remained variable. Partly due to the evident variation in service quality between different clinical teams and also between different parts of the country, as evidence continued to indicate the existence of the so-called 'care by postcode'.

The challenge for everyone was to 'square the circle' between the desire to improve the quality of care whilst also acknowledging and responding to 'rising patient numbers and also living within the expected tight funding' (NHS England, 2014: 25). The *Five Year Forward View* emphasized the need for change and action on several fronts: including a shift in emphasis in prevention and public health; more engagement with communities in decisions about the future of health and social care; efforts to break down the divisions between family doctors and hospitals and greater control for patients over their care.

In 2017, *Next Steps on the NHS Five Year Forward View* (NHS England, 2017b) was published attempting to summarize progress in improving care since the NHS *Five Year Forward View* of 2014. This document promised to improve care focused on urgent and emergency care, primary care, cancer and mental health. This included delivering the four-hour standard in all emergency departments and providing extended access to GP appointments for example. Yet also, in apparent recognition of the inability to achieve certain ambitions within the funds made available by the government – lower priority was given to other 'targets'. Many of these targets were already struggling to be met – for example that patients waiting for less urgent diagnosis and treatment should be seen within 18 weeks. This was claimed by some to be further evidence of declining NHS standards and even failing to deliver commitments enshrined in the NHS Constitution (Ham, 2017).

NHS Long Term Plan (2019)

The *NHS Long Term Plan* (NHS England, 2019a) reflected on some of the areas that the Government believed had been successes since the publication of *Next Steps on the Forward View* in 2017. These included improved data collection in all major accident and emergency departments to enable better tracking of the quality and timeliness of care; an introduction of quality-of-life metrics to track and respond to the long-term impact of cancer; further developing information on the acute and inpatient rehabilitation care of stroke patients and improved technology to free up expensive staff time and provide safety prompts to improve the quality of care.

Some of the main commitments in the Plan going forward were:

- A £4.5 billion uplift to primary medical and community health services in an attempt to improve out-of-hospital care by means of integrated care systems (ICSs).
- Emphasis on a range of clinical priorities including:
  - Children and young people.
  - Cancer, e.g. by 2028, 75 percent of cancers will be diagnosed at stage 1 or 2.
  - Cardiovascular disease.
  - Stroke.
  - Diabetes.
  - Respiratory disease.
  - Mental health.
- Digital technology:
  - Outpatient departments redesigned to reduce face-to-face appointments by 30 million appointments a year.
  - Every patient to get the right to telephone or online consultations.

- Workforce:
  - Critical importance of workforce is recognized – however little specific plans are articulated to highlight a way out of the current workforce problems.

(NHS England, 2019a; contains public sector information licensed under the Open Government Licence v3.0. www.nationalarchives. gov.uk/doc/open-government-licence/version/3/)

The King's Fund (2019b) offered a chastening voice, believing that the 'workforce crisis in health and care is simply too deep and too pressing for any more failed attempts to reform'. The *Interim NHS People Plan* (NHS England, 2019b) claimed that simply training and employing more staff was not enough, and that the 'NHS must also be the best place to work', and thereby aimed to:

- Recruit more staff:
  - Immediately increase the number of nursing students and offer an extra 5,700 hospital and community placements for student nurses.
  - Rapidly increase the number of nursing associates to 7,500, offering a career route from healthcare support work to registered nursing.
  - Launch a new campaign to inspire more nurses to return to the NHS.
  - Quickly grow the number of nurses and doctors recruited from overseas.
- Make the NHS a great place to work:
  - Conduct a major staff engagement exercise immediately exploring issues staff say matter to them, for example career development and progression, access to flexible working and greater support from line managers.
  - Ensure more support and development for frontline NHS managers, from ward to board.
  - Rapidly address current pensions issues which are discouraging experienced doctors and nurses from doing extra work for patients.
- Equipping the NHS to meet the challenges of twenty-first century healthcare:
  - Develop new models of multidisciplinary working to support the *Long Term Plan*'s ambition to integrate primary and secondary care.

- ◦ Launch a national consultation exercise to establish what the NHS, patients and the public require from twenty-first century medical graduates.
- ◦ Devolve significant responsibilities for workforce planning to the emerging integrated care systems.
- ◦ Deliver intensive digital skills training for boards and senior leaders.

The King's Fund (2019c) responded to the Interim NHS People Plan by welcoming the initiatives to recruit more home-grown nurses but counselled that any effects from this would inevitably take a significant amount of time when previous insufficient workforce planning had left patients receiving less than optimum care as the NHS had chronically struggled to recruit and retain enough staff to deliver services. They also welcomed the acknowledgement that the government's education reforms including the abolition of student bursaries had caused damage, but were concerned that there seemed to be little to address this.

Similarly, whilst acknowledging the strong evidence that a motivated and engaged workforce deliver better care for patients, it had to be recognized that staff stress levels were at an all-time high and the levels of bullying and harassment were unacceptable (King's Fund, 2019c).

So, what does this mean for you as a student nurse?

The modern healthcare context requires that student nurses are facilitated by the curriculum and participation in the clinical environment to ultimately achieve a position where they are able to play a unique role as champions of quality, accept managerial and professional accountability for high-quality care and take a lead role in the organization of local health services (Care Quality Commission, 2015; Prime Minister's Commission, 2010).

It is clear that it is the responsibility of all nurses to work with other colleagues to evaluate the quality of their own work and also that of the others in the team (NMC, 2018a: 8.4). To ensure this it is therefore essential that care and treatment be delivered in an environment that promotes professional behaviour and exhibits the values that underpin *The Code* (NMC, 2018a). However, for a student nurse, this can be problematic as all behaviours emerge from the specific context the student nurse finds themselves in, a specific context that can both enable or disable participation in quality care. You may have found yourself occasionally in an environment where learning is difficult for example. As the Francis Report (Francis, 2013) highlighted, learning may not always be a positive thing for students as their experience might include witnessing the negative behaviours and values of those the student is working with, with resultant poor care and negative patient experience. Unfortunately for some students any poor behaviour demonstrated by clinical colleagues can become considered, in some way, normal and appropriate practice and thereby legitimized, maintained and even copied by the student.

This legitimization of poor practice, sometimes as a survival technique by students, can reduce opportunities for poor practice to be recognized, acknowledged and confronted. Unfortunately, however, as Lord Francis and others (Francis, 2013) have highlighted, if quality of care is going to be maintained then it is essential that any examples of poor patient care must be actually recognized and then subsequently challenged. Lord Willis (Health Education England, 2015: 170) reiterated Francis' observation that students and trainees were 'invaluable eyes and ears' in clinical settings and should therefore be encouraged to ask questions and be inspired by their colleagues to act with honesty, integrity and compassion.

--------------------------------- **ACTIVITY 3.3** ---------------------------------

1   Write down five things that you feel impact positively on the quality and standards of nursing care.
2   Then write down five things that you feel impact negatively on quality and standards.
3   Think about and write down how you might contribute to addressing these as a newly qualified staff nurse.
4   Would you expect patients/clients necessarily to have the same opinion on this as nurses?

There are always very practical things that all nurses can do to ensure high-quality standards, thereby ensuring a positive experience for those for whom they are caring. The essential starting point is always putting the patient/client first because patients want to be 'cared about' as well as 'cared for'.

The section below lists some other fundamental contributions that all nurses can make to maintaining standards and ensuring good-quality nursing care. During your various clinical placements, you will have begun to appreciate the contributions that you can make in many of the areas listed below. Students often spend the most time with patients/service users, assisting in the delivery of the fundamentals of care, and therefore can play an essential part in highlighting the specific requirements and requests of individuals, and consequently ensuring more effective communication and subsequent advocacy. As we have seen, students were highlighted as the 'invaluable eyes and ears in hospital settings' (Francis, 2013). Similarly, you may be aware of the latest research and evidence in a particular aspect of care that you can share with your colleagues, practice supervisor, mentor and other staff to help to improve the experience of those for whom you are caring.

Essential contributions you can make to ensure high-quality nursing care:

- Ensure that you are knowledgeable, skilled, competent, and possess up-to-date and expert knowledge.
- Keep patients informed and involved, encouraging involvement in decision-making.
- Respect privacy, confidentiality, and preserve dignity.
- Have a caring and humane attitude.
- Respect your patients' values and beliefs, and treat them equally.
- Advocate for, and listen to, patients.
- Ensure that clinical care is based on sound evidence.
- Identify areas for improvement in patient care and work towards strategies to solve them.
- Ensure effective communication and sharing of good practice across the multidisciplinary teams.
- Contribute to effective leadership where appropriate.
- Recognize that you and every other member of staff have a responsibility for high-quality care and maintaining standards.

Support, supervision and assessment in practice

Being the eyes and ears in clinical practice is inevitably a difficult and potentially traumatic experience for any student nurse. This is especially problematic if there is a lack of high-quality mentorship or supervision whilst in practice. Willis believed that mentorship was not necessarily seen as a 'badge of honour' (Health Education England, 2015: 46) to registered nurses. These considerations led the NMC to announce significant changes to their educational standards and the introduction of new roles such as 'academic assessors', 'practice supervisors', and 'practice assessors' in replacement of traditional mentorship roles. The requirements of staff taking on these roles appeared to be less prescriptive although employers and universities are required to ensure that people who took on the roles were properly prepared and supported.

The role of practice supervisor could now be undertaken by any registered health or social care professional – with the expectation that ALL nurses and midwives should be capable of acting in this supervisory capacity. There is no formal qualification for practice supervisors; anyone on the NMC register, even if they're newly qualified, can be a practice supervisor, as long as they are prepared and understand the new roles and the new standards and receive appropriate preparation and support to ensure they have up-to-date knowledge and relevant experience. Practice supervisors may also be other supported health and care staff as required.

A practice assessor is required to be a registered nurse 'with appropriate equivalent experience for the student's field of practice' (NMC, 2018e). The practice assessor assesses and confirms the students' achievements, overall performance and learning in practice, and with the support of the 'academic assessor' can recommend students for progression.

The third role, the academic assessor, will collate and confirm the student's learning and achievements in the theoretical component of the course.

The six Cs

In 2012, after engagement with over 9,000 nurses, midwives, care staff and patients, a new vision and strategy for nursing – *Compassion in Practice* (DH, 2012) was produced. A major part of the initiative was to clarify and confirm the fundamental and enduring values, behaviours and beliefs that underpin care wherever it occurs, not least as the evidence of poor care in environments such as Mid Staffordshire Hospital and Winterbourne View were felt as a 'betrayal of what we all stand for' (DH, 2012: 7).

Although not new, it was the defining and bringing together of the 'six Cs' that promoted a vision and articulation of professional caring values, put the person being cared for at the heart of care and thereby enabled nurses to be held accountable to those values in the care and services they provided.

1   Care.
    It is claimed that care is the core business of nursing and the organizations in which they work, and although care is presented as a separate 'value' it is hard to consider that nurses could provide effective care in isolation from the values of compassion, competence, communication, courage and commitment (Baillie, 2017). Defining 'care' can be deceptively difficult. Dalpezzo (2000: 261) offered a helpful and comprehensive operational definition of nursing care:

    > Nursing care is a skilled, safe, high quality, holistic, ethical, collaborative, individualized, interpersonal caring process that is planned and designed based on best evidence available, and results in positive patient outcomes, optimization of health, palliation of symptoms, or a peaceful death.

2   Compassion.
    Compassion is evidenced when care is given through relationships based on empathy, respect and dignity – it can also be described as intelligent kindness (DH, 2012). It is important to recognize, however, that compassion – whilst increasingly important in more highly technical, fast-changing care environments – is not sufficient. Compassion without competence may be meaningless or even harmful.

3   Competence.
    Competence can be seen to encompass knowledge, skills, attitudes and personal attributes whilst simultaneously recognizing any contextual aspects of competence including technical, structural and political factors (Bing-Jonsson et al., 2015).

4   Communication.
    Cummings (DH, 2012) highlights that communication is central to successful caring relationships and to effective teamworking. Communication is integral to most of the other values in the 6Cs, and effective communication using verbal and non-verbal skills has a significant evidence base in nursing.

5 Courage.

Courage is often necessary to ensure that nurses feel able to make difficult decisions, raise concerns about standards, safeguard the vulnerable and implement change. It has been argued that courage allows nurses to act ethically and creatively, face challenges and motivate others through role modelling (Lindh et al., 2010). Courage can also be necessary to care for individuals who are suffering where a lack of courage could lead the nurse to distance themselves and thereby indicate a lack of compassion.

6 Commitment.

This value indicates a commitment to quality of care and improving the patient experience, and highlights that 'a commitment to patients and populations is a cornerstone of what nurses do' (DH, 2012).

In the document *Compassion in Practice: One Year On* (DH, 2013b) examples are offered where the strategy and the framework of the 6Cs have helped articulate the values of care staff committed to providing quality care. Jane Cummings, The Chief Nursing Officer of England at the time, believed that the examples also indicated a recognition that no one C was more important than any other and that their strength lay in the combined expression of their values and behaviours (DH, 2013b: 3).

Similarly, an evaluation of the apparent success and positive engagement of the strategy is offered in *Compassion in Practice: Evidencing the Impact* (NHS England, 2016).

Leading Change: Adding Value (2016)

The 6Cs as 'a foundation of our value base' was further reiterated in *Leading Change, Adding Value: A Framework for Nursing, Midwifery and Care Staff* (NHS England, 2017a).

The framework built upon *Compassion in Practice* and was also directly aligned with the *Five Year Forward View* (NHS England, 2014) in that it sought to develop new ways of working, ensure a person-focused approach and break down apparent barriers to quality and provide 'seamless care' across health and social care (NHS England, 2016: 10).

The framework offers 10 aspirational commitments all of which relate to the quality of the care experience. Some of the commitments are more explicit than others, for example:

1   We will promote a culture where improving the population's health is a core component of the practice of all nursing, midwifery and care staff.
2   We will be centred on individuals experiencing high-value care.
3   We will work in partnership with individuals, their families, carers and others important to them.
4   We will champion the use of technology and informatics to improve practice, address unwarranted variations and enhance outcomes.
    (NHS England, 2017a – *Leading Change, Adding Value: A Framework for Nursing, Midwifery and Care Staff*; contains public sector information licensed under the Open Government Licence v3.0. www.nationalarchives.gov.uk/doc/open-government-licence/ version/3/)

The framework envisions nurses as leading change and adding value by generating better outcomes, creating a better experience for the people in their care whilst also making better use of the resources available (NHS England, 2017a: 11). Despite the aspirations articulated in the nursing strategy and subsequent related frameworks, research by O'Driscoll et al. (2018) indicated a limited awareness of the national initiatives 'at ward level' and a degree of professional anger, distress and resistance at what was viewed as a top-down initiative which could only be successful and sustained if there was compassion for the staff themselves (O'Driscoll et al., 2018: e1105). McMahon and White (2017) also believed that although the focus is often on health and social care and the nursing contribution, the so-called 'compassion deficit' is much wider than that and is widespread throughout society in general.

Other initiatives promoting the quality agenda

The NHS Constitution: The NHS belongs to us all (2015)

The first ever Constitution for the NHS in England was launched in 2009 and most recently updated in 2015 (DH, 2015). The Constitution sets out the rights that patients have to care while also stating their responsibilities. The update in 2015 was, in part, to reflect the recommendations of The Francis Report, as well as to highlight the importance of transparency and accountability within the NHS and to incorporate fundamental standards below which standards of care should never fall. It also gave greater prominence to mental health, reflecting the parity of importance between physical and mental health problems (NHS England, 2019b). Although it was criticized in some areas for being a series of optimistic pledges without making clear the consequences for not meeting these pledges (The Patients' Association, 2009), the Constitution has much to say in relation to standards and quality.

The third of the seven principles in the NHS Constitution states:

- The NHS aspires to the highest standards of excellence and professionalism – in the provision of high-quality care that is safe, effective and focused on patient experience; in the people it employs and the education, training and development they receive; in the leadership and management of its organizations; and through its commitment to innovation and to the promotion and conduct of research to improve the current and future health and care of the population. Respect, dignity, compassion and care should be at the core of how patients and staff are treated not only because that is the right thing to do but because patient safety, experience and outcomes are all improved when staff are valued, empowered and supported.

With regards to quality of care and environment:

- You have the right to be treated with a professional standard of care, by appropriately qualified and experienced staff, in a properly approved or registered organization that meets required levels of safety and quality.
- You have the right to be cared for in a clean, safe, secure and suitable environment.
- You have the right to receive suitable and nutritious food and hydration to sustain good health and well-being.
- You have the right to expect NHS bodies to monitor, and make efforts to improve continuously, the quality of healthcare they commission or provide. This includes improvements to the safety, effectiveness and experiences of services. (DH, 2015: 7)

The NHS also commits:

- To identify and share best practice in quality of care and treatments (pledge).

In addition to these legal rights, there are a number of pledges which the NHS is committed to achieving. Pledges go above and beyond your legal rights. This means that they are not legally binding but represent a commitment by the NHS to provide high-quality working environments for staff.

And under the heading 'NHS Values: Commitment to Quality of Care' (DH, 2015: 5):

> We earn the trust placed in us by insisting on quality and striving to get the basics of quality of care – safety, effectiveness and patient experience – right every time. We encourage and welcome feedback from patients, families, carers, staff and the public. We use this to improve and build on our successes.

Clinical governance

You may have read or heard the phrase *clinical governance* before in relation to the quality agenda or strategies being put in place to ensure quality care in one of the organizations you have had a placement on. In the early 2000s and later, clinical governance was a concept central to health policy developments and documents, and although it appears to be less omnipresent nowadays, it remains a useful concept to clarify and focus any initiatives of quality. Clinical governance wasn't a brand new initiative, but a bringing together of several other initiatives under one term.

Definitions of clinical governance

There are many seminal definitions of clinical governance, and one of the most famous was included in the 1998 consultation document *A First Class Service: Quality in the New NHS*:

> A framework through which NHS organizations are accountable for continuously improving the quality of their services

and safeguarding high standards of care by creating an environment in which excellence in clinical care will flourish. (DH, 1998: 33)

According to the Royal College of Nursing (Currie et al., 2003), clinical governance is:

a framework which helps all clinicians – including nurses to continually safeguard and improve standards of care.

Clinical governance is fundamentally about quality of care. It is about making sure that care delivered is safe and patient-centred. Although *all* nurses would probably see this as an important responsibility to aspire to, in many ways, issues of clinical governance can feel very removed from a nurse's daily activity, and therefore it may be quite easy for nurses to feel that clinical governance has nothing to do with them and is simply the responsibility of 'management' – management that is often seen by clinical staff to have different responsibilities and priorities than the day-to-day aspects of patient care. This perception can quite easily be the case for student nurses and newly qualified staff who are unsure of their status and authority, and their role and involvement in clinical governance. Indeed, although there was no overt regulation of health professionals inherent in the clinical governance framework, there was an implied demand that encouraged healthcare staff to think in wider strategic terms about resources and efficiency, indicating a belief that they had previously only viewed their roles at the level of individual health professionals treating individual patients (Crinson, 2009).

However, as we have reiterated, it is important to recognize that all nurses have a significant role to play within the maintenance of standards and quality – and therefore clinical governance – as they have a duty to provide individual care of high quality and are expected to practise this wherever they work. In fact, the majority of nurses know and practise clinical governance daily, as it is embedded in their professional values and general concern for others. Something as simple as ensuring that you have communicated information concerning a patient or client fully and appropriately to a more senior colleague is evidence of adhering to the principles of clinical governance. This apparently straightforward activity helps to ensure a high-quality experience for patients by encouraging consistency, reducing risk, and promoting safety.

———————————————— **ACTIVITY 3.4** ————————————————

If you are not doing so already, you will probably soon be exploring the job opportunities that are available to you on qualification. If there are jobs available in the organization in which you would like to work, try to find out who is the senior clinician responsible for clinical standards and professional development.

Discuss with your practice supervisor or mentor what the current initiatives, priorities, and areas of good practice are for the organization.

Is there any information on the organization's website concerning this?

It is very likely that you will be asked questions related to the quality of nursing care at interview, and this will be excellent preparation, making you 'stand out' at interview (this is discussed in further detail in Chapter 8).

The Care Quality Commission

The Care Quality Commission (CQC) has historically played a significant role in evaluating the clinical governance processes within the organizations that they inspect. It is their role to ensure that the care services in England – hospitals, care homes, general practices, dentists and other services – provide people with safe, effective and high-quality care. A fundamental aspect of improving safety and maintaining standards and quality was the setting up of various organizations to *inspect* practice and health services. Initially, in 2000, this role was undertaken by the Commission for Health Improvement (CHI). The overall aim was to highlight areas in which the NHS was working well and identify areas that needed improvement. Each trust had to ensure that clinical governance systems were in place and to recognize and act on targets. Some of these targets were set within what were then called National Service Frameworks – ten-year programmes that defined standards of care for major medical conditions such as cancer, diabetes and long-term conditions. In 2004, the organization retained its fundamental role in maintaining standards, but changed its name to the Commission for Healthcare Audit and Inspection, or the Healthcare Commission. In 2009 the regulation of health and adult social care in England became the responsibility of the CQC following the integration of The Healthcare Commission, the Commission for Social Care Inspection and the Mental Health Act Commission. All of which had previous roles in the promotion of and drive for improvement in quality in healthcare and public health.

The CQC's role is to make sure care services in England provide people with safe, effective and high-quality care and is a further attempt to address the need to bring the functions of social care and health services much closer together under one independent regulator. Part of the remit of the Commission is also protecting the interests of people whose rights have been restricted under the Mental Health Act (1983; 2007). It is the one 'port of call' for people using these services and their carers and families, and one source of information on standards, safety, and the services that are provided. Such bodies have been questioned due to their apparent 'surveillance' and/or 'controlling' role (Harrison and McDonald, 2008), and their desired impact on the performance of local healthcare organizations has also been questioned (Crinson, 2009). For example, Lord Francis criticized the CQC for failing to hold the NHS care providers to account in his report on the Mid Staffordshire hospital, and believed that while the requirements of quality may appear to be met they can still be given little attention in day-to-day clinical work (Francis, 2013). Similarly, the CQC were forced to defend their processes at a parliamentary hearing, as they had decided not to publish a report which had criticized aspects of care at Whorlton Hall Nursing Home in County Durham, aspects which undercover filming by the BBC later revealed when the recordings appeared to show abuse and intimidation. This resulted in the arrest of several members of staff. The CQC contention is that they were only able to minimize the risk of such cases occurring rather than ruling them out completely given that certain individuals were seeking to behave in such a way (CQC, 2019b).

The Care Quality Commission's definition of quality

The definition of quality in healthcare, enshrined in law and utilized by the CQC, includes three key aspects:

Patient safety
Clinical effectiveness
Patient experience

The achievement of all three aspects ultimately happens when a caring culture, professional commitment and strong leadership in organizations are combined to serve patients. The Care Quality Commission is there to inspect organizations against these elements of quality and hold providers to account for what they are doing to improve quality in their organization or across their local area. The aim and intention of the CQC is, therefore, to improve quality of care (including patient experience) and efficiency, while reducing variation in clinical outcomes.

The Care Quality Commission's 'fundamental standards'

The CQC 'set out what good and outstanding care looks like' (CQC, 2019a) and endeavour to ensure by inspection that services 'meet fundamental standards below which care must never fall' and which everybody has the right to expect.

Let's look a bit more closely at the 'fundamental standards'. The fundamental standards are:

- Person-centred care.
  Care or treatment must be tailored to the individual and meets their needs and preferences.
- Dignity and respect.
  Privacy is ensured when required and wanted, everyone is treated equally and support is offered to maintain independence and involvement as desired in the local community.
- Consent.
  Consent must be given by the individual or anyone acting legally on their behalf before any care or treatment is given.
- Safety.
  Care must always be safe and individuals must not be put at any avoidable risk. Risk must therefore be assessed and care delivered only by appropriately qualified, competent, skilled and experienced staff.
- Safeguarding.
  No one should suffer any form of abuse or improper treatment while receiving care. This might include: inappropriate limits to freedom or unnecessary or inappropriate restraint, degrading treatment or neglect.

- Food and drink.
  Everyone must have enough to eat and drink to maintain good health whilst receiving care and treatment.
- Premises and equipment.
  The environment must be clean, suitable and maintained appropriately and safely.
- Complaints.
  A system must be in place to handle and respond to any complaint with thorough investigation and action taken if problems are identified.
- Good governance.
  Providers must ensure they have effective governance and systems to check quality and safety of care.
- Staffing.
  All staff must be suitably qualified, competent and experienced. They should also be appropriately supported, trained and supervised. Recruitment must be safe and robust and only people who are suitable to their role should be employed.
- Candour.
  Care must be offered in an open and transparent way and if anything should go wrong the provider must explain what has happened, apologize and offer ongoing support as necessary.

The CQC rating of any organization must be displayed in a place where it can be seen with the latest report made available along with any other relevant information offered on the web.

The Care Quality Commission process asks five key questions:

- Are they safe?
- Are they effective?
- Are they caring?
- Are they responsive to peoples' needs?
- Are they well-led?

These five questions are the CQC's 'key line of enquiry' and are used to prioritize and focus the inspection to ensure consistency, and also to focus on the areas that matter most. Visiting services is a fundamental part of CQC's inspection process and allows the observation of care and inspection of records to observe how needs are managed.

The frequency of inspection, size of inspection team and whether the service knows that the CQC are coming depends on the type of service. For example, NHS acute and specialist trusts, NHS mental health trusts and NHS community health trusts are usually unannounced inspections, although the trust may be contacted in specific circumstances simply to ensure senior management are present to answer questions.

NHS GP practices and out-of-hours services, in contrast, are usually given at least four weeks' notice before the inspection starts as this is felt to ensure inspections are not too disruptive to the care of those attending.

Focused inspections are also undertaken. These are smaller than the comprehensive inspections although they follow a similar process. Focused inspections explore areas that the CQC might be particularly concerned about, for example an area of concern that might have been raised during a comprehensive inspection or other monitoring work, or if there is a significant change in the provider's circumstances.

The inspection visit

At the start of the visit the inspection team meet, and explanation is given about:

- Who the inspection team are.
- The scope and purpose of the visit.
- How the findings will be communicated.

The organization can initially present their own view of their performance and then the team will gather views of those who use the services; including complaints and concerns and also information from staff. Records may also be reviewed, policies scrutinized, environments inspected, and care observed.

The CQC attempts to ensure that nurses and other health professionals 'gain a fuller understanding' of the patient experience and what patients need and expect from healthcare, and to give patients more control over their care. This is indicative of how both patients and carers' expectations of healthcare and healthcare professionals have increased significantly over the past decades.

The National Institute for Health and Clinical Excellence (NICE)

NICE has a crucial role in quality improvement. Prior to its establishment, there were no set clear standards of care within the NHS and there was occasional inconsistency and slow uptake of effective treatments. NICE (then known as the National Institute for Clinical Excellence) was originally established in February 1999 to review clinical and cost-effective evidence to support healthcare practice, and to provide advice and guidance to NHS organizations, healthcare professionals, and also the public (Talbot-Smith and Pollock, 2006). In 2005, NICE absorbed the function of the Health Development Agency, which originally had a key role in public health and the prevention of ill health, and took on the extended title of National Institute for Health and Clinical Excellence (although the acronym remains the same). The Health and Social Care Act (2012) established it as a non-departmental public body (NDPB) and confirmed its responsibility for developing guidance and quality standards in social care. As in some other aspects of the NHS, due to its legislative establishment, guidance offered by NICE is officially for England and Wales only with decisions on how NICE guidance applies in Scotland and Northern Ireland being devolved to those administrations.

NICE consists of a group of independent experts responsible for providing evidence-based guidance on health and social care, who make decisions about various treatments based on perceived longer-term benefits versus cost implications. NICE then provides health professionals and the public with authoritative and reliable advice on evidence-based 'best practice' within the resources available.

NICE and the decisions that it has made have often been controversial and the subject of media scrutiny and criticism. This might be to an extent inevitable with the finite resources in healthcare and the high cost of modern interventions, equipment and drugs. Clearly, the NHS cannot fund all treatment and all interventions for all people.

Several of the criticisms levelled at NICE were discussed as early as 2008 in *High Quality Care for All: NHS Next Stage Review* (DH, 2008a), in which it was accepted that NICE appraisal guidance on newly licensed drugs had often taken too long to become available – on occasions up to two years. NICE subsequently put in place a faster appraisal process for key new drugs, which sought to issue authoritative guidance within a few months of the launch of a drug in the UK.

However, NICE attracts, and continues to engender, significant criticisms, not least that the cost-benefit evaluation of new technologies and drugs by NICE remains controversial. This means that it becomes possible to only invest in those innovations that produce the most cost-effective results, and as Bradshaw and Bradshaw (2004) pointed out, this sometimes is seen to deny potentially effective treatments to certain patients simply because they are not seen to be good value for money. Fearon et al. (2018) claimed that fundamentally positivist methodologies – most particularly favouring data from randomized controlled trials – are unable to offer answers to problems that are by their very nature exceptionally complex, and that this approach inevitably included inherent bias such as age inequality and pharmaceutical influence. Taylor and Hawley (2010) highlight that the guidelines generated by evidence-based practices such as clinical trials can be seen as a way to place limits on what is offered and can therefore be viewed as a form of rationing.

Other critics have complained that some NICE recommendations can be considered to be overtly prescriptive, removing the important element of patient choice, and even occasionally being clinically unworkable (Loftus, 2019). The claim is that shared decision-making is one of the important advancements and advantages in modern healthcare and this is being put at risk by some of the guidance prescribed by NICE. Crinson (2009) claims that NICE has actually made very few recommendations to exclude interventions that it had been asked to appraise with regards to patient safety, and yet it has frequently recommended the use of cheaper forms of treatment where more expensive ones were judged to provide little or no benefit. However, paradoxically, according to Appleby and Harrison (2006), costs generally under the auspices and advice of NICE are actually increasing and not reducing. Despite these concerns, it is clear that there have been a number of quality initiatives focusing on standards in different aspects of the patient journey and it appears certain that the role and function of NICE will continue to be reformed and developed, with the aspiration of maintaining its independence and extending its remit to social care (DH, 2019).

Summary

In this chapter, we have explored the role of the nurse in maintaining standards and ensuring quality of care. It is clear that every nurse needs to have an awareness of their unique and individual contribution to this vital area of healthcare. We explored what is often called the 'quality agenda' and the changing responsibilities and expectations of nurses and the public. This 'quality agenda' is here to stay and it is important that, as nurses, we recognize the essential role played by organizations such as the CQC and NICE, the importance and relevance of policies and initiatives such as the NHS Constitution and the 6Cs, and the increasingly lead role that nurses are expected to take in delivering a service that ensures patient safety, quality and dignity. More and more, healthcare is seen as a partnership between health professionals and patients, and increasingly nurses will be called to account for the care that they provide and will be judged against objective and national standards and patient expectations. The chapter offered an overview of many of these challenging, but exciting, initiatives and changes, and an insight into a nurse's current and future roles.

4

ACCOUNTABILITY AND ETHICAL DECISION-MAKING

Graham Ormrod, Nichola Barlow and Rob Burton

THE AIMS OF THIS CHAPTER ARE TO:

- Provide a review of the concept of accountability.
- Discuss the accepted definitions of accountability.
- Specifically explore the *professional*, *personal*, and *ethical* contexts of accountability.
- Discuss the use of a recognized framework to assist in ethical decision-making.
- Explore how this relates to nursing practice for students and registered nurses.

We have also included scenarios highlighting issues of accountability and investigating the nurse's role in the decision-making process with regards to subsequent choices, actions and patient care.

Issues of accountability will also be discussed further in Chapter 5, allowing you to revisit your understanding of accountability more specifically from a legal point of view.

Introduction

Before considering what the literature tells us about accountability, what do you think the term means?

ACTIVITY 4.1

You have almost completed your course as a student and have applied for a post as a registered nurse. During the interview, one of the interviewers asks: 'In your answers you've talked quite a bit about your accountability.

What does this term mean to you?

Before reading any further, write down a couple of sentences about your own understanding and definition of accountability. We will return to your definitions later.

As a final year nursing student, you will have encountered the concept of accountability before and you may think: 'Hey, I know this!' If you do, great – but are you clear on exactly how your accountability changes on registration? Reading this chapter will help you to revisit the issues around this concept in a new light; for those who have not really considered accountability before, fear not – this chapter will also provide a good introduction to what you need to know at this stage of your career. It is important to remember that, to be deemed proficient for entry to the **Nursing and Midwifery Council** (NMC) professional register, all students must demonstrate that they are able to manage the delivery of care services within the sphere of their own accountability (NMC, 2018b).

Definitions of accountability

As you may have found in the exercise above, the concept of accountability has historically been very hard to define. In fact, Jacobs (2004) claimed that nobody is really sure what it means. Similarly, Sinclair

(1995) described accountability as chameleon-like, multiple, fragmented, and subject to continual reconstruction. Authors such as Dimond (2015: 4) do not draw a distinction between the concepts of responsibility and accountability – responsibility seen as being liable to be called to account or being accountable for something. Furthermore, as Melia (2013) highlights, there is also an important distinction to be made between the notion of *moral* responsibility and *legal* liability.

Considerations such as these contribute to the potential lack of clarity of the concept of accountability and the subsequent confusion that may be generated from the complexities of professional practice.

One point that is clear, however, is that all nurses are accountable for their practice. This means that they can be asked to justify their practice or be held to account by others for any actions and/or omissions resulting from their individual practice. The Nursing and Midwifery Council (2018c), in its publication *Delegation and Accountability: Supplementary Information to the NMC Code*, defines accountability as 'the principle that individuals and organizations are responsible for their actions and may be required to explain them to others'.

According to Griffith and Dowie (2019), the registered nurse is accountable to:

- The public, through criminal law.
- The patient, through civil law.
- Their employer, through a contract of employment.
- Their profession, through the NMC via such documents as *The Code: Professional Standards of Practice and Behaviour for Nurses, Midwives and Nursing Associates* (NMC, 2018a).

The differences in accountability are very likely to be the basis of at *least* one question that you will be asked when you go for a job interview, and it is therefore essential that you have a clear understanding of them.

Caulfield (2005) argues that accountability is a key part of the very foundation of nursing. Although as a student nurse professional accountability to the NMC is not as straightforward as for a registered nurse or nursing associate, you are undoubtedly accountable to the patient and public through the law, and also to your university. Moreover in their publication *Raising Concerns: Guidance for Nurses, Midwives and Nursing Associates* (NMC, 2019a), the NMC explicitly confirm that the principles in the guidance apply to student nurses and midwives and nursing associates in exactly the same way that they apply to registered nurses. The professional dimensions of

---

ACTIVITY 4.2

Consider, from your experience in practice, what the major differences and similarities are between the accountability of a registered nurse and a student nurse. Write your thoughts in Table 4.1.

Table 4.1   Differences and similarities between accountability of a registered nurse and student nurse

Similarities	Differences

---

care are identified throughout *The Code* (NMC, 2018a) and the nurse's responsibilities to those in their care are clearly identified, along with the standards of behaviour required from those on the NMC register. Each individual practitioner is reminded that they are accountable for all aspects of their practice, including that which they delegate to others. This has significant relevance not only for the nurse delegating a task, but also for the person to whom the task is being delegated, which is often the student nurse.

Indeed, the NMC (2018b) emphasizes in the standards of proficiency for entry to the register that people must be able to trust that the newly qualified nurse will always safely delegate to others and also respond appropriately when a task is delegated to them. Fundamentally, if a registered nurse has a clear understanding of accountability and acts within the boundaries of *The Code* (NMC, 2018a), they will be able to ensure their professional practice remains ethical, legal, and in line with their professional body requirements.

Caulfield (2005) argued that if accountability is simply seen as being responsible for actions, then this can lead to a negative influence on practice, with practitioners purely concerned with taking the blame when things go wrong. Generally, however, definitions of accountability do speak in some way of justifying practice. For example, one definition speaks of an acceptance of the obligation to disclose what you have done and also the possible consequences of that disclosure (Duff, 1995). This disclosure involves making all decisions explicit so that others can evaluate them. These others include:

- Patients.
- Relatives or carers.
- Colleagues.
- Regulatory bodies such as the NMC.
- Employers.
- Representatives of the law.

The obligation to disclose, or *answerability*, and need to offer *justification* of practice is at the heart of the concept of accountability. Every nurse needs to be aware that they may be asked 'Why did you do that?' or 'Why did you do that in that particular way?' This comment from a third-year student might capture the feelings of many:

> What worries me the most about being qualified is holding the keys and being left on my own.

The idea of 'holding the keys' and thereby being ultimately responsible for drug administration, for example, in some ways encapsulates this image of 'answerability' and very powerfully highlights one of the major differences between being a student and being a qualified nurse, irrespective of the field of nursing that you have chosen.

───────────── **ACTIVITY 4.3** ─────────────

Imagine that you are now working as a registered nurse and part of your responsibilities is to administer medications prescribed by a doctor who usually only visits the care home once a day.

When you come to administer the day's medications, you realize that two of the drugs are known to interact. What would you do and why?

In January 2019 the NMC withdrew the professional standards for medicines management in the belief that it is not within the remit of a professional regulator to provide clinical practice guidance of this type. However, resources are highlighted to support access to accurate information on the safe and effective handling, management and administration of medicines, and it is essential to understand the implications of this information for your practice. For example, guidance offered by the Royal Pharmaceutical Society and the Royal College of Nursing states:

> Before administration, the person administering the medicine must have an overall understanding of the medicine being administered and seek advice if necessary, from a prescriber or a pharmacy professional. (RPS, 2019: 4)

Bearing such guidance in mind, your options would be as follows.

1   Do not give the drugs.
2   Discuss this further with the prescribing doctor, as soon as possible, highlighting the drug interaction and asking for the prescription to be changed.
3   Subsequently administer the medications *only* when you are sure the prescription is correct and appropriate for the patient and the presenting condition.
4   Document events accordingly.

The NMC have reported that many queries it receives arise from nurses' 'uncertainty or lack of awareness about their accountability' (Savage and Moore, 2004: 4). In the example above, the nurse is accountable for their actions in relation to drug administration regardless of advice from other healthcare professionals (NMC, 2018c), and they also have a duty to challenge the doctor's decision, or indeed the decision of any other health professional, in relation to patient care if they are concerned that another approach would be more appropriate. This could be described as 'professional accountability'.

Professional accountability

Accountability is intrinsically linked to the concept of professionalism, whereby there is a requirement to answer to an external governing body. The NMC has had this role in the UK since its establishment in 2002. Its key role is the protection of the public by establishing standards of education, training, conduct and performance, and the maintenance of a professional register that includes the names of all those entitled to be called a registered nurse. Professional accountability gives the NMC the power to control entry onto the register, and also regulates a nurse's right to remain on the register by imposing professional standards and ensuring the nurse's fitness to practise.

The obligations of accountability implied and highlighted in the NMC *Code* (NMC, 2018a) and supporting documents (NMC, 2018c) can essentially be grouped around a central theme: an obligation or duty of care to patients. Professional accountability maintains the patient's trust in the individual nurse and support for the nursing profession as a whole (Caulfield, 2005). Those nurses who meet the minimum standards for registration also have the power to decide whether to remove an individual from the register for misconduct, lack of competence, or ill health. Public protection is the key aspiration of the council, therefore those on the register must have achieved and maintained the appropriate levels of educational and practical expertise.

The role of the NMC is one of protecting the public through the establishment and improvement of nursing and midwifery standards of care. This identifies your accountability in relation to the university and through the law, but not professionally to the NMC until your education is completed and you have been accepted on to the NMC register as a qualified nurse.

ACTIVITY 4.4

The public, employers and registrants can access information on the NMC website (www.nmc-uk.org) and search the register to check whether an individual is registered to practise. This webpage also provides access to NMC publications and guidelines.

Access the website and explore the information available. Think about how the content relates to the idea of professional accountability.

The International Council of Nurses (ICN), a federation of 128 countries worldwide which aims to bring nurses together on a global level, provides nursing advice and influences health policy, and publishes a code of ethics for nurses (ICN, 2012) which identifies the nurse's accountability for nursing practice and the maintenance of competence through continuing professional development. The ICN code of ethics identifies the groups to whom the nurse may have some level of accountability, including people requiring care, the profession, and also co-workers; these are similar groups to those identified previously by Griffith and Dowie (2019).

─────────────────────── **ACTIVITY 4.5** ───────────────────────

The International Council of Nurses (ICN) also has a website (**www.icn.ch**) that contains important and relevant information, guidance, and fact sheets that you may find of interest in the area of accountability, as well as other areas.

Access the website and consider how the content relates to the idea of professional accountability.

Personal accountability

In *Delegation and Accountability* (NMC, 2018c: 3) the NMC confirm that:

> As registered professionals, nurses, midwives and nursing associates are accountable for all aspects of their practice, including accountability for what they choose to delegate, and agreement, or not, to undertake activities which are delegated to them.

This means that you are answerable for your actions and omissions, regardless of advice or directions from another professional.

Prior to qualification

The NMC *Standards for Pre-Registration Nursing Programmes* (NMC, 2018f) emphasize that all students must be 'suitable' for their intended field of nursing practice and continually demonstrate values in accordance with *The Code*, and also have the capability to learn behaviours in accordance with *The Code*. Similarly, the NMC continually emphasize the need to act professionally ensuring public protection at all times. For example it is highlighted that students may jeopardize their ability to join the NMC register if they act in any way that is unprofessional or unlawful on social media (NMC, 2019c). This confirms that behaviour and conduct, inside and outside of the university, in clinical placement and personal life, may impact on the student's fitness to practise and ability to complete the nursing programme.

After qualification

Ultimately, each nurse must answer for their own actions; it is no defence to claim that they were acting on someone else's orders or advice. Nursing is not simply concerned with carrying out tasks, but also involves a process of decision-making informed by specific and/or specialist knowledge. It is necessary for the nurse not only to understand the reasons for the care and treatment given, but also to understand the anticipated outcome. This means that the 'accountable' nurse will not only understand the practical aspects of undertaking a skill, for example, but will also understand the rationale behind it, recognize the possible outcomes of carrying out the related task, and also have the knowledge to assess its relative benefits.

Delegation and accountability: Implications for students and qualified nurses

If a qualified nurse delegates any aspect of care or any task to someone else, especially if that individual is not registered with the NMC, whether a nursing associate, support worker or you as a student nurse, it is the individual, registered nurse's responsibility to make sure that the person is suitably competent, has sufficient knowledge, and is supervised appropriately. The NMC indeed offers specific advice on delegation and emphasizes that delegation must always take place in the best interests of the person for whom the nurse is caring and the decision to delegate must always be based on an assessment of the patient's individual needs (NMC, 2018c).

According to Burnard and Chapman (2005), the above discussion means that while a student, for example, may be responsible for care given to a patient, as a learner, it may not be appropriate to expect them to be accountable because this implies a certain level of necessary knowledge or skill that may not yet have been acquired. However, it is important to recognize that this does not absolve all responsibility from those undertaking the duties. As a student nurse performing any care, you still have a responsibility to the patient and are personally accountable for your actions. Therefore, as a student nurse, you have a responsibility not to take on duties that you are not fully competent to perform, and also have a responsibility to express your lack of competency to the delegating nurse.

A registered nurses' accountability rests on the notion that the task has been appropriately delegated. The student nurse would be responsible for the task, and they must be adequately prepared and work within the employer's guidelines and protocols, and have the authority delegated by the registered nurse.

Accountability and patients/clients

Patients/clients and also family members may ask you what you have done and why, and they are obviously entitled to an explanation with regards to nursing care.

─────────────────────── ACTIVITY 4.6 ───────────────────────

Consider this scenario:

> You are caring for a client with profound learning disability in their own home and you are asked by your mentor to administer medication via a percutaneous endoscopic gastrostomy (PEG) tube, after having checked the medications together. Your mentor tells you to administer them via the tube, saying 'Use a 10 ml flush'.
> In such scenarios, the delegating nurse must be sure that you have the appropriate knowledge, competency, preparation, and skill to undertake the task in line with the employer's guidelines/policy and ensuring patient safety.
> Having received the authority from the delegating staff nurse, you, as the student nurse, are said to be accountable for your actions.
> Where possible, of course, you should also gain consent from the patient.
> The NMC (2018c) states that the ability to delegate duties to others, as appropriate, while ensuring that those delegated to are supervised and monitored is one of the overarching principles of being able to practise as a nurse. It emphasizes that this involves delegating and supervising care safely and appropriately, while remaining accountable.

Historically, this has been described as being accountable 'for' rather than accountable 'to'. For example, Watson (1992) suggested that nurses were not accountable to patients because they have what he describes as an 'informal' relationship. However, the culture in healthcare has changed significantly over the years and is now more one of partnership and equality (DH, 2012), whereby it is now a legitimate expectation of all patients/clients to be able to call nurses, or any other individual, including student nurses, to account for their care.

———————————————— **ACTIVITY 4.7** ————————————————

Consider this scenario:

> You are part of the nursing team caring for a 12-year-old child who has been diagnosed with cancer. She appears very optimistic when you and your mentor meet with her and her parents to discuss the options for care management. She and her parents have researched her condition on the internet and found a website promoting a combination of complementary and alternative therapies as a potential cure. Her parents are less convinced, but do not want to upset their daughter and have not broached this with her. They are told by the consultant that the healthcare team will provide the 'best possible' care and do 'everything' that it can to help her. The girl now wants to know when she can commence her chosen therapies and is convinced that aggressive chemotherapy is not the best approach.
>
> As a registered nurse and recognizing your accountability to the patient, what would you do in this situation?

This type of scenario raises many key issues for the student to learn from. As the standards of proficiency for registered nurses (NMC, 2018b: 31) state, to become a registered nurse a student nurse must take a holistic approach to care at all times and all nursing care should be carried out in a way that reflects cultural awareness and ensures that the needs, priorities and preferences of people are always valued and taken into account.

However, this apparently straightforward aspiration can generate complex dilemmas in practice where the 'rights and wrongs' of the scenario are difficult to discern. It can be even more difficult in the case of children. What is clear in these often very emotional and complicated cases is that a multidisciplinary team approach is essential, with sensitive input and engagement from experts, family, and most importantly the individual child concerned, to manage the complexities of such legal and ethical dilemmas. Ultimately, if it is clear that the patient really knows the implications of her request, and **capacity** is accepted, then her decision needs to be respected. Issues of capacity and decision-making, including the implications of young people and children, will be further discussed in Chapter 5.

ACTIVITY 4.8

Consider this scenario:

> You are visiting a client with mental health problems at home to support with the administration of a prescribed medication. The client declines to take the medication as he feels that the side effects outweigh the benefits. He tells you that his tablets are not helping as they simply make him go to the toilet all of the time. He feels he may become incontinent, making him frightened to go out, because he is embarrassed and fearful that it may happen in public. This leads to the risk of him becoming even more socially isolated than he already feels.

> What would you expect your mentor to do in this situation?

> You would need to consider both their (and your) accountability and how this impacts on the role as advocate.

A possible course of action would be as follows:

1   Listen to his concerns.
2   Discuss your patient's condition and how his medication is helping to treat it.
3   Talk to the prescribing doctor about the patient's concerns to facilitate any possible changes to the medication regimen to reduce any unwanted impact on the patient and his lifestyle. This may include a change of medication or changes to the frequency and administration times.

You have had the opportunity to explore several aspects of the concept of accountability and we have reiterated key principles with regards to the nursing profession – aspects of practice, delegation, and so on. We will now look more specifically at the ethical aspects of accountability.

Accountability and ethical decision-making

Ethical considerations can sometimes seem to have little to do with day-to-day practice, and any discussions of the ethical principles that underpin practice or any moral component of practice can seem more of an *academic* pursuit rather than an underpinning context for everyday practice. However, your modules at university will have confirmed to you that recognition of the ethical values that inform professional practice is as important now as ever. It is no longer acceptable – if it ever was – to leave ethical decisions solely to the medical profession, as might have historically been the case (Mason and Whitehead, 2003). When you qualify, you will immediately confirm your role as a patient advocate and very quickly may have to take a lead role within the multidisciplinary team; both then and in the future it will be necessary for you to have the knowledge and insight to offer informed views on certain potentially complicated ethical dilemmas.

The role of the nurse is constantly changing, as are the views and expectations of the public and society (King's Fund, 2014; Maben and Griffiths, 2008). This change both in role and expectations brings with it a greater likelihood of dilemmas for the nurse. Fundamental questions can be raised such as 'What is good nursing care?' and 'What ought a nurse to do for a patient?' Being described as 'a good nurse' might even change as the context of nursing changes. For example, Florence Nightingale identified a number of essential nursing duties, which predominantly consisted of actions associated with physical care and the environment, while also identifying the importance of nurse education both in the sciences and in human ethics and morals (Bostridge, 2008); in 1944 Pugh described the nurse's most important duty as that of obedience to the physician (Pugh, 1944). More recently the NMC *Code* (2018a) has stated that nurses must respect the skills, expertise and contributions of colleagues and, whilst being supportive of colleagues, this must never compromise or be at the expense of patient or public safety (NMC, 2018a: 8.7).

This may mean challenging the decisions of other professionals including doctors, and these potential challenges indicate the changing context in which nursing is viewed.

Each one of the decisions that you are expected to make requires consideration of certain information. Some of this information may be classed as 'factual' – for example:

- The patient's past medical and nursing history.
- The results of any diagnostic tests or medications prescribed.
- The specific name by which the client would prefer to be called.

ACTIVITY 4.9

Consider this scenario:

> You first meet Bobby, a 35-year-old man with Down's syndrome, when he attends a clinic where you are on placement. Following the assessment process, Bobby discloses some general information about his home circumstances that leads you to believe that he might be vulnerable and at risk of abuse. Although Bobby does not mention anything too specific, he does say that he doesn't want you to tell anyone else as his mother has asked him not to talk about these things to 'other people'. The situation makes you feel concerned, because you feel there is something 'not right' for some reason – although you cannot quite put your finger on it.

Such feelings can point to a real dilemma.

1   How should you respond to such a situation?
2   Should you disclose any information about Bobby to someone, and, if so, to whom?

This type of scenario highlights how purely 'factual' information can only help the decision-making process to an extent. What you, as the nurse involved, *should* do or what you *ought* to do inevitably lead us to different considerations.

Points that you may consider in relation to the disclosure of information that you have about Bobby and his home life will include the following:

1   As a vulnerable adult, is Bobby at risk of harm or neglect?
2   How does Bobby feel about this information being shared with others, such as health and social care professionals?
3   What does Bobby expect you to do with this information?
4   What would the consequences be of disclosure or of non-disclosure?
5   Which course of action would be in Bobby's best interests?
6   What does the law say? (This will be further discussed in Chapter 5.)

In 2011 a BBC television programme exposed the physical and psychological abuse suffered by people with learning disabilities and challenging behaviour at Winterbourne View hospital. The exposé resulted in the closure of the public-funded hospital and the imprisonment of six of the eleven staff who pleaded guilty to criminal offences of neglect or abuse. A subsequent report challenged the UK

Government to produce a Charter of Rights for people with learning disabilities and/or autism and their families, which amongst other recommendations encouraged a supported and resourced shift away from inappropriate institutional care to greater community provision (Transforming Care and Commissioning Steering Group, 2014).

Two years earlier in 2009, the UK ombudsman had highlighted the tragic results that can occur when the rights and needs of vulnerable clients are ignored. The document Six Lives criticized organizations and individuals for failing to live up to human rights principles, especially those of dignity and equality of persons with learning disabilities. (To read the full story, see www.lgo.org.uk and search for 'Six Lives'.)

Also, in the UK, the Royal College of Nursing in various publicity campaigns has emphasized putting dignity at the heart of all nursing care by recognizing the importance of compassion and emotional support as opposed to simply delivering 'technical' nursing (RCN, 2018).

The NMC (2008a), in a series of focus groups consulting on pre-registration nursing education, also stressed that fitness to practise is not just about giving out the wrong drugs, for example, but can be equally applied to staff who are disrespectful to patients and neglect to treat patients with respect and dignity. Particularly vulnerable groups according to the NMC are the elderly, children, people with mental health problems, and the transient population, such as the homeless and asylum seekers.

Within the endeavour to ensure respect and dignity is recognition of an individual's core ethical and cultural values. A member of the focus group convened by the NMC (2008a) highlighted the case in which staff were unaware of the distress caused as they shaved off the beard of a Sikh patient who, due to language difficulties, was unable to prevent it.

─────────────── **ACTIVITY 4.10** ───────────────

1   Have you ever experienced care being provided that you felt compromised a client's values in relation to equality and diversity?

    Reflect on your experience and training in equality and diversity.

2   Do you feel prepared to deal with such situations in your practice?

(Continued)

(Continued)

Discuss with your practice supervisor or mentor the availability of other sources of information and support that might assist you.

3   Are there resources such as booklets that might help to provide a greater understanding of some core cultural issues?

The NMC (2018b) feels that while nurses cannot be expected to know everything about each diverse group, they should have enough basic information available to them to understand the different cultural needs of their patients. Understanding and compassion should be at the heart of all nursing practice, and therefore training and guidance may not necessarily be enough to change attitudes and prejudice. However, feedback from the focus groups set up by the NMC highlighted the need for further training around areas such as:

- Diffusing difficult situations, including:
  - How to cope with a situation in which a patient is being racist toward a staff member.
- Greater understanding of mental health issues for general nurses in particular, in order to:
  - Help staff to recognize mental health symptoms better.
  - Reduce the risk of discrimination due to their behaviour.
  - Subsequently help staff to cope better.
- Greater understanding about specific issues affecting some people with disability.

You might be thinking: 'So why does this matter and what has it got to do with ethics?' It is essential to remember that *every* interaction between you and any service user has ethical implications – implications that carry with them the need to justify practice ethically. In other words, you have to be prepared to be called to account *ethically*.

What is seen to be ethically acceptable is informed by any individual's beliefs and values, which have themselves been influenced by the culture within which they live. These values might be those that are important to the nurse, or the individual patient, or colleagues or society at large, and may well change over time. However, as indicated by the discussion above, there are certain fundamentals, such as equality, fairness, non-discriminatory practices and attitudes, and the support and protection of the vulnerable, which are held as integral and essential to professional practice. So if you recognize the importance of such considerations, how might you help to ensure that these fundamentals are considered in your daily practice? One strategy might be the use of a theoretical framework to focus your thinking and ensure the consideration of each aspect of the specific scenario or dilemma.

A framework to support ethical decision-making

Caulfield (2005) believes that while an *ethical framework* might not provide all of the answers to the complex ethical problems that a nurse might face, what it *can* do is to at least provide the basis for 'principled discussion'.

The four principles approach as a framework

There are several different frameworks designed to help to support discussion and decision-making in relation to ethical dilemmas. One such framework was put forward by Beauchamp and Childress (2019) to help to examine the ethical dilemma raised by a specific situation and thereby facilitate decision-making and ethical practice.

A key point to consider is that nursing students, like all health professionals, are regularly confronted with ethical dilemmas and the framework is useful in this relatively early stage in your career to clarify your thinking, help to resolve dilemmas, and also provide justification for your decisions.

Let's explore further the potential use of a framework to help to clarify our thinking when confronted with dilemmas. The framework suggested by Beauchamp and Childress (2019) suggests that thinking about moral matters can be broken into four interrelated levels of thinking, as follows.

- Level 1: Judgements.
- Level 2: Rules.
- Level 3: Principles.
- Level 4: Theories.

Let's look at this in more detail.

Level 1: Judgements

When *any* situation arises, not necessarily in the healthcare field, those involved, as well as those who witness it or simply hear or read about it, make an initial *judgement* about that situation. This judgement may be quite difficult to articulate: it might simply be a 'gut reaction', or a feeling that something is either 'not quite right', or conversely that something is right or good.

───────────────── **ACTIVITY 4.11** ─────────────────

Imagine an occasion recently on which you heard about something that made you feel uneasy or worried – that you feel should not have happened. This may be something that involves a patient or client for whom you have cared or that you have heard about from a fellow student, or simply something you have heard on a news report.

1   How did this make you feel?
2   Why do you think you felt this way?
3   What made you think something 'wasn't quite right'?

Consideration of the following clinical example may help to further clarify your thinking.

You are asked to assist in the taking of a venous blood sample from a patient for analysis. The patient is very frail and in the last stages of life. The patient's veins are difficult to find. From handover, you know that the patient is to be treated 'conservatively', focusing on the five Priorities of Care (LACDP, 2014) which involves a coordinated individual plan of care delivered with compassion and including symptom control, food and drink, and psychological, social and spiritual support (LACDP, 2014: 7). You ask the registered nurse who is undertaking the procedure why it has been requested and she responds by saying that although they are routine blood tests, on this occasion they have been asked for specifically by the doctor in charge of the patient's care.

Some questions that you may ask yourself are:

- What benefit are these tests to the patient at this time?
- Will the results change the way in which the patient is treated and cared for?

- Has the dying person, and those identified as important to them, been involved in the decisions about treatment?

If the answer to these questions is that there is no benefit, no change in patient management, no apparent discussion with other key individuals has been had, and that the patient may experience unnecessary pain, you may make the judgement that to proceed would be inappropriate or even *wrong*. According to the proposed framework, the judgements that are made in such situations are due to the existence of certain *rules* that state what should or should not be done and thereby provide justification for Level 1 *judgements*.

Level 2: Rules

So what are these 'rules'?

According to Beauchamp and Childress (2019), there are four main 'rules' that generate our judgements. Although these rules are related and in some ways overlap, they can also be discussed individually.

The first rule: Always tell the truth

This is sometimes known as the principle of **veracity**, a principle defined as the obligation to tell the truth and not to lie or to deceive others (Fry and Johnstone, 2008).

A situation may make you feel uncomfortable simply because you realize that there has been some deception and you intuitively feel this to be wrong. This is because the 'truth-telling rule' has been broken.

Telling the truth in a clinical situation is clearly very important. Any therapeutic relationship requires trust and telling the truth goes some way to reinforcing that trust. Trust in a relationship means that everyone concerned will act and perform as expected. Patients should be able to trust that the nurse caring for them is not only competent and working in their best interests, but also open and honest. Therefore when someone asks a direct question about proposed treatment or care, the nurse is under a moral duty not to lie. Telling the truth is fundamental to the trust within that relationship. Similarly, nurses must also be able to trust that a patient will be truthful and fulfil their responsibilities, so the nurse can be confident that any information given is correct and truthful. If this is not the case, then their ability to help might be compromised.

ACTIVITY 4.12

---

1 Is it ever legitimate to tell a lie?
2 How might you justify this ethically?
3 Is there a difference *ethically* between telling a lie and simply avoiding the question?

To help you to answer these questions, let us consider the following example.

> Patient: Nurse – am I going to die?
> Nurse: What makes you ask me that question?

What, if any, is the difference between a response such as this and simply lying to the patient? For example, if the nurse was to respond with: 'No, you are not going to die'.

Let us explore this further by looking at an example from practice in Activity 4.13.

ACTIVITY 4.13

Consider this scenario:

> You are working on a children's ward and a boy, Jamie, aged 13, who has Down's syndrome, asks you what the doctor is saying to his mother and asks if he can go with them to the consulting room. You are aware that the doctor is informing the child's mother of the recent test result, which indicates that he has leukaemia.
> You tell Jamie that he can see his mother later and try to distract him by taking him to the day room to watch a film. You realize that you have not been completely honest with the boy, having deliberately withheld information from him about his condition and the purpose of the meeting between his mother and the doctor, even though he has asked you a direct question. How could you justify not following the 'truth-telling' rule in this case?

Points to consider:

1 You might argue that informing the boy may have caused more distress and do 'more harm than good'. You were therefore acting in his best interests.

2   You might recognize that the best situation would be for his mother to inform him or at least be with him when he is informed.
3   You might feel that due to both his age and Down's syndrome, he would not be able to understand what you are telling him. This might be particularly problematic, especially in the context of the discussions concerning equality and diversity in the previous section.

Issues such as competence and mental capacity will be further discussed in Chapter 5. You may wish to return to this question later to reaffirm your understanding.

The second 'rule': Everyone is deserving of privacy

No one should intrude on the personal space of another, either physically or in relation to their business or personal information. In healthcare settings, privacy is often very difficult to promote and maintain. We know that people highly value their privacy and previous and current campaigns in healthcare emphasize this, including amongst other evidence, the Care Quality Commission adult inpatient surveys (CQC, 2018) and the *Chief Nursing Officer Report on Privacy and Dignity* (DH, 2007a) amongst much other evidence.

Consider the following examples, which might take place in a hospital ward.

Doctors' rounds or reviews are sometimes undertaken when personal care is being delivered. This can make it difficult to ensure that personal space is not intruded upon either due to the environment or the activity of others in that area.

Similarly, when personal issues are discussed with the patient or between staff at the bedside or on the telephone, others may hear private/personal information and details.

Following the rule of promoting 'privacy', therefore, the nurse must do everything possible to minimize these risks by taking the patient away from the bedside to a private area whenever possible. This might be a bathroom, office, or private day room, for example. On the occasions on which examinations and conversations have to take place at the bedside, those who are able to leave, such as visitors, should be asked to do so with due regard always given to the sensitivity of this request and the potentially negative response of those being asked to leave.

Issues of privacy should not be underestimated in any environment, however. These might be equally as problematic in the person's home as in an acute clinical environment, depending on what the home circumstances are.

Remember that issues of dignity and privacy are not only of concern in hospitals or care homes. Below are some examples of feelings highlighted by clients, which could be equally applicable in any care environment, not least in the client's own home.

- Feeling neglected or ignored while receiving care.
- Being made to feel worthless or a nuisance.
- Being treated more as an object than a person.
- Feeling their privacy was not being respected during intimate care.
- Perceiving a disrespectful attitude from staff or being addressed in ways they find disrespectful, for example by their first name.
- Generally being rushed and not listened to.

The third 'rule': We should always maintain confidentiality

According to Avery (2016) confidentiality is possibly the single most sacrosanct principle in healthcare ethics and forms the basis of the professional–patient relationship. Nurses have a duty to protect confidential information and:

> As a nurse, midwife or nursing associate, you owe a duty of confidentiality to all those who are receiving care. This includes making sure that they are informed about their care and that information about them is shared appropriately. (NMC, 2018a: 5)

Does this make you reconsider any of your thoughts with regards to Jamie, the boy with Down's syndrome in Activity 4.13? The NMC is clear that this duty to maintain confidentiality is not necessarily all-encompassing and that there are certain 'exceptional circumstances' in which confidentiality might be broken and information disclosed.

> share information if you believe someone may be at risk of harm, in line with the laws relating to the disclosure of information. (NMC, 2018a:17.2)

However, it is emphasized that should a nurse decide to disclose any information without the permission of the individual concerned, then they are fully accountable for this decision and will need to be able to justify their actions as being in the best interests of the public. The legal aspects of confidentiality and the responsibilities of the nurse are further discussed in Chapter 5.

———————————— ACTIVITY 4.14 ————————————

1   Have you ever felt that you ought to break a confidence?
2   Under what circumstances might this be appropriate?
3   Who might support you in this decision-making process?

Activity 4.15 and the scenario in it may help you to answer these questions.

———————————— ACTIVITY 4.15 ————————————

Consider this scenario:

> You are aware that one of the men whom you are looking after has been diagnosed with a condition that may impact on his ability to drive. While he has a duty to inform the Driver Vehicle Licensing Authority (DVLA) of the changes in his health, he has informed you that he has no intention of giving up his licence, as he feels that this will seriously affect his independence and impact negatively on his lifestyle.
> What might you do?

1   In the first instance, you may try to explain the potential consequences of his choice not to inform the DVLA.
2   However, if you fail to persuade him to inform the authority himself, following discussion with others in the multidisciplinary team, it may be decided to inform the authority, because breaking a confidence may be deemed as being for 'the greater good'. However, this decision should never be taken lightly. Breaking the confidentiality of a person calls into question the whole ethos of the caring relationship and must be undertaken only following significant consideration, appropriate consultation, and with recognition of individual accountability. You also have to tell the patient of your plans to break the confidence.

The fourth 'rule': Always keep promises

This is sometimes called **fidelity** and is concerned with an obligation to keep promises and remain faithful to your commitments. More broadly, it might be seen as upholding principles at the heart of the patient–nurse relationship. Implicit within this relationship are certain promises, including promises to work in the best interests of the patient, maintain confidentiality, obtain **informed consent**, be honest, be responsive to their needs, and take on the role of advocate (Herring, 2018).

One fundamental rule might be that 'breaking promises is wrong'. However, it is possible to argue that it is morally acceptable to break promises when the breaking of the promise produces more good than if the promise is kept. Similar to the professional commitment to confidentiality, it is sometimes argued that breaking promises is morally acceptable when the welfare of a third party is put at risk by the keeping of that promise.

ACTIVITY 4.16
---

1   Is it ever legitimate to break a promise?
2   Under what circumstances might you break a promise to a patient?
3   Has this ever happened to you?

Use the following example to help you to answer these questions.

You are undertaking a drug round with your mentor when a patient says: 'I don't need any pain killers at the moment, but I will need them before physiotherapy. You must promise to bring them at 10 a.m.' At 9.50 a.m., a patient at the other end of the ward becomes emotionally distressed when told that she cannot go home that day as she expected. At 10.30 a.m., you see the patient mobilizing with the physiotherapist. As he passes you, he says angrily: 'You broke your promise.' This comment implies the need for you to justify your behaviour. In other words, you are being called to account.

Any justifications would include the fact that you had acted in a way that reflected your priorities at the time and, in weighing up the conflicting needs of both patients, had addressed the dilemma by assessing where the greatest need lay and acted accordingly – a series of actions that are perfectly justifiable ethically. It is likely that, following an explanation, the person concerned is also likely to agree that your priorities had changed as they are likely to view the situation from the same ethical context.

Therefore, according to Beauchamp and Childress (2019), society generally believes that we should all abide by the rules of:

- Telling the truth.
- Maintaining privacy.
- Maintaining confidentiality.
- Keeping promises.

It also becomes clear that our original *judgements* about a particular situation are made, almost instinctively on occasions, due to the fact that we hold these rules to be true.

So what underpins these rules? Where did these rules come from?

Level 3: The principles

This particular framework offered by Beauchamp and Childress (2019) indicates that the rules are supported by certain key *principles*, of which there are four.

Autonomy

The first principle is respect for **autonomy**. The concept of autonomy implies personal liberty and relates to ideas of independence, self-reliance, freedom of choice, and the ability to make decisions. It does not mean, however, that we can do exactly what we want because it is based on rational thought or reason rather than simply desires or wants. It is worth recognizing that the idea of personal choice is central to current healthcare and healthcare policy and the support of a patient's autonomy coincides with this philosophy (NHS England, 2019b).

Nurses contribute to the autonomy of their patients in a number of ways, not least giving necessary information to promote informed consent.

Historically, John Stuart Mill, a British philosopher of the nineteenth century, argued that the only permissible reason to remove a person's social or personal autonomy is to prevent harm to others (Melia, 2013). However, you may have experienced a situation in which a person has been advised to have treatment and yet decides to refuse this treatment – a decision that may seem illogical, potentially dangerous, and indeed not in their best interests.

——————————————— **ACTIVITY 4.17** ———————————————

What does 'in the patient's best interests' mean?
  Is it:

1   Care/treatment that the health professional considers to be the best for them?

Or:

2   Care/treatment that ultimately respects the individual's autonomy?

Activity 4.18 and the scenario in it may help you to further consider these issues.

——————————————— **ACTIVITY 4.18** ———————————————

Consider this scenario:

  You are caring for a patient who is known to have an alcohol abuse problem; he has been admitted to your unit on a number of occasions following falls at home. He is now mobilizing quite well following his fall and his other chronic health problems are being managed. It is time to clarify the plans for his future care and discharge him from the unit.
  The patient's daughter and a number of the members of the team feel that it would not be safe to discharge him to his home, because previously he has continued to drink, and this could result in further falls and the risk of further injury or being left undiscovered for a long period of time. The patient, however, is insistent that he goes home.
  Should he be 'allowed' home?

Some of the considerations the team may discuss are as follows.

1   Ethically:
    • One should always respect the person and promote their autonomy.
    • One should act in a way to promote well-being and good (known as the concept of **beneficence** – see below).

- One should always attempt to ensure that no harm is caused (known as the concept of **non-maleficence** – also see below).
- One should ensure that the consideration of others is recognized with regard to appropriate use of resources, staff support, and so on.

2 Professionally:
- The NMC directs the registered nurse to act as the patient's advocate, providing person-centred care, maintaining dignity, and showing respect (NMC, 2018b).

3 Legally (as we will see in further detail in Chapter 5):
- No one has the power to take away this patient's right to freedom (Human Rights Act 1998).
- Nor under the Mental Capacity Act 2005 do you have the right to override the decisions of a competent person.

So what should you do in such situations? Clearly, there are many different aspects to consider, however, the key thing for any nurse is that, when called to account, they can justify their decisions with sound ethical, professional and legal reasoning.

Non-maleficence

Another principle is known as non-maleficence. According to the *Oxford English Dictionary* (Waite, 2012), maleficence can be defined as follows.

1 Evildoing; an act of evildoing.
2 Malefic character; harmfulness.

Non-maleficence is therefore the 'absence or lack of' harm or evil.

This concept is generally considered to be the foundation on which healthcare delivery rests, as nurses and other healthcare workers have a duty not to harm patients or clients. On the surface, this seems obvious and even self-evident.

─────────────────── **ACTIVITY 4.19** ───────────────────

1 Can you think of any aspects of nursing care that might be described as 'harmful'?
2 Most procedures carry with them some element of risk of harm, don't they?

(Continued)

(Continued)

3 Who is best placed to define what counts as harmful?
4 Is the patient or client always the best person to decide this?

Use the following example to help you to answer these questions.

You are being assessed by your mentor on your competence at administering medication by intramuscular injection. This procedure carries a number of risks. Some potential risks to consider include:

- Correct drug.
- Correct dose.
- Correct patient.
- Correct time.
- Correct route and site.
- Any issues of informed consent, especially in your role as a learner with relatively limited experience.
- Pain that will inevitably be inflicted.
- Potential for adverse reaction.

Health and safety issues include:

- The potential for a needle-stick injury.
- Correct and safe sharps disposal.
- The reduction of infection risk.
- Any issues of insufficient or poor supervision.

It soon becomes clear that the advice to 'at least do no harm' is far more complicated than might be first thought. It seems almost impossible to avoid doing at least *some* type of harm while attempting to promote, maintain, or restore health. Some of this 'harm' might be quite subtle in relation to the needs and preferences of that individual. It might be psychological and relate to threats to the patient's independence. It may concern an individual's ability to make free choices due to incapacity, for example, or the disclosing of confidential information about a person that may result in distress and failure to respect a person's autonomy.

The question then is: how far does this principle of non-maleficence extend? If it is fair to say that every drug administered has the potential for harmful side effects and if we were to take this principle to its logical conclusion, we would never administer any medication to anyone.

Beneficence

According to the *Oxford English Dictionary* (Waite, 2012), beneficence can be defined as follows.

1 Doing good, the manifestation of benevolence or kindly feeling, active kindness.
2 A benefaction, a beneficent gift, deed or work.

This therefore promotes an obligation to 'do good' and act in ways that promote the well-being of others (Davis et al., 2006).

However, the principle also brings with it potential problems. It highlights that you should always do what is in the best interests of the patient and that the good of the patient may be put before one's own needs as a nurse (Ellis, 2017), thus emphasizing the difference between nursing and many other professions or jobs. There seems to be an implied obligation for *self-sacrifice* for the nurse that may not be expected in other walks of life, which is why, for example, you may have felt the obligation, and indeed the willingness, to stay late after your shift officially ended to help a patient or to complete some aspect of care.

Within nursing, beneficence also relates to considerations of the practical outcomes for the individual concerned, and the balancing of benefits and costs (Beauchamp and Childress, 2019). However, as with the other ethical principles, this is not always self-evident and it is often difficult to determine exactly what will benefit another person most.

Melia (2013) claims that beneficence is not an independent principle, but is inextricably related to non-maleficence, and it is this relationship that justifies care being delivered that might be, on first glance, inappropriate due to the harm that it causes. The administration of medication via a hypodermic needle is clearly harmful in some way, but if the result of non-intervention means certain death from infection, then the morally justifiable act is that which causes the least harm and the most good.

The concept of best-interest decision-making is underpinned by the ethical principles of beneficence and non-maleficence.

Justice

Justice is notoriously difficult to define. It involves ideas of fairness and treating people equally. It relates to giving people what they deserve and/or what they have a right to. However, applying this principle in specific circumstances can be very problematic, as decisions may appear to 'depend on the specific situation'.

Ideas of justice, however, are used to guide our decisions globally, nationally and locally. Justice might be aspired to through government policy decisions and the equal provision of resources nationally. This attempts to ensure that everyone has equal access to services when they need them. These types of considerations also impact on the relationship between individual nurses and individual patients, assuming that all people have the right to be respected and also assuming that all decisions are made on principle rather than emotion.

ACTIVITY 4.20

1 If two people require the same or similar treatment, who should receive the treatment first?
2 How might you justify your decision to prioritize?

Activity 4.21 and the scenario in it highlights some areas that you might consider.

ACTIVITY 4.21

Consider this scenario:

You are undertaking a placement in a health centre and a mother brings her baby to see the health visitor as she is concerned about her development. During the conversation, you get the impression that she is feeling low in mood and has intimated that she has recently experienced suicidal thoughts. When you are asked to make an appointment for her to see the counsellor, you find that the practice nurse also wants the last available appointment with the counsellor for a 72-year-old man. The practice nurse is concerned that, since the death of his wife and with no children close by, the patient is struggling to cope and has expressed a wish to die.

The person who does not get the available appointment may have to wait as long as two months to be seen.

Possible approaches:

1 First come, first served: whoever arrived at reception first to make the appointment gets it.
2 According to merit: who deserves this most? The woman who has a long life in front of her and a baby, or an older man who has no one close left and no one who relies on him, but who has worked hard and contributed to society all his life?
3 According to need – that is, medical need: who needs this appointment most to prevent harm coming to them? Judging this is clearly very difficult.
4 According to outcome: whoever will benefit most from the appointment is given the appointment.

As previously discussed, each of these approaches may be legitimately defended; however, the ethical principles and the overriding ethical theories behind the decision-making are the essential issues in relation to the accountability of the nurse.

Level 4: Ethical theories

According to Beauchamp and Childress (2019), the whole framework of ethical decision-making is underpinned by two main ethical theories generally known as **deontology** and **consequentialism**. A specific type of consequentialism called **utilitarianism** is also often described.

- Deontology.
  - Deontology speaks of a person acting according to certain given principles – that which is their *duty*. An act is good or bad simply by the fact that it conforms to a set of rules that lay down our duty or obligation. Therefore the consequences of the act are almost immaterial.
- Consequentialism.
  - Consequentialism, on the other hand, judges the rightness or wrongness of an act only on the grounds of whether its consequences produce more benefits than disadvantages. It promotes a calculation of the benefits and disadvantages of the consequence of an action.

- Utilitarianism.
    - Utilitarianism, put simply, is a type of consequentialism in that a person ought always to act in a way that produces the *greatest amount of good for the greatest amount of people.*

These ethical theories are very complex. What might these fundamentally theoretical standpoints mean in practice? How might they help your decision-making in the *real world*?

Let us revisit a previous example. You are undertaking a drug round with your mentor when a patient says: 'I don't need any pain killers at the moment, but I will need them before physiotherapy. You must promise to bring them at 10 a.m.' At 9.50 a.m., a patient at the other end of the ward becomes emotionally distressed when told that she cannot go home that day as she expected. At 10.30 a.m., you see the patient mobilizing with the physiotherapist. As he passes you, he says angrily: 'You broke your promise.'

How might the 'rights and wrongs' of this situation be assessed from the point of view of the ethical theories?

1 Deontology.
2 Consequentialism.

A *deontologist* may argue that the rule of keeping promises overrides other considerations. Therefore they might feel obligated and would have a duty to maintain their promise. Clearly, this becomes less straightforward in reality as they may also hold the belief that you should always help someone in distress. Two 'rules' or 'obligations' clash here and create a *dilemma*.

A supporter of *consequentialism* would justify their practice by working out the alternatives first and the *consequences* of each alternative. Their decision-making would be driven by assessing which action resulted in the best consequences for those concerned.

Such discussions show how integral ethical thinking in the form of principles and theories are to nursing practice. As we shall see in the next chapter, the law and/or professional advice such as the NMC *Code* (2018a) will not necessarily offer you specific answers to the complex dilemmas that you will inevitably face as a nurse. In fact, as we have seen in relation to the NMC's withdrawal of their previous standards for medicines management, there appears to be an acknowledgement – probably appropriately – that specific clinical practice guidance is not within their remit. However, it remains clear that dilemmas that raise questions about whether a nursing intervention is morally acceptable and ethically right require thorough exploration and analysis to help to provide clarity and rationale and justification for practice.

Summary

This chapter has highlighted and confirmed the key role that nurses play as advocates for patients, particularly in their lead role in the multidisciplinary teams in which they work. This role involves a recognition and acceptance of the *accountability* essential to professional practice, with a requirement for nurses to be able to justify their individual practice. The significant differences in the accountability of students and registered nurses was also highlighted along with the potential complexity of the delegation of activities and being answerable for any subsequent actions or omissions.

The complex professional and personal context inevitably involves both registered nurses and student nurses being challenged by certain ethical dilemmas. It is argued that the use of an ethical framework can provide the basis for 'principled discussion' of the intricate aspects of any situation and can then consistently and appropriately inform any subsequent action. The particular framework explored in detail argues that initial *judgements* are justified by a set of *rules* that state what should or should not be done. These rules are further supported by four main ethical *principles* – autonomy, beneficence, nonmaleficence and justice – and the whole framework of ethical decision-making is underpinned by two main ethical *theories*: deontology and consequentialism.

5

ACCOUNTABILITY, DECISION-MAKING AND THE LAW

Graham Ormrod, Nichola Barlow and Rob Burton

THE AIMS OF THIS CHAPTER ARE TO:

- Explore the legal context of accountability and its relevance for student nurses in their transition to becoming staff nurses.
- Review specific legal concepts and definitions.
- Explore the differences between criminal and civil law.
- Further investigate the concept of negligence and its relevance to nurses.
- Discuss the concepts of consent and capacity in a legal context.
- Confirm the practical and everyday relevance and importance of the law to the nurse's role.

Introduction

In the previous chapter, we explored the concept of accountability, particularly from an ethical point of view, and highlighted the importance of this in everyday nursing practice. The ethical context of society can change, and the things that society deems good, right, or proper can change as years pass. The law might change accordingly, as the law represents the rules that reflect the values of a society at that particular time in its history. The function of the law, therefore, clearly relates in some way to the current moral context of society. The law can, for example, state what is acceptable as *good* behaviour and place *duties* on individuals to act in the best interests of others. It also requires individuals to behave in a *fair* way and insists on equal treatment of every member of the community. These points have obvious *moral* components and similarities.

ACTIVITY 5.1

David Jones, aged 55, has had type 1 diabetes since he was 10 years old. The disease has taken its toll and David is now registered blind, although he can vaguely see shapes, and has severe cramps and pain in his lower legs. This prevents him from going out to work or to socialize as he would like. He feels that he is a burden on his wife and two children. Whilst you are assisting in his care, he tells you that he is considering going to a clinic abroad to assist him to end his life. He also reminds you of your duty of confidentiality and says that you must not tell anybody this.

1   In relation to the scenario above, consider how you think ethical accountability is related to legal accountability?
2   Are they the same?
3   In society generally, how do you think ethical values relate to the laws that govern that society?

Such scenarios indicate how legal, ethical and professional issues are invariably intertwined whilst at the same time remain fundamentally different. They indicate some of the difficult moral questions about modern life and the potentially changing moral landscape both nationally in the UK and also internationally. Only time will tell if this ongoing *ethical* debate will eventually be reflected in *legal* changes.

Professionally, however, it is worth remembering that the Nursing and Midwifery Council (NMC, 2018c), while confirming the need for the student to ensure confidentiality, also emphasizes that it is essential that a student consults and refers to a registered nurse when clinical decisions need specialist knowledge. Similarly, the NMC provides guidance for registered nurses and student nurses alike concerning the potential conflict of the need to ensure confidentiality whilst also feeling the need to raise concerns not least in relation to a patient's vulnerability (NMC, 2019a). Your university may also provide you with guidance, advising that as a student, you should seek advice from your practice supervisor, mentor or tutor before disclosing information if you believe someone may be at risk of harm.

Similarly, following the publication of the Crown Prosecution Service (CPS) guidelines, *Suicide: Policy for Prosecutors in Respect of Cases of Encouraging or Assisted Suicide* (CPS, 2014), and ongoing debate in the professional and mainstream media, the NMC felt it necessary to reiterate its statutory duty and remind all nurses that *the law on assisted suicide had not changed.*

What is the law?

Let's first review a few fundamentals. You might think that the healthcare context is more *litigious* or *legalized* than in the past, as there may appear to be an increasing number of healthcare cases being heard in court. An understanding of the law as it relates to nursing is therefore essential, as knowledge of the law helps in understanding the scope of nursing practice and the responsibilities that come with being a registered nurse, as well as providing insight in how to prevent any potential legal problems before they happen. It is essential, however, not to get too anxious about the possibility of becoming embroiled in legal action! From your discussions with colleagues during your training, you may conclude that *every* nurse knows of 'someone' who has been sued for negligence and 'struck off' or removed from the NMC register. Rest assured that this is far from the truth: as we shall see, it is still very rare for nurses to become involved in legal processes and the vast majority of nurses go through their career without such an unfortunate experience.

According to Caulfield (2005), the law is a set of rules and penalties agreed by society. Another definition claims that the law is the framework that a society develops to limit lawlessness, thus allowing it to function in a way that is predictable and acceptable to its members (Jones and Jenkins, 2004).

Scottish law

Scotland has a different court system from that of England and Wales. Scots law is the law of Scotland. It is a unique system with ancient roots and has a basis in Roman law, combining features of both civil law and common law. Thus Scotland has what is called a pluralistic legal system. Since 1707, Scotland has shared legislature with the rest of the UK, but both Scotland and England retained their fundamentally different legal systems, although there is some English influence on Scots law. In recent years, Scots law has also been affected by European law.

The Court of Session is the supreme court and the Sheriff Courts are the regional courts. The main division in Scots law is between *public law*, involving the state, and *private law*, in which only private persons are involved. Public law covers, among other areas, criminal law. Private law or the 'law of persons', including children and adults, is often simply part of the law of the land: for example, murder and theft are not defined in statute as offences, but are dealt with under common law. The majority of discussion within this chapter will relate to English law, but reference will be made appropriately on occasions to the differences in the two countries.

The two main types of law

The two main types of law that affect nurses to be discussed in this chapter are *criminal* law and *civil* law. What are the main differences between criminal law and civil law? According to Griffith and Dowie (2019: 11):

> a breach of the criminal law can be followed by prosecution in the criminal courts, whereas liability in civil law is actionable in the civil courts and may or may not be a crime. There is no necessary moral difference between the two.

Let us explore the differences a little further.

Criminal law

Criminal law is concerned with the relationship between the *state* and the *individual* (Caulfield, 2005). This type of law essentially settles disputes between individuals and society as a whole. It deals with offences that transgress rules of society and is a means of enforcing society's rules on an individual. To break the laws of the land allows the state to punish the offender by means of arrest by the police and prosecution by the state in the name of the Queen as head of state. Guilt under criminal law invariably results in some form of punishment. Punishment can be in the form of:

- Fines.
- Probation (which can include conditions such as attendance at a training centre or hospital order under various sections of the Mental Health Act 2007 or Mental Health (Care and Treatment) (Scotland) Act 2015).
- Community service.
- Suspended sentence (with or without supervision).
- Prison.

One of the main differences between criminal law and civil law is what is known as the *burden of proof*. In criminal law, the prosecution has the burden of proving to the satisfaction of the jury that the accused is guilty 'beyond all reasonable doubt'.

Civil law

Unlike criminal law, civil law regulates relationships between *individual citizens* rather than between the *state* and an individual. An action is brought by a person, who has suffered harm, known as the claimant or plaintiff, against another person or organization, known as the defendant. This is often the area of the law that concerns nurses most as they feel they may be accused of *negligence* and of causing harm to a patient or client.

The *burden of proof* in cases of civil law rests 'on the balance of probabilities' rather than 'beyond reasonable doubt'. What this means in practical terms is that the accusation has to be deemed more likely to be true than not. If an accusation of negligence is proved 'on the balance of probabilities', then, again unlike in criminal law, this wrong is redressed by awarding *damages*, and financial compensation is given in place of a punishment, such as imprisonment (Griffith and Dowie, 2019).

Vicarious Liability

It is important to recognize and understand the concept of *vicarious liability* at this point. Vicarious liability is defined as the indirect liability of an organization for negligence by its staff while acting in the course of employment. An employer has certain responsibilities to their staff: a National Health Service (NHS) trust, for example, has responsibilities towards the nurses whom it employs. These responsibilities may include creating an environment in which the general working conditions are appropriate and equipment is available and working properly. Similarly, the employer has a responsibility to ensure that staffing levels are adequate, and staff are competent and know what they are doing. This all relates to the concept of vicarious liability. As the employer is responsible for the environment and ultimately the competence of its employees, it is invariably the employer/trust that is sued if any employees are accused of negligence. Therefore, the employer would take on any liability *vicariously* as long as the nurses were working within an appropriate scope of practice and within any appropriate guidelines. It is also true to say that your employer will undoubtedly have more money than you!

────────────── **ACTIVITY 5.2** ──────────────

1   Do you know how to access relevant guidelines, policies, or procedures in your placement area? It is important, and could be very interesting, to find some of the key policies within your current placement.
2   Do you know of any that specifically relate to students while undertaking placement learning?
3   For example: what is the policy in relation to student involvement in the administration of controlled drugs?

Find this policy, read it, and discuss any implications for your learning experience with your practice supervisor.

It is worth remembering that the NMC, in *Future Nurse: Standards of Proficiency for Registered Nurses* (NMC, 2018b), stress that students must be able to recognize the laws, policies, regulations and guidance that underpin the prescription, supply, dispensing and administration of medicines and must exercise professional accountability in ensuring the safe administration of medicines to those receiving care.

Elements in an action of negligence

Let us look a little more closely at the concept of negligence, which can cause anxiety for nurses. Put simply, the elements involved in any action of negligence can be summed up in three key points (Griffith and Dowie, 2019), as follows:

- A *duty of care* is owed by the defendant to the plaintiff.
- There is a breach in the *standard* of the duty of care owed.
- This breach has caused *reasonably foreseeable harm*.

--- **ACTIVITY 5.3** ---

1 What is your understanding of the term 'duty of care'?
2 How does this relate to the relationship between a nurse and a patient/client?
3 Make a list of those to whom you feel the nurse may owe a duty of care.
4 Discuss this with your practice supervisor and/or personal tutor.
5 Did their list match yours?

Concept summary: Duty of care

It is not always easy to decide when a nurse owes a duty of care to another person. For example, if you are looking after a child, you clearly owe that child a duty of care. However, where does the duty of care lie in relation to the parents, both the mother and/or father? This might not be quite so clear, especially if there is disagreement with regards to which treatment is in the child's best interests. This may be further complicated by the rare, but tragic, 'right to life' decisions (see for example: www.bbc.co.uk/news/uk-england-london-42862431), particularly those that generate opposing views from the mother and father, for example in the case of the mother and father who opposed each other in court over whether life support for their severely ill son should be turned off (see www.bbc.co.uk/news/uk-england-merseyside-43152332).

These are just two examples of where things may not be as clear as initially thought. Remember that the plaintiff or claimant must show that a duty of care was owed for any accusations of negligence to be further pursued.

The standard test of duty of care in law was laid down in the case of *Donoghue v Stevenson* (1932) AC 562, and enshrines the philosophy of the 'good neighbour principle' (Griffith and Dowie, 2019). Famously, the specifics of this case were that, having bought and drunk half a bottle of beer, someone (the eventual claimant) claimed to have discovered the decomposed remains of a snail in the bottle and then chose to sue the manufacturer, rather than the cafe owner, arguing that they owed a duty of care to the consumer who bought their products to ensure that such a thing should not happen.

Lord Atkin subsequently pronounced:

> You must take reasonable care to avoid acts or omissions which you can reasonably foresee would be likely to injure your neighbour. Who then in law is my neighbour? The answer seems to be persons who are so closely and directly affected by my act that I ought reasonably to have them in contemplation as being so affected when I am directing my mind to the acts or omissions which are called in question. (Cited in Griffith and Dowie, 2019: 44)

Put simply, this means that a duty of care exists if you can see that your actions are reasonably likely to cause harm to another person. Therefore, simply by virtue of your relationship with a patient, you owe a duty of care to them.

In Scots law, *delict* – a Latin word sometimes translated as 'a wilful wrong' – is, among other things, the responsibility to make reparation caused by breach of a duty of care, whether deliberate or accidental. Scots law is different in many respects and concentrates more on general principles and less on specific wrongs. However, the landmark decision in this area for Scotland, as for the rest of the UK, was the Scottish case of *Donoghue v Stevenson* (1932) AC 562.

So do you have a duty of care to other service users and carers, relatives, and so on? This may become less clear in the complex healthcare situations in which you find yourself.

What about situations that arise outside work, being witness to an accident for example?

Duty of care outside of work

Presently in the UK, there is no *legal* duty to volunteer help in such circumstances, as there is no *pre-existing* duty of care. It is interesting, however, that this is not necessarily the case in all other countries. Morally, it might be argued, you have a duty of care to assist. If we agree that *all* individuals ought to adhere to the principles of **beneficence**, **non-maleficence**, justice and **autonomy** as discussed in Chapter 4, then, within a civilized society, it might be argued that such a duty of care is owed simply by virtue of being a fellow human being.

Therefore, in such circumstances, the nurse owes no greater duty of care than anyone else who might be at the scene. From a professional point of view, the NMC has previously insisted that the nurse should stop and assist as best they can with regards to their competence, although this is slightly less explicit in the current *Code* (NMC, 2018a). Therefore, although the nurse has no legal duty to stop and give care, it could be argued that she does have a professional duty. Depending on the circumstances, it might be reasonable to expect the nurse to do no more than comfort and support the injured person and to reduce the potential for further harm; if a nurse chooses to walk away from an emergency situation, they could be called to account for this.

So, if you do stop and become involved, then you thereby take on a duty of care and would be expected to employ an appropriate professional standard of care. You would be judged against what could reasonably be expected from someone with your knowledge, skills and abilities when placed in those particular circumstances, and would have to demonstrate that you had acted in the person's best interests.

As Dimond (2015) points out, if you move the victim in a car accident and this causes spinal injury, then you could be sued for any further injuries that you have caused. It would have to be shown that you should have anticipated the dangers of moving a person when a spinal injury was possible and also that the victim was not in greater danger by being left where they were.

─────────────────── **ACTIVITY 5.4** ───────────────────

The examples above highlight the complex issues of the nurse's role and responsibility while off duty. It might be interesting to discuss such issues further with colleagues and friends.

1   For example, should a nurse stop at the scene of an accident?
2   Should this be a legal requirement or is it more of an ethical or professional responsibility?
3   How might this differ from the responsibilities of a member of the general public?
4   Would you expect the response to be different from nursing students, qualified nurses, and your friends who aren't nurses?

───

One thing that is clear is that 'being a nurse' brings with it certain responsibilities that many other careers do not. Nurses have an obligation to be of good health and good character, and part of the ways of assuring this is the necessity to undergo a Disclosing and Barring Service (DBS) check.

The Disclosing and Barring Service

The DBS allows organizations such as hospitals, schools and universities in which staff, volunteers or students work with children or vulnerable adults to check police records and, where appropriate, information held by the Independent Safeguarding Authority (ISA). The two levels of DBS check are:

• Standard disclosure.
• Enhanced disclosure.

Both are available in cases in which an employer is entitled to ask exempted questions under the Exceptions Order to the Rehabilitation of Offenders Act (ROA) 1974.

Standard disclosure checks show current and spent convictions, cautions, reprimands and warnings held in the police national computer system. Enhanced disclosure, as in the case of student nurses, is the highest level of check available to anyone working in regulated activity with children or vulnerable adults. This disclosure contains the same information as the standard disclosure, but with the addition of:

- Any relevant and proportionate information held by the local police forces.
- A check of the new children and/or vulnerable adults barred lists where requested.

Similar systems are in place in Scotland. Disclosure Scotland has a role in enhancing public safety by providing employers or organizations with criminal history information about individuals applying for posts. More information can be found at: www.disclosurescotland.co.uk/about-disclosure-scotland/

The Nursing and Midwifery Council indicate that the public may not differentiate between nursing and midwifery students and registered practitioners, and therefore refer students to *The Code* (NMC, 2018a). This indicates that a student's personal life should be equal to that of a registered professional, and therefore may have an impact on:

- Their fitness to practise.
- Their ability to complete their programme.
- The willingness of the university to sign the declaration of good health and good character that enables the student to become a registered nurse.

The examples of inappropriate behaviour offered by the NMC include such wide-ranging issues as aggressive, violent or threatening behaviour, cheating on course work or plagiarism, and misuse of the internet and social networking sites. The implications of misuse of social media indicate the ever-changing potential for students to be accused of inappropriate behaviour. The NMC (2019c) advise:

- Be informed.
- Think before you post.
- Protect your professionalism and your reputation.

Although still very rare such accusations can undoubtedly have a profound and negative effect on a student's career aspirations and also confirm that these obligations continue after registration.

Standards of care

So, if we now have greater clarity with regards to the concept of duty of care, let's explore a little further the second element in any accusation of negligence: the concept of *standard of care*. The test to decide whether the standard of care has been broken is based on 'the reasonable man'. (You will note that discussions with regards to the law are often very gender-specific – that is, the law often appears only interested in 'men' and also often relates to specific professions, such as medicine. Unfortunately, or fortunately, however, the law relates equally to us all!) So the 'reasonable man' in the case of nurses means that the nurse acted to the standard expected of a *hypothetical* reasonable nurse in that same situation, or behaved to the standard expected of a reasonable student at that point in their training. It is interesting to note that the law does not speak of acting as the *best* nurse might have done or even a *good* nurse, but simply a *reasonable* nurse.

This test of the standard of care is often known as the 'Bolam test', after *Bolam v Friern Barnet Hospital Management Committee* (1957) 1 WLR 583. Any nurse would be deemed to have acted appropriately if they had:

> Acted in accordance with the standard of ordinary skilled man exercising and professing to have that special skill. (Cited in Griffith and Dowie, 2019: 47)

In other words, the Bolam test means that where a nurse acts in a way that would be supported by other nurses as being appropriate or *reasonable* practice at that time, it is likely that the court will find that the nurse did not act below the standard of care expected. The court would only deem that the nurse had 'failed' the Bolam test if this was seen as '[a] failure to act in accordance with a practice accepted as proper by a responsible body of medical men skilled in that particular art' (Griffith and Dowie, 2019: 51).

This does not mean that if a nurse chose in very particular circumstances to deviate from standard and 'normal' practice, this would automatically be deemed negligent or wrong, as there may well be appropriate reasons for this in very specific circumstances. This decision to act outside normal practice may have been made following great consideration and delivered subsequently in a most careful or caring way, even though it unfortunately resulted in harm to the patient. However, the great wealth of policies and procedures that support nursing practice are there for a very good, hopefully evidence-based, reason and nurses choosing to take actions outside any standard guidance do so on the understanding that they might well be asked to defend their practice as 'reasonable' in the future.

This standard will have implications for you throughout your career, especially if you are eventually in a role that requires extended or specialist education and practice. Nurses working at a 'higher' level of practice, such as nurse specialists or nurse consultants, for example, will be judged against the standard expected of others working at that level of practice. This may therefore result in a nurse being judged against the standards of care traditionally delivered by a doctor.

In a climate of changing public and professional expectations and the continuing blurring of professional boundaries and responsibilities, standards will inevitably change accordingly. This reinforces the importance of ensuring competence and proficiency before undertaking any aspects of care, no matter how experienced you are.

As *The Code* (NMC, 2018a) emphasizes, you should always recognize and work within your limits of competence and:

> ask for help from a suitably qualified and experienced professional to carry out any action or procedure that is beyond the limits of your competence. (NMC, 2018a: 13.3)

─────────────────────────── **ACTIVITY 5.5** ───────────────────────────

1   Have you ever been put in a position in which you felt that you were working outside your level of competence or felt inadequately supervised?

Such situations can sometimes have tragic consequences, as seen in the case of a student who misunderstood the instruction of her supervising nurse, resulting in a fatal drug error: http://news.bbc.co.uk/1/hi/england/merseyside/7664404.stm

2   How would you advise a more junior student to handle such a situation?

It is also important to ask your practice supervisor and staff from the university for advice if you find yourself in a situation in which you feel that you lack proficiency or do not know what you are doing. The golden rule is do not put patients at unnecessary risk.

It is extremely important that you inform your practice supervisor or university lecturer immediately if you believe that you, a colleague, or anyone else may be putting someone at risk of harm (NMC, 2019a). Just as for qualified nurses, you have a responsibility to report poor practice and/or abuse. This is often called 'whistleblowing' and can cause significant upset and anxiety for the student nurse.

The NMC (2019a) clearly sets out the role for both student nurses and registered nurses on raising concerns concerning safeguarding the health and well-being of those in their care. This guidance indicates what actions nurses and students should take in situations where patients or members of the public are perceived to be at risk. The Royal College of Nursing (RCN) in the UK also recognized the seriousness of poor standards going unreported and provided detailed guidance in its initiative *Raising Concerns* (RCN, 2017b).

The nurse's responsibility in highlighting poor practices again indicates the importance of recognizing and understanding local policies and procedures for safeguarding and protecting the vulnerable in your care, and whistleblowing if necessary to ensure that agencies such as social services or the police are involved as appropriate. The NMC (2019a) and RCN (2017b) indicate serious concerns should initially be disclosed 'internally'. This means discussing with your practice supervisor, mentor or tutor first and using local clinical governance and risk management procedures and whistleblowing policies where appropriate. However, clearly this may not always be possible, especially if the poor practice involves your mentor or a senior member of staff, and in such cases your university tutor will be the obvious initial option for support. In the unlikely event that this remains an inappropriate option, talking through with a trusted independent person will help you to clarify whether further action needs to be taken. Available policies for whistleblowing will support and perhaps clarify your thinking and you should always be mindful of the potential for breaking confidentiality in such difficult and often traumatic circumstances. Indeed, according to Gallagher (2010), balancing the obligation to report concerns that prevent further harm to patients with the obligation to maintain confidentiality is one of the most challenging ethical issues in relation to whistleblowing. This is just one aspect of the complexity of context that can occasionally appear to show nurses seemingly failing to intervene, raise concerns and effectively respond to prevent the occurrence and continuation of poor patient care (Roberts, 2016).

Let's get back to the law. It is important to recognize that, fundamentally, the law does not see inexperience as any justification for poor standards of care. A student nurse providing care is judged, legally, by the same standards as an experienced nurse. On first glance, this may seem a little unfair. However, we would all agree that a learner driver is not allowed to drive on the pavement simply due to their inexperience! Certain levels of competence and standards of proficiency are still legitimately expected.

Professionally, as far as the NMC is concerned, it is the registered nurse who is accountable for what they choose to delegate to a student (or any unregulated member of staff), and they are therefore professionally accountable for the consequences of your actions and omissions (NMC, 2018c), and this is why, as a student, you must always work under appropriate supervision and recognize your own accountability. Remember that you can always be called to account by the law or by your university for the consequences of your actions or omissions as a student.

It seems fair to say that patients are entitled to be cared for in a competent way at all times irrespective of whether they are being cared for by a student on their first day or a staff nurse of 20 years' experience. This again emphasizes the importance of:

- Only undertaking care when you are competent.
- Ensuring appropriate supervision at all times.
- Calling for assistance if you are unclear about any aspect of care.

─────────────────── **ACTIVITY 5.6** ───────────────────

A student nurse is caring for a patient whose care plan indicated that she had serious difficulty with her balance, which made it necessary for her to have assistance when standing or walking and when transferring. The student nurse had also been told this by her mentor at handover report.

The student nurse had assisted the patient to the bathroom and subsequently helped her up from the toilet. The student then walked away and left the patient standing with her Zimmer frame in the bathroom, while she propped the door

(Continued)

(Continued)

open and adjusted her wheelchair, and waited for the patient to walk to the wheelchair on her own. The patient took a step forward, fell backwards, and was injured.

1   What do you consider to be the main legal issues here?
2   Is the student nurse negligent?
3   What is the legal position of the mentor?

Some points that may help you to answer the above are as follows:

- From a legal point of view, any negligence claim would undoubtedly be made against the trust or care home rather than the individual nurse.
- Failing to give proper appropriate attention to a patient's need for assistance while ambulating is negligence.
- The healthcare facility would be held to the same legal standard of care for a student nurse's error or omission as for the same error or omission by a registered nurse.
- Had the student received training to assist patients with ambulation and transfer?
- Testimony from appropriate colleagues might establish that it is reasonable to expect a nursing student to have the competence and experience to safely support a patient in these circumstances.
- It might be deemed reasonable to expect a student to have had mandatory moving and handling training, for example.
- The nursing student's practice supervisor may be called to testify with regards to her delegation, supervision, communication and record-keeping. Should the student have known whether the patient needed someone close with her at a safe distance at all times to ambulate?

Caulfield (2005) does acknowledge that the courts will accept that junior staff who have articulated any concerns about their levels of proficiency, competence and inexperience – for example, if you ask a more senior member of staff to check your work – are more likely to be recognized as having met their expected standards of care. This also highlights the continuing need for all nurses to assertively challenge instructions that they believe to be inappropriate or incorrect.

Reasonably foreseeable

One of the basic principles of the law of negligence is that precautions can be taken only against reasonably known risks (Griffith and Dowie, 2019). A case of negligence would only be successful if the claimant could prove that what happened could have been foreseen or predictable. The court will ask whether a reasonable person in the defendant's position would have foreseen that the claimant might be injured. If they could not have foreseen injury or damage to the claimant, then the claim will inevitably be unsuccessful.

In Activity 5.6, in which the patient fell while being cared for by a student nurse, was the fall 'reasonably foreseeable'?

In such cases, considerations could include the following:

- What was included in the patient's care plan? As emphasized by *The Code* (NMC, 2018a), keeping clear and accurate records is an integral part of nursing practice, and is essential to the provision of safe and effective care.
- Had a mobility assessment been undertaken?
- Had advice been taken from physiotherapy colleagues, if appropriate?
- Was the patient appropriately confident and aware of the proposed plan?
- What was the student's previous experience and level of proficiency?
- Was the level of supervision sufficient?
- Was delegation appropriate in such circumstances?

Exploration of the above and other aspects of the scenario would help to confirm whether this unfortunate accident was, indeed, 'reasonably foreseeable' or not.

Cause

Not only has the outcome to be reasonably foreseeable, but a *causal* link between the actions of the nurse and the harm suffered by the plaintiff has also to be proven. Put rather bluntly in the eyes of the law, unlike the NMC, it may not matter how badly a nurse behaves as long as there is no injury. The law is not only interested in the behaviour of the nurse, but crucially also the consequence of that behaviour. This is often known as the 'but for' test. In other words, *but for* the action of the nurse, acting in a way that breaks the standard expected, then no harm would have been caused (Griffith and Dowie, 2019).

Is the injury measurable?

The final consideration in negligence cases is whether the injury is measurable in some way. This is to enable calculation of the financial compensation, if required. In many cases of healthcare negligence, as with many patients who complain about their care, the claimant is often simply asking for an apology or an assurance that such practice will not be repeated. However, should financial damages be deemed appropriate, they are essentially an attempt to place the victim, as far as is possible, in as close a position as that in which they would have been had the incident not happened (Herring, 2018).

Accountability: Consent and capacity

As was discussed in the previous chapter, the underpinning ethical principle of consent is the promotion of autonomy. The concept of consent is at the heart of the nurse–patient relationship and, on a day-to-day basis, this relationship is often developed on the assumption of implied consent. However, as a qualified nurse, you will need to be continually mindful of the many difficult issues associated with gaining appropriate consent. For example, any mentally competent adult has the right in law to consent to any touching of their person. If they are touched without consent or other lawful justification, then they have the right of action in the civil courts of suing for trespass to the person, under Section 18 of the Offences Against the Person Act 1861, which relates to grievous bodily harm. In fact, those who provide treatment without consent are more usually prosecuted under the offence of battery, which is a relatively less serious crime. There is no requirement for proof of damage, and any non-consensual touching can result in a case being brought (Tingle and Cribb, 2013). However, the gaining of consent is the main form of defence to an action of trespass and will usually prevent a successful action for this accusation (Griffith and Dowie, 2019).

The role of the registered nurse in ensuring appropriate lawful consent

So, what is the registered nurse's role in ensuring that they act in a legally appropriate manner in line with the NMC *Code* (2018a)? How might this differ from your role when you are a student?

As we have seen, the International Council of Nurses (ICN) and the NMC identify the importance of obtaining consent from patients before conducting any type of intervention or care activity (ICN, 2012; NMC, 2018a). The NMC (2018a) states that, as a registered nurse, you must obtain consent before engaging in any aspect of treatment and care and that it is important that registered nurses always respect the patient's right to decline any treatment offered. As a registered nurse, you must be able to demonstrate that you have acted in the patient's best interests in any situation, particularly in an emergency. As we have seen previously these standards also apply to you as a student nurse.

The principle of patient autonomy means that every competent adult has the right to refuse treatment. A person who acts autonomously is self-directed, free from the interference of others, and is able to process information, understand, deliberate and reason, enabling them to make independent choices (Beauchamp and Childress, 2019). This highlights the crucial consideration of **capacity** in all aspects of consent.

Patients who lack capacity *can* be treated without consent, although slightly different rules apply depending on the reason for the patient's incapacity. The introduction of the Mental Capacity Act 2005 means that statute law rather than common law now governs the treatment of some of these patients.

The Mental Capacity Act 2005

The Mental Capacity Act 2005 provides healthcare professionals with a clear legal framework for ensuring that consent obtained from patients is valid. It also highlights the required course of action when the patient may be temporarily or permanently unable to provide consent (Figure 5.1 provides an overview of the Act's main areas).

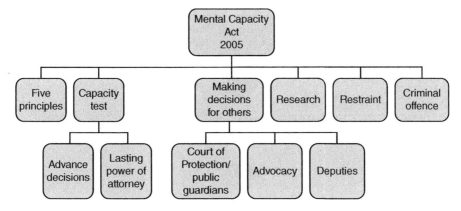

Figure 5.1 The Mental Capacity Act 2005: Overview and structure (adapted from Richards and Mughal, 2006)

The Mental Capacity Act 2005 provides a set of good practice principles that encompass all aspects of consent (see Figure 5.2).

Obtaining consent

Consent can be obtained in a number of ways, all of which are equally valid. It may be given in an expressed way, either through word of mouth or written, or it may be implied – that is, the actions of a patient will suggest that they are consenting to the treatment to be given. However, written consent is considered the best evidence in proving that consent was given (Dimond, 2015).

It is important to remember that consent must always be gained for *all* nursing interventions, assessment and care, and not simply limited to those procedures that constitute medical treatment.

Examples of the various types of consent are given below.

1 Implied consent: You approach a patient to take a blood pressure recording and, as you approach, he rolls his sleeve up and holds out his left arm ready for you to take the measurement. His action therefore *implies* consent.
2 Verbal consent: When you wish to take a urine sample from a patient, you might obtain verbal consent from the patient by simply explaining why you need the sample and asking if they understand.
3 Written consent: This type of consent is usually obtained prior to an invasive procedure such as surgery. The consent will be obtained on the form chosen by the organization providing the

Always assume that an adult has capacity unless otherwise established
(Burden of proof lies with those making the assessment)

All possible efforts must be made to promote capacity

What appears to be an unwise decision must not lead to an assumption
that a person lacks capacity (respecting the views and beliefs of others)

When making decisions or acting on behalf of a person who lacks capacity

Any act done or decision taken under this Act must be a 'best interest' decision

Acts and decisions must be those that ensure that the
restrictions of a person's rights and freedom of action are minimized

Figure 5.2 The principles within the Mental Capacity Act 2005

© Mental Capacity Act 2005. Contains public sector information licensed under the Open
Government Licence v3.0. (www.nationalarchives.gov.uk/doc/open-government-licence/version/3/)

treatment and requires that the person taking consent explains
the procedure and the possible benefits, risks and alternatives,
thereby allowing the patient to make an informed decision prior
to signing the consent form.

Concept summary: Capacity

To make an informed decision, it is important that the person fully
understands the implications of this consent. This is often called
capacity. When obtaining consent, capacity to give this consent always
needs to be assessed.

Where there is any doubt about the person's capacity, then a test for capacity must be performed. This test is performed by the person requiring consent unless this is disputed for some reason (see Figure 5.3). In such circumstances, it may be taken to the Court of Appeal.

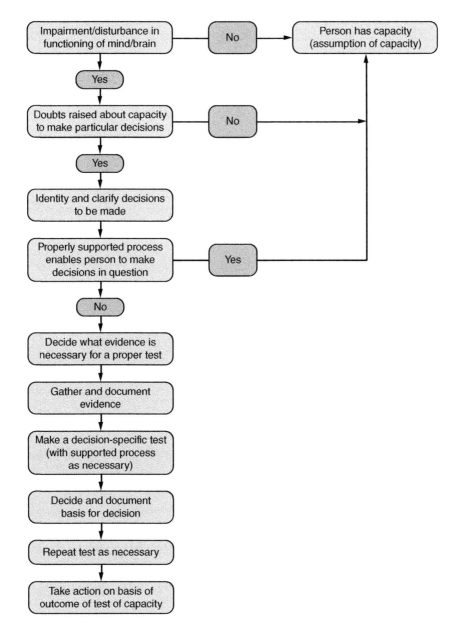

Figure 5.3   Flow chart of the assessment of capacity (Church and Watts, 2007)

Reprinted with kind permission of Cambridge University Press

Where a person is found to have capacity, their wishes must be respected unless others are put at risk. Wherever possible, there is a duty to support the person in the decision-making process to facilitate autonomous decision-making. This support might include:

- Ensuring that information is provided in a format that the person making the decision understands.
- Providing all of the appropriate information in order that they can weigh the variety of probabilities.
- Ensuring the provision of time and support for deliberation.
- Answering any further questions appropriately.
- That a means of communicating the decision must also be facilitated – for example, if a person no longer has the ability to express their decision verbally, other means may be used to support communication, such as picture boards, using closed questions, allowing for nods of the head or hand-squeezing in response, etc.
- The use of interpreters, which is recommended as appropriate, as is the use of specialist hearing equipment if required.
- The provision of written information, which can also help the patient to retain the information long enough to make the required decision.

As the patient's **advocate**, the nurse may need to play a central role in support of this process.

Best-interest decisions

Where the person is found *not* to have capacity, then a 'best-interest decision' is made. The Mental Capacity Act (2005) provides clear guidance of how this decision should be made, including that:

- All relevant circumstances must be considered.
- Whether the person might have capacity in the future, and if so when.
- The person's previously expressed and present wishes.
- The person's significant and relevant beliefs and values.
- Factors that the person would consider if able to do so.
- Consultation of significant others if possible and appropriate (which might include family, religious leaders, social workers, who can provide information on the person's known beliefs and views).

- Encouragement and support to enable the person to participate if possible.

Once all circumstances have been considered the least restrictive option must be preferred.

─────────────────────── **ACTIVITY 5.7** ───────────────────────

You wish to provide care that you know will help improve a patient's condition and have a positive impact on their life. They, however, report that they will not accept the treatment as they believe the treatment has been tested on animals and their conscience would not allow them to consent to this.

1   As a student nurse, what would you do in this situation?
2   Would your actions change as a registered nurse?

───

Here are some points that may help clarify your decision-making in Activity 5.7.

1   The NMC *Code* (2018a) states that, as a registered nurse, you must respect the patient's beliefs and values. The Mental Capacity Act 2005 emphasizes that a decision that might be considered by some as an unwise decision does not mean that the individual concerned does not have the capacity to understand the consequences of that decision.
2   If, however, there is doubt about the patient's ability to understand the information provided and the consequences of the decision then the test for capacity may be applied; if they are deemed to have capacity then you must respect the decision. If the patient is found not to have capacity then a 'best-interest decision' may be made.

The use of restraint/restrictive practices

Any decisions made on behalf of another person must always be the *least restrictive option* available and the consequences should be kept to a minimum. Practices that might be viewed as restrictive can be confusing and complex. The Care Quality Commission (CQC) inspection findings post-Winterbourne View (Transforming Care and Commissioning Steering Group, 2014) described confusion and concern among staff in the awareness and use of restrictive practices. This confusion can result in an over-reliance on physical restraint rather than other more positive behaviour supports and management of the environment that makes it less likely that someone might behave in a way which could be seen as challenging. It is clear that physical restraint should be used only in very specific circumstances, however other forms of restrictive practice that staff might use without appropriate consideration for the positive rights of the individual might include: bed (cot) sides, use of lap belts on wheelchairs etc., use of 'when required/prn' medication, locking doors, restriction of free movement within the environment, only allowing a person a certain amount of time to watch television and so on (RQIA, 2014).

Patients/clients refusing treatment is a very difficult situation to deal with and can be very distressing for all concerned, especially for less-experienced staff or students. This is particularly the case if any form of restraint (particularly explicit physical restraint) has to be used. These situations are inevitably upsetting, and it is not acceptable that employers allow nursing students to be put in a position of making decisions about restraint because of a lack of qualified nurses. The RCN define restrictive practices as 'those that limit a person's movement, day-to-day activity or function' (RCN, 2017b).

Such practices are not inherently wrong, harmful or illegal and *may* be justified in certain circumstances as part of a comprehensive therapeutic plan according to the RCN (2017c) – for example, when the individual is:

- Displaying behaviour that is putting themselves at risk of harm.
- Displaying behaviour that is putting others at risk of harm; prohibiting family contact for safeguarding reasons for example.
- Requiring treatment by a legal order, for example under the Mental Health Act 2007.

It is important to recognize that these decisions may need to be made in many different settings, whether that be in a mental health or forensic environment, critical care, continuing care, or care delivered within the community in someone's own home. It is interesting that the use of certain devices of restraint that might be quite common in some countries might be seen as unacceptable in others, although the debate about their appropriateness continues (Morgan, 2010).

Clients who were confused when restrained may later remember and value nurses' explanations of what was happening to them, particularly with regards to the reassurance that the nurses were trying to keep them safe. Therefore, if a client cannot give **informed consent**, you should always explain the rationale behind what you are doing, helping to achieve understanding and agreement as far as possible. If you suspect that restraint is being used inappropriately, you should report this immediately to your practice supervisor, mentor and/or your personal tutor.

Advanced directives

Advanced directives are directives made by individuals when they still have full decision-making capacity and they give guidance to those providing care as to the present or future wishes of that individual should certain specific circumstances occur. It is important to recognize that nothing can override an appropriately written and legally sound advanced directive.

However, a directive can only be viewed as legally binding in very specific circumstances. For example, if the directive expressly refers to long-term care following a stroke (when the patient may no longer be able to communicate their decisions and wishes), then it will not apply in relation to long-term care or treatment where the person has dementia. It will, however, indicate the person's fundamental values and beliefs and therefore will contribute to discussions prior to the making of any best-interest decision.

Where the advanced directive relates to life-sustaining treatment, this must be documented very clearly and unequivocally. The directive must be signed and also witnessed by another person. It is also important to recognize that advanced directives can be withdrawn and altered at any time while an individual has capacity.

——————————————— **ACTIVITY 5.8** ———————————————

You are caring for a woman who has been admitted following a road traffic accident, and her family provide you with an advanced directive that she had asked them to give to the hospital staff if she were ever admitted to hospital in a condition in which she was not able to make her own decisions. The advanced

(Continued)

(Continued)

directive states that when the degenerative disease that was diagnosed four years ago becomes so advanced that she cannot care for herself, or if she is unable to eat or drink, then she does not want her life to be prolonged or any attempt to resuscitate to take place.

While in your care, the patient suffers a cardiac arrest. What would you do?

In such situations, unless a decision regarding resuscitation has been agreed upon by the healthcare team and the patient, if they are able to participate, resuscitation would need to be commenced. In this instance, the advance directive is in relation to a specific disease and there is no indication that her condition is such that her quality of life has deteriorated to the extent detailed in the advanced directive.

Points to remember

It may be a good point here to recognize the potential upset and anxiety that such scenarios can cause for students. Never be afraid to ask for help as a student nurse or once you are qualified and registered. There is a lot of help available if you feel you need it and the golden rule should be to ask your university tutor or clinical practice supervisor straight away, so that they can provide the support and advice you may need. This early support should reduce the possibility of the matter becoming more serious later on. Your university and your clinical placement provider will also provide student support services, such as confidential counselling, occupational health services, advisers, and student groups or unions. The NMC also has a confidential helpline to talk to expert advisers, and the RCN also offers advice and advocacy should you be having a difficult time at university or on placement.

The role of independent mental capacity attorneys

So what happens if someone no longer has capacity? An independent mental capacity attorney (IMCA) makes decisions on behalf of an individual who no longer has the capacity to make that decision independently (Richards and Mughal, 2006). The IMCA must provide support for the individual concerned and gather any information that is relevant to any decisions. In order to do this, the attorney has the right to see all relevant health and social care records to ascertain the individual's wishes and gain clarity concerning possible alternatives.

There is a statutory duty upon NHS organizations to appoint such an advocate in specific circumstances. These circumstances might include when the person involved has been found not to have capacity to make decisions related to:

- Any serious medical treatment, including the taking of a biopsy.
- Any intention to detain the individual in hospital for greater than 28 days, or eight weeks in the case of a care home.
- Any change of accommodation to another hospital where the stay will be greater than 28 days, or eight weeks in the case of a care home, and the person has no relative, friend, or unpaid carer who is appropriate to consult in determining their best interests.

(Dimond, 2016)

──────────────── **ACTIVITY 5.9** ────────────────

You are working in a local authority care home that provides care for 17 people with learning disabilities and mental health problems. The building needs upgrading to improve the facilities. The home needs to be closed for several weeks and all residents will need to be placed somewhere temporarily. All but two of the residents have close family who are able to support them with decision-making in relation to the temporary move. One resident has the capacity to make the decision; the other, however, does not.

1 What is an appropriate course of action in these two cases?
2 What will your responsibilities be as a registered nurse?
3 Are they any different from those of a student nurse?

Points to consider:

- Registered nurse.
  As a registered nurse, in the case of the patient who has capacity, the NMC *Code* (2018a) requires you to 'ensure you gain consent'. You can achieve this by ensuring that the patient has all the required information to facilitate informed consent and that you promote their autonomy by *advocating* for them when appropriate.

- Student nurse.
  Remember, as a student nurse, you are also both legally and ethically accountable and the NMC (2018a) states that you must treat patients as individuals and respect their dignity. Where the patient does not have the capacity to make the decision, a 'best-interest decision' would be made incorporating the patient's current and previous views if they are known, involving the health and social care team and, if they have no family, perhaps close and long-standing friends of the individual. If these are not available, then the organization that plans to move the patient will be required to appoint an IMCA.

Lasting power of attorney

A lasting power of attorney (LPA) is another means for people to plan ahead and can be appointed by an individual who at the time has capacity and the ability to forward plan in relation to financial management for their future health and social care. The lasting power of attorney only becomes effective when capacity is lost, and the appointed attorney must then be consulted when any health and social care decisions are made. This is to ensure decisions are in the person's best interests. It is important to recognize the distinctions between the two different lasting powers of attorney.

- **A lasting power of attorney – property and affairs** essentially allows a person to appoint somebody to look after their money and related affairs. This effectively replaces the old enduring power of attorney.

So while a will ensures that a person's estate can be distributed according to their wishes when they die, a lasting power of attorney – property and affairs protects their assets by authorizing somebody chosen by them to deal with their property and affairs on their behalf, should they become unable to manage them themselves, while they are alive.

- **A lasting power of attorney – personal welfare** allows a person to appoint one or more attorneys to make decisions on their behalf about their personal welfare and healthcare. This includes whether to give or refuse consent to medical treatment or deciding where they might live, decisions that can only be taken on their behalf when they lack the capacity to make them themselves.

The duties of the attorney include:

- A duty of care.
- A duty not to delegate authority.
- A duty not to take advantage of the position.
- A duty to act in good faith.
- A duty to maintain confidentiality.
- A duty to keep their money separate from that of the person for whom they are the attorney.

Issues of withholding or withdrawing treatment, donation and best interests

Just as with some of the complex situations mentioned above, some decisions are made *solely* by the courts. These include the withholding or withdrawing of life-sustaining treatment, organ and bone marrow donation, non-therapeutic sterilization, and where there is dispute relating to a best-interest decision.

Decisions relating to the withholding or withdrawing of life-sustaining treatments, for example, occur frequently in healthcare practice, and such decisions require both the consideration of a number of principles and assessment of the possible outcomes of any course of action. Clearly, this can be very complex and is rarely straightforward. Where an individual has capacity, the Mental Capacity Act (2005) requires that the individual's autonomy, beliefs, values and wishes be respected. However, if the individual concerned does not have capacity at the time, then certain processes would be initiated.

In cases of withholding and withdrawing life-saving treatment:

- An advanced directive in writing and witnessed would take precedence.
- If there is no advanced directive, a lasting power of attorney would be consulted.

- Failing these contingencies and depending on the individual circumstances a best-interest decision will be sought *or* application made to the Court of Protection.

ACTIVITY 5.10

What about consent and capacity where children are concerned?
   Consider the following scenario.
   Barney, a 6-year-old boy, is admitted to the ward for insertion of grommets. His parents insist that he is not told any details of the surgery, so he is not able to be fully informed or prepared for theatre.

Consent, capacity and children

Such a scenario clearly raises many issues and to resort to the law in such cases appears an overreaction. However, the principles enshrined within the law can help and guide our plans and interventions in such cases.

The Mental Capacity Act 2005 applies to adults – in this case, those over the age of 16 (Dimond, 2016). However, young people under the age of 18 are not able to refuse *life-saving treatments*. They are, however, able to consent or refuse other treatment, as identified within the Family Law Reform Act 1969 or Family Law (Scotland) Act 2006. Younger children who fully understand what is involved in the proposed procedure can also give consent. 'Gillick competence' is often the name given to the competence of a minor.

Gillick competence

In 1982, Mrs Victoria Gillick took her local health authority (West Norfolk and Wisbech Area Health Authority) and the Department of Health and Social Security to court in an attempt to stop doctors from giving contraceptive advice or treatment to under-16-year-olds without parental consent. The case went to the High Court, where Mr Justice Woolf dismissed Mrs Gillick's claims. The Court of Appeal reversed this decision, but in 1985, it went to the House of Lords and the Law Lords (Lord Scarman, Lord Fraser and

Lord Bridge) ruled in favour of the original judgement delivered by Mr Justice Woolf:

> whether or not a child is capable of giving the necessary consent will depend on the child's maturity and understanding and the nature of the consent required. The child must be capable of making a reasonable assessment of the advantages and disadvantages of the treatment proposed, so the consent, if given, can be properly and fairly described as true consent. (Willmott, 2010)

The eventual outcome was that the consent provided by the young girl was deemed lawful as she was found:

- To understand the doctor's advice.
- Not to be able to be persuaded to inform her parents.
- Likely to engage in sexual activity, irrespective of the prescription.
- Likely to do so without contraception, which might adversely affect her physical and mental health.

Therefore, the decision to prescribe contraception was found to be in the child's best interests (Griffith and Dowie, 2019). It is important to note that while Gillick competence allows a minor to consent to treatments provided that they are found to have capacity to do so, they are not able to *decline* treatment that is *life-saving*.

Where the child does not have capacity to make the decision, the consent of the parent or legal guardian is sought, and if this is not possible a 'best-interest decision' is made. Where there is a need for ongoing decision-making or a dispute, a deputy is appointed through the Court of Protection. Similar provision is offered in Scotland under the Age of Legal Capacity (Scotland) Act 1991.

Persons with learning disabilities

Clearly, individuals who have learning difficulties will all have different levels of understanding and each case therefore requires individual assessment. If their capacity is in doubt, the 'test for capacity' would be applied.

Persons with mental health problems

Patients detained under a section of the Mental Health Act 2007 are held regardless of their capacity to make decisions. The order under which they are held will be simply to detain them for assessment or to provide treatment in relation to the *specific* mental health problem that they are experiencing. This does *not* mean that they do not have capacity generally. As such, valid consent must be obtained for any intervention other than the conditions set out in the detention order, if the nurse is to act legally, ethically, and within *The Code* (NMC, 2018a).

ACTIVITY 5.11

A patient has been detained under the Mental Capacity Act 2005, Section 3, and the decision has been taken to detain him for electroconvulsive therapy, because he is in a severe depressive state and other conventional treatments have proved ineffective. However, he refuses to undergo a barium enema to investigate recent changes in his bowel habit.

   What is the best course of action for you as a nurse?

Remember that although the man is detained under the Mental Health Act 2007, this is not in relation to the condition affecting his bowel and, as such, these investigations and treatments require specific informed consent. You would first need to *ensure capacity*.

   If there is doubt with regards to capacity to consent, then the test for capacity should be applied. If it is confirmed that the patient has capacity, information must be provided in a form that he can understand, and time and support given to allow him to consider the information and provide the opportunity for him to communicate his decision. As a nurse, you have the responsibility within the law to facilitate this. As a registered nurse, you are professionally accountable. You must uphold people's rights to be fully involved in decisions about their care and treat people as individuals and respect their dignity (NMC, 2018a).

- If the man is found to be lacking capacity, you must first establish if he is likely to recover capacity, and if this is likely following treatment for the depression, and intervention is not urgent, *you should wait until capacity is regained.*

- If capacity is not likely to be regained or if it is not possible to wait, then a *best-interest decision should be made.*

Adults with Incapacity (Scotland) Act 2000

The Adults with Incapacity (Scotland) Act 2000 provides a similar framework for safeguarding the welfare and managing the finances of adults who lack capacity due to mental disorder or inability to communicate. It allows other people to make decisions on their behalf subject to certain safeguards. The main groups to benefit from this Act include people with dementia, people with a learning disability, people with an acquired brain injury or severe and chronic mental illness, and people with a severe sensory impairment.

Power of attorney is also a similar means by which individuals, while they have capacity, can grant someone whom they trust the powers to act as their continuing (financial) and/or welfare attorney.

The Act allows treatment to be given to safeguard or promote the physical or mental health of an adult who is unable to consent. The principles apply to medical treatment decisions as to other areas of decision-making.

Principle 1: Benefit

Any action or decision taken must benefit the person and only be taken when that benefit cannot reasonably be achieved without it.

Principle 2: Least restrictive option

Any action or decision taken should be the minimum necessary to achieve the purpose. It should be an option that restricts the person's freedom as little as possible.

Principle 3: Take account of the wishes of the person

In deciding if an action or decision is to be made, and what that should be, account must be taken of the present and past wishes and feelings of the person, as far as this may be ascertained.

Principle 4: Consultation with relevant others

Take account of the views of others with an interest in the person's welfare.

Principle 5: Encourage the person to use existing skills and develop new skills

Further information can be gained here: www.gov.scot/collections/adults-with-incapacity-forms-and-guidance

Research and the issues of capacity and consent

You may think: 'Why include this section in this book?' While you are unlikely to begin undertaking research in the early stages of your nursing career, research and **evidence-based practice** play a central role in professional practice. Similarly, you may be caring for a patient who has been asked to be involved in research, and they may ask for your guidance and advice. The following information will help you to protect the rights of the patient and give you an insight into pertinent considerations should you be interested in pursuing research yourself in the future.

All research that involves human participants, including cases in which tissues or organs are intended to be retained for research or education, requires ethical approval from local and/or national ethics panels. This includes identifying how freely given and informed consent will be obtained from the participants. To be deemed to have capacity to consent to be involved in research, like consenting for any other procedure, a participant must be able to demonstrate the four aspects shown in Figure 5.4.

For further information, see www.myresearchproject.org.uk

This site requires you to log in, however it is possible to access the 'help' section without doing so, which contains interesting and relevant information.

Particular complications occur when research subjects no longer have, or may never have had, capacity to consent to participate in research. These are often groups of the most vulnerable people, such as children or those who have learning disabilities and mental health

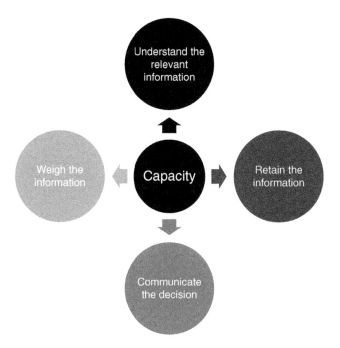

Figure 5.4 Components of capacity (adapted from Mental Capacity Act 2005)

© Mental Capacity Act 2005. Contains public sector information licensed under the Open Government Licence v3.0. (www.nationalarchives.gov.uk/doc/open-government-licence/version/3/)

problems. Despite the difficulties, however, it would be morally wrong to avoid research that involves these groups, as research is crucial to continuously improving and developing health and social care practice (Dimond, 2015). Moreover, as we have seen, the NMC *Code* (2018a) identifies the importance of delivering care that is based on the best available evidence and ensuring that any healthcare advice is evidence-based.

The Mental Capacity Act 2005 sets out seven precise conditions for research involving participants who do not possess the required capacity to consent. The purpose of these conditions is to protect the welfare of the individuals involved (Dimond, 2016).

These conditions are that:

1 The research is related to their condition.
2 Their condition is an impairment or disturbance of the brain.

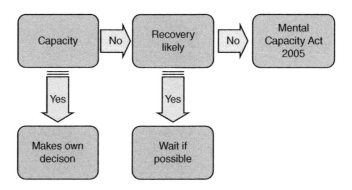

Figure 5.5 When to consult the Mental Capacity Act 2005

3 There is reasonable belief that the research would not be as effective if carried out on those with capacity.
4 The research must have potential to benefit the individual and not impose a burden that is disproportionate.

Or that:

1 It is intended to provide knowledge of the cause or treatment.
2 If point 5 applies, but not point 4, the risks to the individual are reasonably believed to be negligible.
3 There are reasonable arrangements in place for ensuring that the requirements of consulting carers and additional safeguards are met.

The decision-making path for patients/clients whom you consider may not have capacity, and therefore when the Mental Capacity Act may be invoked, is shown in Figure 5.5. It is very likely that you will be involved in caring for people who need to consent for certain interventions or treatments.

Summary

This chapter has explored various aspects of the law in relation to professional practice and how this may impact on your current and future experience. You should now understand the major differences between criminal law and civil law. We explored in detail the area of negligence that can cause anxiety for students, explaining the elements in any accusation of negligence. These include proof, *on the balance of probabilities*, that a duty of care was owed, that the standard of that duty of care was not breached, and if it was, that this breach did indeed cause reasonably foreseeable harm.

The complex issues of consent were further discussed – particularly in relation to those deemed to be without capacity, and how ensuring informed consent is paramount in providing good health and social care while acting within the law. Essentially, the underpinning principle that informs this and other current healthcare practice and the law is having respect for persons.

You must always assume that those for whom you are caring have capacity unless it is proved otherwise using the test for capacity. The Mental Capacity Act 2005 is a structured legal framework to protect those who are vulnerable and may not have capacity to make all of their own decisions, while also providing each person with the opportunity to plan for the future when, for whatever reason, capacity may be temporarily or permanently lost.

Here is a recap of some of the main points that you will need to consider.

- No treatment may be given to an individual unless the patient has consented to treatment.
- If nurses proceed with treatment without the patient's consent, they are vulnerable to an accusation of battery. However, this assumes certain circumstances.
- For consent to be valid, the individual must have capacity and understand what is involved in the proposed treatment.
- They must also be fully informed of the advantages and disadvantages of the proposed treatment, including the risks involved, whether any alternatives are available, and the possible consequences of the treatment.
- Consent must be given freely without coercion or under real or implied threat.
- If the person is unable to offer valid consent, the principle of 'best interest' would be utilized. This is a complex concept, but includes

such considerations as the welfare, interests, values and known wishes of that person.

- The decision-making must take into account the patient's values and preferences when competent, their well-being and quality of life, and relationships with other family members, carers and friends.

6

LEADING, MANAGING AND WORKING IN TEAMS

Rob Burton and Graham Ormrod

THE AIMS OF THIS CHAPTER ARE TO:

- Explore issues of transition to the role of newly qualified nurse and being in charge.
- Explore theories of leadership.
- Explore theories of management.
- Outline strategies to help a newly qualified nurse to be in charge.

Transitioning to the role of newly qualified nurse

One of the first things that you will need to get used to as a newly qualified nurse is being in charge. This may mean being in charge of the care of a single person, or group of people, as well as being in charge of the whole care environment, including all staff and other multidisciplinary team members. To do this, you will not only need to understand the care needs of the clients, but also to understand and be able to demonstrate skills of leadership and management. It is recognized that you should have a period of preceptorship and supervision on qualifying, but there may be times during this period in which you do have to lead or manage teams.

What does 'being in charge' mean? And what does it take to make the transition from being a student nurse to finding that you are the one who is responsible for yourself and the welfare of the patients, staff, visitors, and anyone else in the care environment? The focus of this chapter is on what you need to know and what you might need to do when you are leading and managing in a care setting early on in your career.

We will discuss the concepts of leadership and management, how to apply them in a new role, and how to feel confident and competent to do so. By identifying the different concepts and looking at how they can be applied, you will be able to analyse workplace situations and decide on the best leadership/management approach. Wong et al. (2013) found from their study that nursing leadership is essential in the creation of environments, management of staff and resources, and development of care processes which ultimately lead to improving patient outcomes.

Being in charge as a nurse

As a registered nurse you may be assigned responsibilities for patients in your clinical area and the staff working alongside you in order to:

- Ensure the safety of people in your care.
- Deliver required care.
- Delegate tasks in a team.
- Deal with staff issues.

The Nursing and Midwifery Council (NMC, 2018b) standards of proficiency for entry to the register as a qualified nurse state that nurses should be able to lead nursing care and work in teams. Nurses should understand the theory underpinning principles of effective leadership, group dynamics, human factors and strength-based approaches and apply this to teamworking and decision-making. They should understand the principles and processes of performance management, and exhibit leadership potential by demonstrating an ability to manage, support and motivate individuals, and interact confidently with other members of the care team.

Therefore, in the final year of training, you need to take as many opportunities to be in charge of a shift (under supervision) in your field of practice as possible to help you to achieve these aspects.

Activities 6.1 and 6.2 describe typical situations in which you may find yourself as a newly qualified nurse, whether in a busy hospital setting, in a community nursing team, or community home setting. These are common experiences that need the person dealing with them to show leadership qualities and to manage the situation well.

─────────────── **ACTIVITY 6.1** ───────────────

Visiting patients

You are a third-year student in your final placement prior to qualifying, working in a health centre. Your practice supervisor is a community nurse and, after three weeks of being introduced to a group of patients in the community with various health problems, your practice supervisor decides that you can take responsibility (under supervision) for visiting six patients, working with two healthcare assistants and one student.

1   What would your priorities be in this situation?
2   What would you need to consider?

In a scenario like the one above, you should concentrate on the skills identified within the NMC (2018b) standards of proficiency, particularly 'lead nursing care and work in teams'. Some of these aspects have also been discussed in earlier chapters and include ensuring that the environment for care management is safe for patients, clients and staff, and making effective decisions related to managing risk. You would need to clearly communicate with the other staff members you are working with, as well as with other members of the interdisciplinary team involved in care. It is your responsibility to ensure that these communications take place and your responsibility to delegate duties to others. It is here where your leadership qualities are tested. The principles of delegation are also discussed in Chapter 4, and delegation requires leadership qualities and skills. For example, you will have the responsibility for recording and managing the information related to your clients and communicating this to colleagues, thereby also demonstrating some management skills.

You will also have to manage your time and the time of those allocated to you to ensure that the care priorities are met equitably and competently among your clients. As the NMC (2018b) states, nurses should be able to demonstrate proficiency by 'acting as a role model' for best practice and delivery of care, demonstrating accountability for appropriate delegation and supervision of care by others in the team, and communicating and collaborating with the wider multidisciplinary team. The next scenario would require you to demonstrate all these aspects but would test your leadership responsibilities even further.

––––––––––––––––––– ACTIVITY 6.2 –––––––––––––––––––

Shift management

As a qualified nurse, you take a phone call as you commence the late shift in a busy care area. The morning staff are completing their duties for the day, and there is another member of the late shift just arriving. The environment is bustling with activity. You listen to the other person on the end of the phone; it is the nurse manager who was supposed to be in charge of the area for the late shift. They tell you that they are unable to come in on duty as there has been an emergency with their young daughter.

1   What considerations would you make after receiving this phone call?
2   What action could/would you take?
3   How have you seen such situations handled before?

    The answers are hinted at in the following paragraphs.

As a student nurse, you would probably have had a qualified nurse with you on duty to whom you could turn for advice, or who could deal with the matter themselves. Therefore, you could have looked over your shoulder and confidently handed the issue on to them to deal with. But, now, you are qualified and currently the most senior member of staff on duty for the late shift. There is no one else for you to hand the matter to: you are the one who must deal with this situation.

For a newly qualified nurse, this can be a stark realization. The other qualified nurses, healthcare assistants and others in the team are looking towards you now with an expectation that you should do something about this. Your leadership abilities are now open to scrutiny.

A nurse in the situation described in Activity 6.2 would have little choice but to take on a leadership role, even if that were to mean informing more senior staff of the situation. However, in some services such as small care homes or in primary healthcare settings, there might not be anyone more senior that you can turn to. This may seem daunting at first but dealing with such issues is part and parcel of the responsibilities of newly qualified nurses and, rest assured, becomes easier to deal with, as practice helps you to recognize that there are standard approaches to many of these situations.

Definitions of leadership and management

We now look at the terms 'leadership' and 'management' in more detail to demystify them and to help you to recognize that there are structures and approaches that can be utilized to deal with potentially difficult events that occur daily.

The terms need to be closely scrutinized because they are different concepts that are often confused and misinterpreted as having the same meaning. Courtney et al. (2015) suggest that the concepts of leadership and management have a symbiotic and synergistic relationship. Leadership is not always seen as the function of management, and leadership cannot necessarily replace management. The two roles are complementary.

Marquis and Huston (2012) point out that for nurses to function effectively the two concepts should be integrated. Can you be a leader without being a manager? Can you be a manager without being a leader? Northouse (2016) describes leadership as: 'a process whereby an individual influences a group of individuals to achieve a common goal' (Northouse, 2016: 6). This might come about by a nurse acting as a role model and being able to create change by communicating with and motivating others, without necessarily being placed in a position of authority. In contrast, management, as described by Mullins and Christy (2016), is:

> the process through which efforts of members of the organization are co-ordinated, directed and guided towards the achievement of organizational goals. (Mullins and Christy, 2016: 620)

They suggest management takes place within organizations through prescribed roles, focuses on aims and objectives, is achieved through the efforts of other people and uses systems and procedures. Leaders are not necessarily managers as they may not have prescribed managerial roles, but it is argued that managers should be able to demonstrate leadership.

From the above statements, there are elements of responsibility for you related to **tasks** and **outcomes** and also elements related to communicating, **dealing with** and acting as a **role model** to people in the service.

ACTIVITY 6.3
---

1   Considering Activity 6.2 above, how would you describe the role and responsibilities of the nurse taking the call?
2   What are the leadership and management aspects as outlined in the above definitions (Northouse, 2016; Mullins and Christy, 2016)?

Although there is some overlap between the two concepts, they clearly have different properties and dynamics (see Figure 6.1).

Leadership

The word 'Leadership' derives from the Old English word *læden* (of Germanic origin), which means 'travel', 'show the way', 'be ahead of' (Chantrell, 2004: 297). This suggests some kind of journey with someone guiding the way. 'To lead' can be defined in the following ways (Collins Dictionary, 2014):

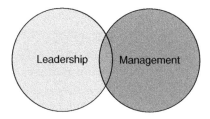

Figure 6.1   The overlap between leadership and management

- To guide, control or direct (a group of people): to be the person who makes decisions that other people choose to follow or obey.
- To show the way to (someone or something that follows), especially by going first.
- To induce.
- To cause to act, think, feel, or behave in a certain way.
- To initiate the action of something.
- To influence.
- To be in front, be first, or be winning.
- To be the first, or foremost.
- As the position or the function of someone who is a leader.

This dictionary definition gives us a broad overview of leadership behaviours. The nurse in Activity 6.2 must make decisions, initiate actions, show the way, and influence and direct others. In taking the call, the nurse is also in the position of acting as leader with a function to fulfil, whether by choice or purely by circumstance. However, the definitions above may not capture the complexity involved, as leadership involves further elements such as establishing rapport, empathising with others, being trustworthy and fair. Leaders develop vision, inspire and challenge (David and David, 2015).

Leadership is concerned with leading (showing the way) and, by implication, causing others to follow. It is important to recognize what role you are taking on in terms of leadership or 'followership' at any given time. Courtney et al. (2015) state that leaders need to build and develop others. To do this they should focus on people, have perspective and develop a power base by demonstrating knowledge and credibility. This can be achieved by:

- Demonstrating competence.
- Fair treatment of followers.
- Showing genuine concern for the welfare of those being led.

Activity 6.2 shows just how those words could apply to a newly qualified nurse. Even though there is a current requirement for newly qualified staff to have a period of preceptorship (DH, 2010; HEE, 2017; NMC, 2006), unforeseen circumstances can still occur. This means that the practicalities of preceptorship are not always so easy and there may not always be others to turn to. The newly qualified nurse then needs to act in order to meet the needs of those in their care, the staff, and others working and visiting the environment.

In a systematic review by Whitehead et al. (2013), being supported by a preceptor in order to set and achieve professional goals was a major factor in newly qualified nurses staying in the profession. Being given objective feedback on the performance of tasks assists in this. Developing leadership ability is one of the important skills that newly qualified nurses need to acquire, even when supported in a preceptorship period.

Your co-workers are important as a source of reward in nursing. You need to gain respect through your actions, as other members of staff will be observing how you react and the decisions you make. If you can deal with such an issue fairly and confidently, you will be held in high esteem. Emotional intelligence is an important factor here, so dealing with such challenges effectively is a necessity, as Goleman et al. (2002) suggest that the leader in any group is the one to whom others look in order to provide assurance, clarity, or to do the job. The saying 'lead, follow, or get out of the way' could be a useful piece of advice here. However, in situations such as that in Activity 6.2, there is little scope for the nurse to be a follower or to get out of the way.

Before going any further, it is appropriate to reflect on one of Rob's own experiences of working with colleagues with regards to management.

When I entered my first role as a staff nurse many years ago, I saw the charge nurses and managers of the areas where I worked and was in awe of them. At that time, I thought I would never be able to gain the skills that would be needed to manage. I also believed they were the leaders and that we had to follow their say on everything.

However, as my journey progressed, I was lucky enough to work with many excellent managers (and some not so excellent, mainly due to their lack of emotional intelligence and adopting an authoritarian approach only). I was *once advised that to become a leader and be in charge you need to be a role model. That is to 'walk the talk'. On reflection I realized the 'poor' managers I have experienced since then were not able to do this.*

Another aspect and valuable lesson learned from one of my previous managers was to trust the people you are working with. This particular manager gave me tasks (probably beyond my scope at the time) and left me to report back. One of these was on devising a whole new strategy for rostering staff. I presented my findings after much research. This was then discussed with the whole staff team. Many debates were had, and many many options put forward, before the manager made the decision on keeping the same system. Although my proposal was finally rejected, I had been given the trust and support of my manager and was shown gratitude for completing the task even though it was dismissed in the end. This same manager could also be very authoritarian when needed, showing flexibility to deal with short-term emergencies and long-term strategies.

I learned that to be a leader you do not necessarily have to be in a formal role, and that you can put forward ideas, demonstrate new approaches and lead others as long as you can be creative, supportive and willing to accept rejection at times. Since then I have had many leadership roles with no formal authority over the teams of people that I have had to manage (some of them in higher positions than myself). However, by setting priorities, delegating duties, taking advice, supporting others and being prepared to be assertive I have managed to develop my roles, responsibilities and project management within senior leadership positions.

--- **ACTIVITY 6.4** ---

1   What skills do people in leading roles need?
2   What actions do you think the nurse taking the call in Activity 6.2 could take?
3   What actions have you observed being taken by nurses in this kind of situation?

Scully (2015) suggests that a crucial element is the relationship between the 'leader' and the 'followers', in that colleagues need to be enlisted, supported and inspired in order to make transformations via reciprocal relationships.

Some leadership characteristics:

- Developing supportive relationships.
- Acting as a role model.
- Communicating effectively.

- Maintaining team dynamics.
- Explaining roles, responsibilities and expectations.
- Making decisions.
- Delegating.
- Being knowledgeable.

These characteristics are translated into standards of proficiency by the NMC (2018b), which include providing rationales of care, multi-disciplinary teamworking and assigning of duties where appropriate, as well as managing performance.

You may have worked with qualified staff who appear to make the shift run smoothly and efficiently. You may find that those who do this more successfully are also those who develop and maintain good relationships with clients, staff, and interdisciplinary team members. They are people who are seen to make decisions rather than agonize over them (no matter how unpopular the decisions may be), but, most importantly, they demonstrate that they can show the way and are prepared to be involved in some of the tasks that they would expect other team members to complete. If these aspects are demonstrated, the person can create an aura of trust-worthiness and reliability. The phrase 'leading from the front' can be taken literally!

Management

The origin of the word 'management' derives from the Latin *'manus'* for 'hand' and was originally expanded to mean how to handle a situation, related particularly to managing a horse (Chantrell, 2004). This was then extended to controlling/handling other types of situation and person. According to Marquis and Huston (2012), the management process is related to meeting the organization's goals by controlling such aspects as finance and human resources. The central focus of management could be considered as being directing, control and coordination. In nursing there are many levels of management from Chief Executives to team leaders. These are important factors to be considered whilst caring for patients or service users in health and social care settings. Even on a day-to-day, shift-to-shift basis, many aspects of coordination are needed to ensure the smooth running of any service and best outcomes for all.

The definitions below give an indication of how management is viewed in the modern world (Collins Dictionary, 2014):

- The members of the executive or administration of an organization.
- The skilful or resourceful use of materials, time, etc.
- To be in charge of; to administer.
- The technique, practice, or science of managing or controlling.

Leadership and management: The theory

It is now necessary to look at the theory underpinning the practice of leadership and management with a view to analysing how these can be applied in the role of the qualified nurse. Some of the key theories will be discussed below, bearing in mind that this is not an exhaustive list. The concept of leadership theories will be explored first.

Leadership theories

According to Murray (2017: 46), leadership is 'A process of influencing others through effective relationship skills'. From this definition, it is implied that leadership resides within a person rather than a position as in management. Therefore, the theories that encompass leadership tend to relate to individuals and their personalities, behaviours and styles. Personality, or trait, theories will be considered first.

Trait theory

Weiss and Tappen (2015) suggest that there are many theories of leadership with no clear 'winners'. However, trait theory implies that there are characteristics often recognized in leaders, raising the question of whether leaders are born or made. Trait theory, evolving from 'great man' theory, suggests that leaders had particular recognizable traits or characteristics such as being tall, male, white, well educated, and wealthy, but these can be deemed to be dependent on social norms and cultural drivers of the time, which is clearly a weakness in this theory. Most early studies focused on historical leaders to determine the characteristics considered necessary to be a leader (Marquis and Huston, 2012). During the development of Europe from the Middle

Ages there was a need for structure, hierarchy and authority within the emerging state hierarchies (Pidgeon, 2017). This therefore led towards identifying traits from political, religious, militaristic leaders and members of the aristocracy, hence the beliefs regarding traits mentioned above. The trait theory isolates characteristics that differentiate leaders from non-leaders. The flaw, however, is the dismissal of those of low status and ignoring females as leaders (Cutler and Steptoe-Warren, 2014).

Some other traits identified in this theory are drive, honesty, integrity, being able to inspire followers, charisma and self-confidence (Pidgeon, 2017). Grossman and Valiga (2016) point out that trait theory did not always truly identify universal leadership characteristics applicable to all leaders, although there was some correlation. However, the focus on traits associated with people born to be leaders shifted as leadership began to be applied to wider, less traditional fields.

Pendleton and Furnham (2016) discuss trait theory in terms of what is described as the 'five factor', or the 'big five', model of categorizing leadership traits as personality traits. They suggest that leaders are more likely to be stable, extroverted, open and conscientious than their followers.

The 'big five' model of categorizing leadership traits. Surgency/ extraversion:

- This is related to the energy with which a leader demonstrates their enthusiasm and positive emotions and beliefs towards a task. This could also be considered as a drive and willingness to be at the front.

Conscientiousness:

- This is related to being focused on the job in hand. Achievement and dependability are inherent traits.

Agreeableness:

- This is an ability to relate to others, providing trust, warmth and kindness.

Adjustment:

- This is the ability to deal with issues in a rational manner without becoming anxious or emotionally distracted.

Intelligence:

- This is related to openness to experiences, creativity and imagination, and being perceptive and thoughtful.

ACTIVITY 6.5

Think of someone you have worked with who you consider an effective leader.

1   Which of the 'big five' traits did they have and how did they demonstrate them?
2   Is there anyone who you have considered to be a poor leader? What were their traits? How did they compare and contrast with those of the effective leader?
3   What traits do you feel you have that might highlight your leadership potential?

The big five traits might be better described as behaviours or habits. This is because individuals may not be able to do anything about their height, weight, gender, age or attractiveness (traits sometimes associated with leaders), although they could further develop skills and abilities that may improve their leadership qualities. Abilities such as conscientiousness, reliability, agreeableness, being able to communicate well, developing problem-solving strategic skills and intelligence can all be worked on and developed, and are still popular to an extent considering leaders are often 'head hunted' to turn around 'failing' organizations. In his famous book, *The 7 Habits of Highly Effective People*, originally published in 1989, Stephen Covey suggests that there is a '**character ethic**' and a '**personality ethic**' that defines individuals in relation to interpersonal and leadership situations. The 'character ethic' includes integrity, humility, patience, industry and justice, to name but a few. The 'personality ethic' differs in that it focuses on public images, attitudes, and skills related to processes of human interaction. Basically, this concept is related to promoting positive imagery and developing and maintaining public relations.

It could be argued that the character ethic is based on '**intrapersonal behaviours**' and the personality ethic on '**interpersonal behaviours**' (Covey, 2013). According to Pendleton and Furnham (2016) it is logical that a leader's personality impacts on those around them which then influences their performance. Covey (2013) suggests that the character ethic is the primary driver in leadership and the personality ethic is secondary to this. Therefore, habits or behaviours that develop the character ethic help to develop both. Covey describes habits as internalized principles and patterns of behaviour. These include:

- **Knowledge** – of what to do and why to do it.
- **Skills** – how to do it.
- **Desire** – wanting to do it.

By utilizing these habits, individuals can move from *dependence* to *independence* to *interdependence* in achieving leadership goals. As discussed in Chapter 2, your transition is likely to take you through a variety of stages, including shock and an ongoing adjustment to different levels of competence requiring you to gain further knowledge and skills and retain the desire to continuously develop. This applies to being a leader too.

ACTIVITY 6.6
---

1 What 'habits' have you noticed in some of the people whom you considered to be leaders in healthcare areas?
2 What behaviours would you class under character ethic and which would you classify under personality ethic?
3 What habits do you feel you have that can be linked to these classifications?

Grossman and Valiga (2016) suggest that leadership skills develop as a result of experiences that form the individual. We can see that this is a move away from traits and personality into behaviours and attitudes. They suggest that true leadership occurs when you can find ways to develop and improve your leadership skills in relation to contextual situations.

A newly qualified RNLD's experience:

When I first qualified as a nurse, I went to work in a registered nursing home for seven adults with learning disabilities and complex needs. Once there, I was often the shift leader and found that most of the challenging issues that I faced were related to managing the shift team. As the only qualified nurse on shift, I had to delegate duties to unqualified staff, many of whom had worked within the home and/or company for several years. I had to overcome a significant age difference in conjunction with my newly qualified status – 'proving my worth' was my most difficult task.

Sheena Hiller

In 'proving her worth', the nurse in the situation above demonstrated her ability to deal with others and get them on her side, demonstrating a move towards interdependence. This is a situation in which most newly qualified nurses find themselves as they transition. Those seen to lead from the front, making confident, efficient decisions that are effectively communicated, will gain the trust of fellow staff members. This requirement is highlighted by the NMC (2018b) when it requires nurses to demonstrate effective interprofessional working while respecting the contributions from all team members.

So far, leadership has been discussed as a range of attributes inherent in the person, as aspects related to character or personality, habits and behaviours. It is now necessary for us to consider aspects related to leadership styles.

Leadership style theory

Murray (2017) suggests leadership styles are related to behaviours and things that leaders do, as opposed to their characteristics. Style theory is different to trait theory, as it proposes that there can be differences in approaches adopted by leaders. Different actions of leadership relate to different styles of leadership.

Marquis and Huston (2012) state that a major contribution to leadership style theory was made by Kurt Lewin, who identified three major styles of leadership: **authoritarian**; **democratic**; and **laissez-faire**.

- **The authoritarian style** is characterized by a downward flow of information, control, coercion, commands, decision-making and giving of rewards or sanctions.
- **The democratic style** is characterized by two-way communication, encouraging the sharing of ideas and decision-making and the use of constructive criticism.
- **The laissez-faire style** allows individuals to be empowered to complete the tasks. The work is delegated and the member is trusted to carry it out successfully. Communication flows up, down and across the members of the team; little direction is given, and criticism is withheld.

Cope and Murray (2017) suggest that these styles reflect whether the leader is **task focused** or attentive to the **relationship** with followers. In a healthcare workplace, there are a range of differing daily situations. Some of these situations need more direction from the leader than others, therefore requiring quick responses or task completion. In health settings where acute situations arise, such as dealing with people with traumatic physiological needs, or perhaps where patients might be displaying aggressive/violent behaviours, you may notice there is a need for powerful direction from the leader. In such situations the authoritarian style of leadership would be recommended as action needs to be taken quickly and efficiently.

Decisions need to be swiftly made and each team member needs to know, or be told, exactly what their roles and responsibilities in the situation are. In such circumstances the team is dependent on the leader for direction. Barr and Dowding (2016) point out that effective communication from the leader is important and the leader exercises power whilst making decisions. There is no room for ambiguity when instructions and directions are being given. There is not enough time for questioning or discussing options, so decisive decision-making is necessary. The communication should be clear and effective. Good communication is also the basis for the other styles.

You might employ a democratic style within nursing when working practices are being reviewed or developments considered. Marquis and Huston (2012) suggest that this style is effective when cooperation and coordination between groups is necessary. It is useful as a method for empowering members of the team and valuing their contribution. However, the democratic style can be less effective than the authoritarian style due to the time it takes to coordinate ideas and opinions. The danger is that some decisions may have to be a compromise to suit all. Here, team members are encouraged to express their own views to the leader for consideration.

The laissez-faire style of leadership requires the person leading to hand over, or delegate, power in the situation to those considered as subordinates or followers. The team is left to manage the situation itself. Tasks are delegated with the confidence that those carrying them out are able to complete them effectively. Basically, it could be argued that this style may be demonstrated when newly qualified nurses are delegated to lead teams in a clinical environment in the absence of more senior staff. This requires trust in the abilities of the person in charge. It is important for you to remember that ultimate accountability should lie with the person who makes the decision to delegate to a junior worker, although the latter will still have their own professional accountability to consider (NMC, 2018c).

The style theory represents two different interpretations of leadership that you may need to consider: **fixed** and **flexible**. The 'fixed' interpretation would align to the trait or behavioural characteristics of the person, suggesting that they always operate in that style. This may or may not be successful. It may also affect their popularity in the team, as it could lead to admiration, antipathy or even fear of the person. They may be effective, but at the cost of their relationship with the team. Alternatively, they could be popular because of their style, but be ineffective as a leader if they do not achieve outcomes.

The alternative 'flexible' interpretation suggests that, as a leader, you should be able to adjust to the circumstances faced and utilize whichever style is recognized as being most effective in that particular kind of situation. This fits a behavioural model and focuses on the adaptability of the person.

ACTIVITY 6.7

Think of some of the people with whom you have experienced working who have been designated or described as leaders. Identify characteristics of those who you believe had leadership styles that were authoritarian, democratic, or laissez-faire.

(Continued)

(Continued)

Identify times and situations that you recognize as requiring the different style(s) to be adopted.

1   Which style do you associate most with yourself?
2   What situations have you been in during your course that demonstrate the necessity of using different styles?

In developing an understanding of style theory, it is important to recognize that the style depends on the interrelationship between several factors, including:

- The person considered to be the leader.
- The individuals considered as followers or subordinate/ teamworkers.
- The purpose or task/outcomes needed.

This is similar to Adair's (2010) notion of the interrelationship between the **task**, the needs of the **individual**, and the needs of the **group**. The leader needs to assess these needs and maintain the balance or development of each (see Figure 6.2.).

According to Pendleton and Furnham (2016) there are some important historical authors with ideas related to style theory. They discuss the work of McGregor who suggested that there are two types of worker who need handling with different approaches from the leader. This is the famous **theory X** and **theory Y**. Basically, theory X represents workers who are unmotivated, mainly due to tasks that are unfulfilling, therefore requiring the leader to be authoritative,

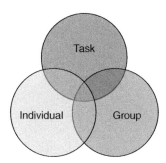

Figure 6.2 Adair's (2010) effective leadership considerations

with a need to provide extrinsic rewards (or punishments) in order to encourage participation. Theory Y represents a workplace in which the workers enjoy going to work and the rewards are intrinsic, therefore requiring less direction and demonstrating independence or interdependence as Covey (2013) outlined. Weiss and Tappen (2015) discuss the concepts of 'concern for production' or 'concern for people', suggesting that both are needed for successful outcomes. Productivity is optimized when both are addressed.

The process of leadership, therefore, can be complex when considering styles. You need to understand the work environment, the outcomes required, and the tasks essential for meeting them. Individuals need to be understood, as well as the dynamics of an effective working group or team. The context is important as you need to be able to adapt styles that fit the situation, ranging from being authoritative to democratic or laissez-faire.

Contingency/situational theory

Building from style theory, contingency theory relates to the application of the styles mentioned above and their deployment in specific situations and contexts. Thompson and Glasø (2015) outline the work of Hershey and Blanchard in developing situational leadership theory. This theory proposes a taxonomy of styles from directing to delegating in order to match specific contexts and situations. Situational leadership arises out of contingency theory which focused on the behavioural styles discussed above such as authoritarian, democratic and laissez-faire. Blanchard (Blanchard and Ken Blanchard Companies, 2010) suggests that those who stick to one style exclusively are only a fraction of the leader they could be, particularly if they take up an extreme position or style. In situational leadership the level of skill of the person(s) being led defines what style should be used. He suggests there are four styles of leader and that these should be utilized to recognize the requirements of the task in hand and the individuals that are being led. The styles are:

- Directing.
- Coaching.
- Supporting.
- Delegating.

Therefore, there is a formula for finding the right style between meeting the supportive needs of the workers and ensuring the task is completed. The qualities of the followers need to be considered along with the level of skill they have plus their level of motivation. Therefore, a balance is needed between support and direction provided by the leader. For example:

- Someone with a high level of motivation and a low level of skill will need directing (bottom right in Table 6.1).
- Someone with a low level of motivation and a low level of skill will need coaching (top right in Table 6.1).
- Someone with low level of motivation and a high level of skill will need supporting (top left in Table 6.1).
- Someone with a high level of motivation and a high level of skill will need delegating to (bottom left in Table 6.1).

The key point is that your leadership style should be flexibly adapted to meet the needs of the individual and the situation faced. These styles can also be applied in the completion of a task/skill or new project. In the early stages, there will need to be clear direction from the leader. This is followed by a period of coaching during which the skills of others are developed. The stage of supporting is then applied in terms of ensuring resources and skills are maintained. Finally, when the leader is confident that everything is in place, the followers can be entrusted to make independent decisions based on their level of skill and therefore have tasks or duties delegated to them. Delegation

Table 6.1 Situational leadership (Blanchard and Ken Blanchard Companies, 2010)

	Low direction	High direction
High support	*Follower behaviour*	*Follower behaviour*
	Low level of motivation High level of skill	Low level of motivation Low level of skill
	Leader style	*Leader style*
	Supporting	Coaching
Low support	*Follower behaviour*	*Follower behaviour*
	High level of motivation High level of skill	High level of motivation Low level of skill
	Leader style	*Leader style*
	Delegating	Directing

is highlighted by the NMC (2018b) as a required standard of proficiency, so it is important to be aware of the right kind of situations in which to do so.

ACTIVITY 6.8

Think of a responsibility that you have had to undertake as part of a team at some point. Identify the stages of the task at which the behaviours of directing, coaching, supporting and delegating were applied.

1   What strategy (directing, coaching, supporting, delegating) did the leader employ at these stages?
2   What worked well at each stage?

You may have been involved in developing a new method of reporting in the workplace or implementing a specific plan of care for a client which needed to be communicated to the care staff to ensure its success, or you may have been involved in introducing and learning how to use a new piece of equipment. A shift leader often finds themselves making decisions about delegation of duties as it is impossible to carry out all duties associated with successfully managing a shift alone. Therefore, the notion of situational leadership is particularly important – especially depending on the skill levels of the supporting staff on a given shift. Some days there might need to be more direction, others will require more delegating.

When delegation is used, you may have to relinquish some control to more junior staff, yet you may then need to focus on other developments, such as the support or coaching of other staff and the completion of further tasks.

In answering the above question, it may be useful to think of it in terms of time and responsibility. Some aspects will be urgent, which need dealing with, and others, although important, may not be quite as pressing, but will still need to be dealt with in the long run.

Contemporary theories of leadership

Transactional and transformational leadership theory

According to Marquis and Huston (2012), the transactional leader concentrates on 'day-to-day' operations and is closely associated with the role of the manager. Transformational leadership is about empowerment, inspiring the workforce, and acting as a positive role model – perhaps almost like the coach in situational leadership.

Wong and Giallonardo (2015) outline the basic components of transactional and transformational leadership:

- **Transactional.**
  The leader's behaviour depends upon reciprocal transactions with followers aimed at achieving task completion, with rewards being contingent upon performance.

- **Transformational.**
  o   Idealized influence.
      This aspect is related to the 'charisma' of the leader and the influencing factors that this brings in terms of admiration and respect from followers.

  o   Inspirational motivation.
      This relates to how the leader models desired behaviours, therefore creating meaning and challenges for the followers.

  o   Intellectual stimulation.
      This relates to how the leader engages the followers to be creative, and problem-solves in relation to the challenges presented in the workforce.

  o   Individualized consideration.
      This relates to the ability of the leader to identify and show concern for the development of individual members of the team.

ACTIVITY 6.9

Having read these factors, consider the situation below.

A nurse has just completed a consecutive run of five night shifts. Arriving on duty, the shift leader finds that the nurse has made a medication error, which fortunately has not resulted in any harm to a patient. Consider this in light of what transactional and transformational leadership responses would look like.

In a transactional leadership approach, the perception might be that this is a crisis situation and that the nurse needs some remedial intervention or sanction. Alternatively, a transformational leader would listen to the nurse and ascertain any developmental needs and education or skill development that they may need, then take steps to ensure that the nurse is supported with these.

Wong and Giallonardo (2015) suggest that transformational leadership creates healthy work environments based on support and genuine open and honest communication. A transformational leader will develop meaningful dialogue with others in order to resolve workplace issues and improve patient care. Look at the situation below.

Have you seen examples of this in practice settings?

Statement from a registered nurse

A recurring issue in my workplace is debate about the duty rota. The manager permitted flexibility, so staff would often swap shifts (sometimes without the agreement of the person being swapped). As a shift leader I sometimes had to negotiate these arrangements between staff members.

As mentioned above, as a transactional leader you might make a unilateral decision and state that person A or person B must do the shift. This might be a necessary tactic if all else fails. However, transformational leadership requires that you as a leader are empowering, fair, and that you consider individual needs. Therefore, it is necessary to gather the facts. In doing so, a mediator role can be adopted by the nurse in charge. The best result would be that as a leader you then present the facts as they stand, and check that all parties understand and agree that this is a fair appraisal of the situation.

However, as a leader you may also need to explain the constraints and provide boundaries on what must be achieved and by when. In doing this, the followers may find a solution themselves, thus transforming the working environment. The leader can still make the final decision (transactional leadership) if there is no satisfactory result, yet by taking a transformational approach, this should lead to decisions that eventually are advantageous for all.

Magnusson et al. (2017) identified issues for newly qualified nurses in delegation and decision-making. The newly qualified nurses demonstrated a number of approaches such as: 'doing the job themselves' to avoid delegation and conflict; 'justifying the decision' (defending their position); acting as a 'buddy' (leading to seniority not being recognized); acting as a 'role model' (demonstrating behaviours but not clearly delegating tasks); and acting as 'Inspector' (this ensured tasks were completed but did not save time due to constant checks of the tasks. Therefore, gaining trust while leading the workforce can be a delicate balance and quite a challenge. This is applicable to newly qualified nurses from all fields of practice. Allan et al. (2015) highlight that delegation and decision-making are important aspects affecting the newly qualified nurse's transition and that through support mechanisms and structured preceptorship the skills learned can be applied.

Management is a different concept from leadership as it mainly relates to the role or position that is ascribed to a person. Pidgeon (2017) suggests they are inherently separate concepts with leadership focusing on people, motivation, influence, achievement and facilitation, and management focusing on tasks, directing and controlling, demanding results and being involved in the work. Therefore, not all leaders are managers, but managers can benefit from developing leadership skills in order to focus on both the hearts and minds of their workers.

Therefore, these aspects can be considered in respect to a care environment in which nurses might be part of the workforce. What roles do staff have that require a leadership element? Think of roles of staff from lower bandings to those with higher bandings. In the NHS, a newly qualified nurse is likely to be at band 5, so may have some supervisory, planning, and organizing responsibility for those from lower bands and students.

─────────────────────── **ACTIVITY 6.10** ───────────────────────

Seek out the job descriptions from your organization or one you would like to work in and look at the expectations and responsibilities from senior nursing positions and those below it. Make a note of the requirements that relate to having responsibility for the supervision and management of those on lower scales.
   What kinds of decisions are made at each level?

───

An example may be that a support worker may have to make very small decisions in providing care to individuals while following prescribed plans of care. These may also need to be communicated to a shift leader. A shift leader may have to decide which staff to delegate certain duties to and decide which tasks gain priority. They also need to be able to report to senior staff about day-to-day issues affecting the running of the care environment, thereby contributing to larger-scale change processes.

The senior staff may not have many direct care responsibilities (although in some smaller units this may be unavoidable), but they need to maintain the integrity of the service and have wider responsibilities, including budgeting/finance, the service users or patients, staff environment and others involved. They will have to report these aspects at an organizational level. Therefore, it can be seen that, at all levels, the leader has to make specific decisions while providing broader information in an upwards direction from which more senior staff can make decisions about the level below.

Weiss and Tappen (2015), suggest that as a leader you should set priorities, think critically, solve problems, respect and value individuals, communicate skilfully, communicate future vision, and develop self and others. Barr and Dowding (2016: 8) break this down into three main approaches:

1   Set direction (mission, goals, vision and purpose).
2   Build commitment (motivation, spirit and teamwork).
3   Confront challenges (innovation, change and turbulence).

We would suggest therefore, in accommodating the theories already discussed, that the key elements in leadership in creating small-level or grand-level change are:

- Knowing where you want to go (goal/outcome).
- Deciding when and how you are going to get there (strategy formulation).
- Communicating this vision to others (communication).
- Filling others with enthusiasm for this vision (motivation).
- Causing the first steps to happen/take the first steps (action).

To see how these aspects can be applied to a broader situation, let us return to Activity 6.2, in which you take a call informing you that the senior nurse will not be turning up for the late shift, and consider what you need to do.

Goal/outcome

The goal is clear: the care area needs to be run in such a way that minimum standards are met, all individuals in the environment are safe, and optimum achievement occurs within the constraints given. You now have the perfect opportunity to demonstrate your leadership skills and to demonstrate your ability to solve the problem in the fairest way possible. You will no doubt have a strong internal desire to ensure that your first experience of leadership is successful.

Strategy

You now need to assess the practicalities of what needs to happen and decide on what would constitute a successful shift. One of the very early decisions needing to be made is whether, and how, a replacement should be sought for the one missing member of the team. It may be that, in considering the tasks, the workload could be shared among the remaining staff. You may volunteer to provide cover for a short while until you (or someone senior) can organize someone else. You may have some identified people who can be contacted in such circumstances; there might be staff in nearby services who perhaps could be spared or moved, or you may need to contact outside agencies. In contacting senior staff, it is sometimes best to have either completed these actions first, or if you need permission for further action (such as being allowed to provide overtime), to let them know of your intended actions and that you seek their approval.

Communication

All members of your team need to be made aware of the situation in the swiftest way possible and made aware of what you propose to do as a result. You will be able to gauge their concerns from their verbal and non-verbal responses. Remember the staff nurse who felt that she had to prove her worth to junior staff? In such a situation there is an expectation from junior staff for swift action. There is also a need to communicate with senior staff. However, this may need to be carefully judged. If there are actions that you can take to remedy the situation and report your actions to them rather than pass the problem directly to them without any thought or action, this will be much better received.

Motivation

Having listened to the concerns, you are now in a position to propose what you would like to do, giving your reasons and linking these to the concerns and reasons given by the other staff. Any perceived obstacles to achieving the vision need to be identified and, if possible, removed at this point. You need to consider how you can maintain the morale of the staff in what could obviously be considered a negative situation in which some or all staff may have to do extra work.

Action

It is important that you do something, even something that may be a small action but which represents for others that you have been decisive and that you are working to resolve the situation. This could simply be to begin the communication process to attempt to replace the missing staff member. In the end, it does not matter if you succeed in this initial action; what is important is that you do something that all those involved regard as being important. Finally, you need to record your actions and decisions.

Arnold and Underman Boggs (2016) highlight some aspects involved in decision-making.

- Identify the significant problem.
- Clarify the concepts.
- Integrate data and identify any missing data.
- Generate options and alternatives.
- Evaluate and take action.

By seeking alternatives, you may be able to offer solutions with which the other people involved will agree. Agreement should be brokered using this technique by finding out how your proposal or action can be attractive to the followers, either by generalizing or specifying what is required.

You will be more successful in motivating the others if you make them aware that you are seeking beneficial outcomes for patients. The other staff members are likely to care very little about whether or not you succeed, but they certainly will want to feel that they have succeeded in their own right. Knowing that you and they are working towards the same end goal is a real motivating factor. Remember – if you do not know what to do, you can always ask the question: 'Who could help me find out what to do?' It is important to note, however, that whatever actions you take must align with your employer's policies and procedures.

Authentic leadership

According to Fallatah and Laschinger (2016), authentic leadership is a relatively recent theory of leadership which is becoming more applicable in healthcare settings. It is based on ethical, transparent and open approaches with followers. It focuses on four main aspects of self-awareness, balanced processing, relational transparency and internalized moral perspective. Ibarra (2018) suggests authenticity is the gold standard for leadership and relies on the leader being true to themselves, maintaining coherence between what they feel and what they say or do, and making values-based choices. It is important to be aware of this in joining a workplace and being in charge as first impressions are quickly formed and can affect perceptions and performance. Ekström and Idvall (2015) point out that newly qualified nurses need the guidance of an authentic leader during their transition in their role.

Bamford et al. (2013) highlight that authentic leadership is crucial to retaining nurses within the workforce and delivering high-quality care. By demonstrating self-awareness and trueness to self, combined with an ethical approach, the authentic leader builds respect, credibility and trust amongst followers. This requires a certain amount of visibility, being prepared to demonstrate that you are competent in the workplace, and that you understand the context and complexities that occur within it. Basically, being able to 'walk the walk' as well as 'talk the walk'. The approach suggests placing the right person in the right job, which results in increased work engagement and outcomes as the person, the job and the values are aligned. Figure 6.3 shows some basic attributes in authentic leadership.

Kramer and Crespy (2011) highlight that leadership functions can be shared amongst group members. This suggests that legitimacy and position are not necessarily prescribed for, or placed within a leader, but change in relation to who is best placed in terms of talent and approach in response to the specific situation. Kramer and Crespy (2011) suggest that authentic leaders will empower groups with authority and responsibility to make decisions often resulting in enhanced performance.

Alexander and Lopez (2018) found that authentic leadership is an important factor in providing healthy working environments.

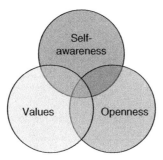

Figure 6.3 Authentic leadership

Dirik and Seren Intepeler (2017) suggest that authentic leadership improves patient safety. By having an open communication system and network, bridges can be built between senior managers/leaders and the personnel on the ground. However, Ekström and Idvall (2015) point out that newly qualified nurses can find their leadership role challenging if their responsibilities are vague, the mandate is not clear and there is insufficient support. These need to be addressed for newly qualified nurses' leadership abilities to be developed. According to Laschinger et al. (2015), evidence suggests positive relationships between authentic leadership and increased performance, trust, job satisfaction, patient safety, work engagement and lower ratings of burnout.

Rao (2013) also suggests another term of 'soft leadership' which is built around several characteristics encompassing the notion of partnership with the people involved in whatever the task or organizational goal is. It relates to the ability of the leader to empower the partners and allow them to make mistakes.

George et al. (2018) suggest the following is needed to become an authentic leader:

- Learn from your life story.
- Knowing your authentic self.
- Practising your values and principles.
- Balancing your extrinsic and intrinsic motivations.
- Building your support team.
- Staying grounded.
- Empowering others.

―――――――――――――――――――― **ACTIVITY 6.11** ――――――――――――――――――――

Reflect on your experiences in clinical settings.

1 How did those in charge demonstrate 'authentic leadership'?
2 How could you recognize their self-awareness, their values and their openness?
3 What kinds of outcomes did you notice for yourself, other staff and patients?

Clinical leadership

This aspect of leadership is an approach that is about specialization in specific areas of healthcare. Barr and Dowding (2016) suggest it focuses on facilitating evidence-based practice and improving patient outcomes. They propose that it is required to respond to the health demands of society for the future. The NMC (2018b) requires nurses to be proficient in promoting health and well-being. The clinical leadership aspect revolves around the client/service user and their specific needs by focusing on antecedents, attributes and consequences of certain health issues within populations (Barr and Dowding, 2016).

Mannix et al. (2013) state that clinical leadership is important in ensuring quality patient care, and creating healthy working environments and job satisfaction. Their study suggests that clinical leaders need to demonstrate clinically competent technical and practical skills, high-level communication skills and being supportive of colleagues to create healthy working environments.

Marquis and Huston (2012) outline that a clinical nurse leader should use evidence-based practice at the point of care in services, seeking quality improvements and managing microsystems of care for individuals and families. Therefore, a clinical leader may not be directly managing or leading specific staff teams but may need to advise and prescribe care approaches that should then be implemented by the teams involved. It is therefore not deemed an administrative role; rather they are accountable for the care approach provided and must design, implement and evaluate care whilst coordinating, delegating and supervising that care.

Chávez and Yoder (2015) suggest that the term clinical leadership is related to separating the leadership of clinicians at the bedside from those in organizational administrative positions. In order to develop this, they need to attain leadership status and maintain it. As a clinical leader you would achieve this through demonstrating clinical ability, effective communication and coordinating skills, innovation and change management, and the ability to become an integrated member of the healthcare team.

Both clinical leadership roles and management/leadership roles are available to all qualified nurses in their careers. Ailey et al. (2015) suggest that technological and supportive investment is needed to empower nurses to demonstrate such leadership skills in order to improve healthcare outcomes. There are different ways in which you can exploit these opportunities. Pepin et al. (2011) suggest that there are different levels of leadership for a nurse wishing to be a clinical leader to aspire to:

- Awareness of clinical leadership.
- Integration of clinical leadership in action.
- Leadership with patients, families and colleagues.

However future healthcare systems and the nursing profession may be organized, there will always be a requirement for nurses to demonstrate leadership skills at all levels within it to create small-scale and large-scale changes that impact on the care of individuals. As mentioned earlier, although leadership and management can be considered different concepts, they are inextricably linked, and the theories do overlap.

It is now important to focus on some theories of management.

Theories of management

Heizer and Render (2014: 43) suggest that the management process consists of:

- Planning.
- Organizing.
- Staffing.
- Leading.
- Controlling.

This process derives from classical management theory studied by scholars such as Fayol and Taylor where research into industrial organizations was first conducted. Marquis and Huston (2012) suggest that these scientific management theories have changed little over time and are still recognized in healthcare management today. Management requires a different set of skills and attitudes to leadership, although there is some overlap. The added dimension is the fact that responsibility for the effective functioning of the healthcare setting (and, at higher levels, the organization) lies with the manager. Marquis and Huston (2012) highlight how the human relations theory of management evolved where management began to focus on people and their motivation/satisfaction, such as the task versus relations debate mentioned in the previous section. Wood et al. (2016) describe a manager as being a person responsible for the completion of work in an organization accomplished through the performance of one or more people. Therefore, they aim for two key aspects: task performance and human resource maintenance.

Mullins and Christy (2016) argue that management is a great responsibility as it requires making sure things happen through processes, systems and management styles. Attention must be paid to the work environment, systems of motivation, developing job satisfaction and rewards/sanctions. They suggest that it pervades all aspects of an organization and is related to achieving the goals and objectives of the organization whilst ensuring the satisfaction and expectation needs of the employees. Therefore, it is a process common to all functional aspects in an organization. Moore et al. (2017) point out that as managers have responsibility for both human and capital resources, they are vital to the success of healthcare organizations. Deyo et al. (2017) suggest a nurse manager should have the following competencies:

- **Communication and relationship building.**
  - The manager is a figurehead and organizational representative, needing to lead staff and liaise with external parties. They need to be able to influence others.
- **Knowledge of the healthcare environment.**
  - The manager needs to organize the work design, measure and monitor outcomes from this and provide metrics for performance.
- **Leadership.**
  - The manager creates the vision and strategy for change, whilst evaluating ideas, objections and viewpoints.

- **Professionalism.**
  - The manager needs to demonstrate advocacy for patients, staff and the organization.
- **Business Skills.**
  - The manager needs to be involved in strategic planning, ensuring effective use of resources and maintaining financial stability through appropriate budgeting.

———————————————— **ACTIVITY 6.12** ————————————————

Duties and responsibilities

The above principles can broadly be translated as managing *tasks, clients and relatives, staff* and *resources*. Think of an average shift you may have experienced in an acute setting, a community residential or care home, or as part of a community team, and then make a list of the types of duties or responsibilities with which you would generally need to deal if in charge, under the headings of:

- Tasks.
- Clients.
- Staff.
- Resources.

Even though it may be a few years before you consider managerial positions or aspects in your career, it is always beneficial to understand the principles involved and to be aware of the contributions that you can make.

As mentioned above, one of the first roles of the manager is in planning. There are two main types of planning: strategic and operational. Strategic planning leads to the development and implementation of the vision, mission and objectives of the organization. Operations management is related to how the objectives are operationalized and managed at the ground level.

Strategic management

David and David (2015: 39) state that strategic management is:

> The art and science of formulating, implementing and evaluating cross-functional decisions that enable an organization to achieve its objectives.

They highlight that strategic management consists of three stages:

- Strategy formulation.
- Strategy implementation.
- Strategy evaluation.

The formulation stage requires the development of a vision and mission, identifying strengths, weaknesses, opportunity and threats (often known as a SWOT analysis), establishing long-term strategic goals and generating strategic approaches to follow. Strategy implementation is the action stage where resources and personnel are mobilized to address the strategic priorities. Strategy evaluation is the stage of review where the progress of the strategy and the objectives of the organization are checked (David and David, 2015). Note how this is very similar to the nursing process of assess, plan, implement and evaluate. The main difference is the level at which it is implemented. You might use the nursing process with a patient, yet as a manager this process occurs across the whole of the organization, and must be communicated to each unit or section of the organization and the workforce.

ACTIVITY 6.13

Workplace mission statement

In your current workplace, seek out the current vision, mission statement, philosophy and objectives.

1   How are they written?
2   How realistic do you think they are?
3   Do they become realized in the work you are involved in on the ground?
4   What is the reporting mechanism for you to provide feedback on the strategy?

You may find as a qualified nurse that you have to rise up the career ladder before being able to make fundamental decisions about the nature of the organization for which you work, but you can have a direct influence on the culture of the organization by the ways in which you perform your duties and act as a role model. Gallo (2007) suggested a development ladder of four stages that a nurse may go through once qualified (Figure 6.4). As a newly qualified nurse, the main area of your influence is likely to be at stage 1 or 2. However, with adequate training, expertise and experience, the other steps can be achieved. Doria (2015) argues that promotion to a leadership position such as charge nurse usually depends on demonstrating clinical proficiency and role modelling. However, management brings with it many challenges as it requires constant reprioritization of competing tasks.

By gaining a promotion your contribution is also important in at least informing the strategy: by highlighting what those necessary changes need to be on the front line and how current initiatives are currently operating. You may be nervous as a newly qualified nurse, but your opinions, if expressed appropriately, may still have some weight. Some areas appreciate the benefits that a fresh pair of eyes can bring. Indeed, having just completed three years of education in a

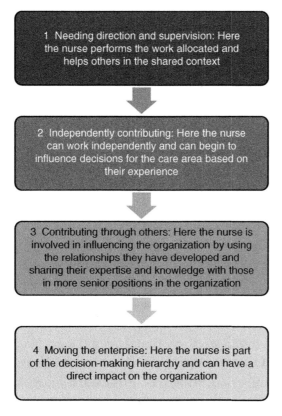

Figure 6.4 Four stages through which a nurse may go once qualified

Reprinted from Gallo 2007, 'The new nurse manager: A leadership development program paves the road to success', *Nurse Leader*, 5(4): 3, with kind permission from Elsevier

variety of settings, you may have the advantage of experiencing some useful approaches and initiatives that may not have been thought of by the staff in your current work or clinical placement. By sharing these, you can have an impact and contribute to the strategic development of the organization.

Daly et al. (2015) suggest that to demonstrate good strategic management the nurse needs to be able to understand organizational challenges, including climate and culture. They need to be able to plan strategically for change. They need highly effective communication skills, particularly in negotiation and conflict resolution. And finally, they must have an ability to influence others and gain support for meeting objectives. Here, you should be able to spot that the nursing process they use in caring for their patients (assess, plan, implement, evaluate) could be applied to strategic thinking in the work environment. In Egan's (2014) major work, *The Skilled Helper*, he suggests that there is a need to identify the 'What's going on?' (present state), 'What do I need or want?' (desired state) and the 'Way forward' (resources required) to get to the position of setting and meeting outcomes. This is another example of strategic thinking if applied to the work environment.

Operations management

This aspect is related to the day-to-day running of services, with the focus being on ensuring that satisfaction of the stakeholders is achieved by delivery of a quality service. Barr and Dowding (2016) describe it as issues around the service's clinical and operational performance (such as managing capacity and quality derived from its policies). It is about turning the organizational strategy into action at the point of delivery. However, the important aspects of operations management are keeping the client as the central focus and utilizing the best evidence to create, deliver and monitor efficient and valued care. Barr and Dowding (2016) point out that quality is basically being **effective** and **efficient**. So, for a qualified nurse delivering care, this means you need to ensure that the care provided is to the highest possible standard, using resources in an efficient, cost-effective manner.

As a qualified nurse you will be the interface between the organization, service and the clients. As well as having technical competence, you will need to understand the importance of communication with patients, junior staff, other professionals and senior staff within the organization. Stevens et al. (2017) highlight how the failure of operations management can impact on services and organizations. They suggest that nurses on the frontline are crucial in providing information related to areas that need attention. These failures are often within the processes and systems designed for accessing equipment and resources, liaising with other multidisciplinary team members and the time taken to solve these issues. Communication is the key to all of this, including ensuring effective use of information technology.

Communication needs to operate in both upward and downward exchanges. In most cases, it is obvious that patients/service users need to have their needs met. You need to communicate effectively to let service users know the steps that will be taken in moving towards the goal to be achieved (as nothing can ever be fully guaranteed). This means highlighting what is realistic in the situation. In discussions with your senior managers, you need to inform them of the situation as it is at ground level, to request the appropriate resources and support needed to ensure optimum care delivery. Doria (2015) supports the notion that communication is a key factor in becoming a manager. In terms of operations management there may need to be difficult conversations held with some people. Networking and collaboration is crucial in ensuring services are delivered effectively.

Organizational structural management

Marquis and Huston (2012) suggest that within an organization there are formal and informal structures. These are used for methods of communication, channels of authority and decision-making processes. It is about how rules, processes and procedures are decided on in the organization and how these are communicated throughout the workforce. It is about the division of labour and how this is managed. Formal structures are related to highly planned, controlled visible work structures. The informal structures are hidden and often unplanned, being based on relationships rather than across lines of authority.

As a newly qualified nurse, you might not be involved in the large-scale decision-making and organizing of the structural aspects of the service in which you work, but you will be involved in aspects on a micro level, such as being in charge of a team in the day-to-day running of the care area. In this role, you may have to decide on how workload and tasks are distributed among the staff team. These decisions may have to be taken on the actual day once all staff are assembled and the duties required are recognized, or it may be that there needs to be more mid- and longer-term planning in which you may become involved, such as the allocation of responsibilities.

An effective healthcare provider will need efficient communication systems at all levels. Marx (2014) argues that nurse managers have to ensure effective communication occurs in the working environment in relation to the organization's goals. A nurse manager needs to convey the philosophies, strategy and directives from senior management, whilst maintaining supportive relationships with the nurses regularly working directly with patients. This requires dialogue, listening, and answering questions. The communication structure can be affected by the hierarchy in the organization, by workload distribution, cultural and environmental factors. Stein-Parbury (2018) suggests that communication is at the heart of quality patient care. She suggests that organizational characteristics that promote communication channels increase job satisfaction and ultimately the quality of patient care. In a work environment this means recognizing autonomy, creating control over nursing practices, collaboration with other professionals and effective written communication. If you are in charge of a shift or a work area, you need to communicate with the team under your supervision. This means that there is a need for a visible style of management to foster open communication, without being oppressive and reducing the **autonomy** of trusted workers where relevant.

Barr and Dowding (2016) argue that a number of activities must be achieved in being a leader or manager. So, if you are in charge you need to be aware of:

* Setting and achieving of goals for the day.
* Communicating the goals to the team.
* Defining the tasks required.
* Planning the work.
* Bargaining for and mobilizing resources.
* Delegating the work and responsibilities.
* Monitoring the performance and reviewing progress.

------------------------------- **ACTIVITY 6.14** -------------------------------

Imagine that you are responsible for a group of six clients in a community nursing home. These are divided into separate areas in two groups of three. You are allocated one support worker to assist you.

1   What steps could you consider demonstrating for effective communication and addressing the factors listed above?

In the above scenario, you would have to provide the support worker with discrete instructions on what tasks are required, with which group of clients, and delegate some of these to them. You then need a mechanism for them to report back to you. You might seek their opinion on some approaches but will still need to make appropriate decisions. You may organize some times when you are able to observe them in order to provide support and assistance where necessary. Most important is the notion that the support worker can access you if needed.

Another factor that impacts on structural management is the large-scale introduction of information technologies in healthcare environments as a way of improving communication systems to improve teamwork. Bichel-Findlay and Doran (2015) suggest that it is difficult to create any transformation in healthcare delivery without sufficiently advanced technologies and a culture that supports it. They discuss the use of health informatics, which is a science and practice around health information that makes data and information available to the healthcare delivery team in a prompt and accessible manner. However, this does change the role of the nurse somewhat in ensuring that the information system is used correctly and that it serves the patient, as well as the wider team and organization. Nurses are often the greatest users of health informatics technology across multidisciplinary teams (Bichel-Findlay and Doran, 2015).

In this case, training in the use of such technologies is important for you, and the supervision of others while under your management becomes a crucial role. It is important therefore that you use the hierarchical structures to ensure that information about the effectiveness of such systems is communicated to senior management personnel.

ACTIVITY 6.15

Think of the practice settings in which you have been involved.

1   What types of technological equipment and approaches did you experience?
2   What were the benefits and disadvantages of these?
3   Is there another technology that you use (such as a mobile phone with various applications) that you think would be useful in the workplace?
4   How do you think you could introduce this to a working environment?

Human resources (HR) management

Organizations providing healthcare employ a wide range of individuals within the teams in their healthcare settings. Having the appropriate skills and knowledge to carry out the organization's goals is critical. Townsend et al. (2015) state that ward or service managers have a responsibility for delivering the goals of the organization and in doing so managing the employees within their area. They are the lynchpin in providing an effective working environment. Usually, HR management is deemed to be an organization-wide role, but managers at all levels make HR decisions about the workforce that reports to them. Truss et al. (2012) highlight several functions of human resource management (usually situated within the human resources department, but also to be enacted by managers at all levels). These functions include administrative aspects related to employees, being a champion for employees, acting as a change agent and being involved in the strategy or the organization or service. As a newly qualified nurse, this might appear daunting and outside your remit. However, you will be responsible for making or communicating decisions that may affect junior staff, whilst maintaining approaches that are relevant to meeting the goals of the organization. These may include decisions related to development and change, reducing costs, and maintaining standards and quality. You may be involved in some of the tasks of human resource management such as orientating new staff, training them and appraising their performance.

To have good HR management, certain considerations need to be borne in mind. According to Barr and Dowding (2016), these are:

- Workforce planning.
- Recruitment and selection of appropriate staff.

- Induction, training and development.
- Performance management and appraisal.
- Employer well-being and support.
- Outsourcing.

ACTIVITY 6.16

To understand the above processes, it might be useful for you to consider them from your own experiences. Therefore, reflect for a few moments, then write a list of aspects that you have experienced or would expect in your own employment in relation to the above bullet points. For example:

1 What were the recruitment processes?
2 How were you inducted and how were your developmental needs identified?
3 How has your performance been appraised?

Therefore, if, as a staff nurse, you are required to carry out specific tasks, you may need to alert senior staff to the amount and skill mix of staff needed to carry out such tasks. You may be required to train, teach, and educate others in the work environment. There will also be times when you need to alert staff to any deficiencies in their work (while remembering that it is also important to alert them to the positive aspects of their work).

Duty rotas

One of the aspects you may need to deal with as you progress in your role is the organization or, more realistically, the reorganization of a duty rota. It is usually the responsibility of more senior staff to provide the rota for the service area. Marquis and Huston (2012) argue that the manager should ensure minimum staffing levels and skill mix for each shift to meet patient and organizational goals. This is sometimes a decentralized process with the manager having more control over a discrete team of staff, or a centralized process where the rostering is viewed organization-wide. If you find yourself having to create a nursing roster you will discover that this includes managing annual leave, study leave and the involvement of agency staff where necessary. In relation to annual leave and study leave, these should have been agreed and planned as far in advance as possible, so should be recorded on the rota in the first instance. These are usually placed in a diary or request book and agreed by the manager of the service. This then needs to be followed by ensuring there is adequate senior or qualified cover as necessary and stated by the care manager in line with policy. Next, the numbers and skill mix of staff need to be met within the rota.

However, day-to-day occurrences happen such as sickness, or a sudden request for a change of shift, or changes in work demands, which may require the rota to be amended. Such amendments may have to be made by you if you oversee the shift or if a manager delegates the task to you. If you are involved in developing or amending the rota, it is important to be as fair as possible in ensuring equality in shifts, meeting the needs of staff with family commitments and meeting requests of staff. Remember, if staff feel that they have been provided with a favour that suits them, then they should also be willing to return the favour at some point. What should not happen is that some people always get favourable shifts at the expense of others, without thorough negotiation. Staff who have been provided with favours in having their requests accepted should recognize that this will not always be the case and that they are expected to work the shifts prescribed to them within reason. In the authors' experience, completing a rota can appear to be an easy task on paper, but remember that we are dealing with people and that your decisions will need to be communicated clearly. The ability to show flexibility while meeting the requirements of the service is paramount.

Marquis and Huston (2012) highlight that staff shortages can occur on a day-to-day basis. The range of ways to deal with this are usually already decided at managerial level, but may include closed unit staffing, where staff from an area not on shift are contacted to cover. This is usually agreed by all the team as a recognized approach. There may also be some scope for providing overtime. If this is necessary, it may be appropriate for you to contact the budget-holder before making any decisions to allow this. There is also the option of contacting agency or pool/bank staff to cover and, again, you may need to alert the budget-holder before sanctioning this. The important thing is to act as soon as the staff shortage/difficulty becomes apparent.

Management and supervision

The infrastructure and its rules have been set in place and it is now important that the workforce adheres to these in order to meet the strategic vision of the organization.

Systems of audit and discipline and reward need to be put into place and utilized by the workforce. Marquis and Huston (2012) suggest that performance appraisal is an important managerial role. This requires that the person identified as manager objectively collect data through a formalized system, maintain the appropriate documentation, set goals and action plans, and establish mechanisms for review and feedback. Further management roles and functions relate to health and safety, risk management, and policy development. It is about resolving unsatisfactory situations within the work environment, problem-solving and decision-making.

Within this aspect of management, there might arise issues related to power and authority. This can occur due to a number of factors across physical, psychological, sociological, political and emotional domains. These include factors such as age, gender, position experience and skill. As a newly qualified nurse with responsibilities on a day-to-day basis for management of care areas, be that in hospital wards, clinics, residential and care homes, or as visiting community nurses, these aspects need to be addressed. Marquis and Huston (2012) suggest that although power usually comes with the position or status of the employee – in this case, the nurse – it can be gained by utilizing several skills, including:

- Maintaining energy.
- Demonstrating a positive professional persona in all situations.
- Working hard and being seen to be doing so.
- Knowing when to ask for help and from whom.
- Understanding the culture of the organization.
- Continually developing skills and expertise.
- Maintaining a broad vision.
- Being flexible.
- Demonstrating assertiveness (while avoiding aggressive and bullying tones).
- Having a sense of humour.
- Ensuring others are empowered.

Dealing with complaints

As well as having to deal with staff being late, other professionals and delegating workloads, other aspects with which a newly qualified staff nurse must regularly contend include dealing with complaints or conflicts with staff. Oxtoby (2015) highlights how complaints are an important reminder that the patient is central to your working practice. In dealing with complaints you need to understand what practice, standards and guidance are being followed and what the procedures are for handling complaints arising from deviation from this.

To address such issues, focusing on people, being positive, and being professional are important. This means that you should be able to be aware of others, find solutions, and stay loyal to the core values of the profession and employers. All care services have a complaints procedure that states exactly the steps that should be taken. Gage (2016) argues that most patients and relatives do not want to make formal complaints. It is much better for issues to be resolved locally in a fast and effective manner and nurses are in the front line for this role.

The most important aspect is communication. Relatives may make a complaint because they believe that their loved one is not receiving the level of service that they would expect. Whether the complaint is valid or not, it does need to be seen to be dealt with. You may need to explain the circumstances of the situation, because an explanation may suffice in helping the relative to understand why certain things are happening. You should alert them to the procedure for dealing with complaints if they wish to continue their claim. The formal procedure may need to be invoked if your explanation does not satisfy their concern. It may be necessary to alert your immediate line manager or senior staff of the complaint and it most definitely needs to be recorded.

Oxtoby (2015) highlights that resolution should include remedial action such as an apology, a financial remedy, plans to ensure mistakes are not repeated, staff training and changes to policy and procedures. Most of these will be a result of going through a formal complaints procedure.

Dealing with conflict

You should be able to coach and influence, give constructive feedback, deal with conflict and motivate others. Dealing with staff conflict may be a regular aspect of your role as a qualified nurse. This may be as simple as staff disagreeing with you or each other, or the wider members of the interdisciplinary team. The main thing is that this is dealt with quickly and professionally. A golden rule, which has been stressed in this chapter throughout, is to not ask staff to do something that you would not be prepared to do yourself or might have done yourself at some time. Speedy (2015) points out four levels on which conflict can occur:

- Intrapersonal (conflict within the individual).
- Interpersonal (individual-to-individual conflict).
- Intergroup conflict.
- Inter-organizational conflict.

Arnold and Underman Boggs (2016) remind us that the priority in conflict resolution is to maximize service users' health in a safe manner. Clear communication is a priority in such circumstances. They highlight principles that need to be addressed in conflict management. You need to understand your own personal response to conflict, and you need to know the context and develop an effective conflict management style.

The aim is to create a state of negotiation to resolve the problem. First, it is vital that such conflicts should not take place in front of patients, relatives or others. The parties should be politely asked to move to a private area in the work area. Arnold and Underman Boggs (2016) suggest the following steps:

- Identify the conflict/issue; acknowledge whether or not you have the capacity to resolve the issue.
- Know your response to conflict; take responsibility for your response.
- Separate the issue from the people involved; use a no-blame approach.
- Stay focused on the issue; clarify the situation including antecedents, situation and consequences.
- Identify options; be prepared to listen to others' alternative solutions.
- Negotiate and agree a solution.
- Summarize.

From these strategies it is clear that you need the parties to clearly agree, clearly disagree, or clearly agree to differ (as long as the difference is clearly identified). You may have to assertively request that they put differences aside and continue in meeting the service goals in order to provide safe, secure care for patients/service users. You may have to separate them or reassign tasks. It cannot be stressed enough that clarity of goals and their communication are of the utmost importance.

Acting quickly is something that junior staff will associate with you and a way in which you can start developing respect as a leader in their eyes. If these informal mechanisms are unsuccessful, then you may need to refer to senior staff.

Barr and Dowding (2016) suggest that it is important to develop good working relationships with others to manage conflict. Conflict occurs because of differences in perception of the situation, often arising from many different causes such as hidden agendas, lack of resources, work design and tasks, role overlap and unfair situations.

To summarize, management may not directly be the first remit of the newly qualified nurse and these concepts may be more applicable to organizational management – but they can still be considered in the day-to-day running of a care environment.

First, if you are in charge of a care area, you need to have in place a strategy for the day. There will be prescribed activities and duties related to individuals or the environment that must occur on that day only, along with any other contingencies that may arise. Therefore, at the start of the day, the nurse needs to set out their strategy of how these would be best addressed and handled.

Second, in setting out the strategy, there is the need to fully understand the operational management and maintaining of standards that is required. You also need to fully understand the structural nature of the organization and how this filters down to the day-to-day running. Therefore, the nurse in charge will delegate tasks and duties to the workforce and issue commands on how to feedback on these to ensure everything is in order.

There are issues of HR management, such as ensuring that staff with the right skills are deployed to the right duties and that they are given feedback on their performance and assisted where necessary. The issues of management and coordination are therefore important throughout the day; the nurse needs to understand what events are happening, including any that are unforeseen, and they then need to demonstrate flexibility and positive decision-making skills before reporting back on the day to senior staff.

Teamworking

Teamworking has been implicitly mentioned throughout this chapter. This section will discuss some issues related to ensuring effective collaboration within nursing teams and other professionals.

The NMC (2018b) standards of proficiency state that nurses should expect to provide leadership in multidisciplinary teams and be accountable for appropriate delegation to others. There are responsibilities in establishing and monitoring safe delivery of care. They are responsible for ensuring the smooth functioning of interdisciplinary teams and group dynamics. The NMC (2018b) recognize that teamwork is an important consideration for nursing within their leadership proficiencies as they need to monitor, evaluate and communicate care outcomes to others in the team. They need to ensure effective use of digital technologies and ensure they contribute to organizational change.

Firstly, there must be good understanding of the principles used in team nursing. Marquis and Huston (2012) suggest that the care for a group of patients is conducted with nurses and ancillary staff under the supervision of a professional nurse. This relies on excellent communication and supervision and is usually employed if there is a high proportion of ancillary staff involved in delivery.

Lewis and McGowan (2015) suggest that transitioning to be a qualified nurse can be a stressful experience. Their clinical confidence, dealing with other professionals and the responsibility of maintaining safety all contribute to this. Hence, the period of preceptorship nurses normally have can act as a bridge to provide support to overcome these stressors.

King et al. (2017) suggest that collaborative working is a multi-faceted concept with many overlapping terms such as multi/inter/trans/joint disciplinary/professional/agency working. They define it as occurring when:

> …two or more professionals from different professional groups are required to interact to ensure that appropriate care is delivered to a service user. (King et al., 2017: 1)

Fealy et al. (2015) state that nurses bring their expertise to the table with other professionals within their working contexts. You should articulate your discipline-specific contribution in words and actions to give an impression of a clear professional identity whilst working with other professionals to provide optimum care.

Barr and Dowding (2016) highlight that such approaches require skills and competence in this area. Effective collaboration is based on:

- Patient-centred goals.
- Openness.
- Collaborative decision-making.
- Clear communication channels.
- Good conflict management and good leadership.

This can be affected by differing interpretations, differing values and differences in power/authority. So, the first aspect is to ensure that you make yourself clear. This means that clarity is necessary in the requests that you make, the information that you request or provide, and the instructions that you give. If you relate them to the patient needs and the goals of the organization this should help. Mullins and Christy (2016) highlight that effective teams exhibit shared goals, values, norms, are committed to each other, participate, communicate information and express agreement/disagreement. However, there can be some conflict between teams due to differing role perspectives and competition from individuals outside of their own profession which can be overcome by reiterating the goals of the organization and services and each profession's contribution to it.

Collaboration means sharing while maintaining your own boundaries. There are several mutual benefits of learning from sharing with other professionals. Speedy (2015) suggests that collaborative practice is crucial for achieving optimal patient, healthcare worker and organizational outcomes and is an essential aspect in the role of the nurse. Therefore, taking steps such as socializing (in a professional sense) with other disciplines helps to show that you are willing to listen to them. You can gain awareness of what and why they are carrying out certain tasks/approaches. However, there is also a need to utilize assertiveness skills to maintain your own authority in such arenas. This again boils down to clarity: creating clear goals/outcomes, clearly communicating these, and being clear about the potential consequences or benefits of the actions requested. Once again, making decisions and suggesting them to others is a good way of leading from the front. It shows that you can take the initiative, which will instil trust in others. For example, you will need to have a working knowledge of the care environment, the patients/service users within it and the planned events during your shifts.

By understanding how teams function you can adapt specific roles to ensure effective teamworking. This is based on the concept of Belbin's team roles (Isaac and Carson, 2012). As mentioned earlier, Adair (2010) highlighted that leadership requires ensuring that the task, individuals and the team are attended to. Similarly, Belbin highlights different factors and roles required in creating effective teamwork. The main aspects are roles related to thinking, action and people. These are broken down into further roles which can be seen in Table 6.2.

The notion is that teams are made of different people and someone needs to assume these roles at different stages while moving through processes designed to meet outcomes. Some individuals have specific skills, so can be delegated to roles and functions that reflect their particular strengths in relation to the team roles.

Summary

This chapter has looked at the major theories related to leadership, including trait, style, situational, transactional and transformational,

Table 6.2 Belbin's team roles (Isaac and Carson, 2012)

Team role			Function
Thinking	Plant	PL	Creative, imaginative, free-thinking. Generates ideas and solves difficult problems.
	Monitor evaluator	ME	Sober, strategic and discerning. Sees all options and judges accurately.
	Specialist	SP	Single-minded, self-starting and dedicated. They provide specialist knowledge and skills.
Action	Shaper	SH	Challenging, dynamic, thrives on pressure. Has the drive and courage to overcome obstacles.
	Implementer	IMP	Practical, reliable, efficient. Turns ideas into action and organizes work that needs to be done.
	Completer finisher	CF	Painstaking, conscientious, anxious. Searches out errors. Polishes and perfects.
People	Coordinator	CO	Mature, confident, identifies talent. Clarifies goals. Delegates effectively.
	Team worker	TW	Co-operative, perceptive and diplomatic. Listens and averts friction.
	Resource investigator	RI	Outgoing, enthusiastic. Explores opportunities and develops contacts.

Reproduced with kind permission of Belbin

authentic and clinical. The important aspect to remember is that leadership is related to your people skills. It is about your ability to observe the situation, identify problems and create solutions within teams. It is about taking action, leading by being seen to be involved, and doing some of the tasks that you would expect others to do, as well as giving clear directions and instructions.

Theories of management have been discussed, demonstrating how the organizational goals are aligned and that strategies are put in place to maintain them. It is about formal mechanisms and infrastructure, and how these are maintained or developed. It is about the day-to-day running of services by following the policies and procedures set in place by employing organizations and professions. It is about formally dealing with people at all levels of an organization reporting up from the ground floor.

Overall, it is hoped that this chapter has shown that there is a great deal of overlap of concepts related to leadership and management. Management may be a role achieved by position, whereas leadership demonstrates interpersonal power and influence. Managers should, as far as possible, be leaders, but leaders do not necessarily have to be managers. As a newly qualified nurse, these aspects may be challenging, but by transferring skills gained in other areas of life, observing others, asking questions, and practising by getting involved, they are skills that can be developed and integrated as you progress in your career.

- **Leadership** is related to achieving goals through people. It is about dynamic relationships, goal-setting, strategy and action.
  - ○ Leadership encompasses theories related to traits, styles, contingency, situational flexibility and being authentic.
  - ○ Clinical leadership relates to extending roles, developing approaches and decision-making across nursing and interdisciplinary teams to achieve positive outcomes for patients/service users.
- **Management** is related to making sure that goals are achieved.
  - ○ It is related to developing organizational structures and systems to accomplish this.
  - ○ It encompasses managing resources effectively and supervising people effectively.

- **Teamwork** is related to ensuring collaboration with other nurses and wider healthcare professionals to meet organizational objectives and provide optimum care for service users. It is about effective communication and collaboration by adopting specific roles and functions to provide effective individual and team cohesiveness whilst focusing on the objectives.

7

LEARNING, TEACHING AND ASSESSMENT IN PRACTICE

Rob Burton and Graham Ormrod

THE AIMS OF THIS CHAPTER ARE TO:

- Identify the practice learning and teaching, practice assessor supervision and assessment responsibilities of the newly qualified nurse.
- Explore the NMC proficiency standards (NMC, 2018b), the framework for nursing and midwifery education (NMC, 2018d) and standards for student supervision and assessment (NMC, 2018e).
- Explore theories of learning and teaching and help the reader to learn how to apply them in practice.
- Explore practice assessor supervision and assessment and help the reader to learn how to apply them in practice.

Introduction

Qualified nurses need to possess a wide variety of skills. These include the seven platforms of proficiencies outlined by the Nursing and Midwifery Council (NMC, 2018b): being an accountable professional; promoting health and preventing ill health; assessing needs and planning care; providing and evaluating care; leading and managing nursing care and working in teams; improving safety and quality of care; and coordinating care. As they further their career, there are also expectations that the nurse will need to provide **practice supervision** for student nurses and also eventually aim to act as a **practice assessor** to assess them in relation to their progressive competencies and confirmation of their final **proficiency** to practise. Indeed, a large professional responsibility of a qualified nurse is related to the development of themselves and others around them to share their 'skills, knowledge and experience for the benefit of people receiving care and your colleagues' (NMC, 2018g). As a final-year student or recently graduated student, you will hopefully appreciate the huge input that qualified nurses have had in your nursing education and the value that a good practice assessor supervisor and practice assessor has made to your placement experiences.

As a newly qualified nurse, you will not become a supervisor or practice assessor overnight, but you will need to be involved in some teaching of others. This chapter is designed to help you to prepare for teaching, supervision and assessing others in practice. We will look at setting learning outcomes, identifying learning needs and acting to meet them. Learning opportunities present themselves in practice every day and it is up to the nurse to seize those opportunities readily when they arise. Therefore, theories of learning, managing learning environments and teaching strategies will be discussed so that the nurse can understand their role in developing others more clearly. The Nursing and Midwifery Council (NMC) produced two documents in 2018: the first on the standards framework for nursing and midwifery education (NMC, 2018d), and the second on standards for student supervision and assessment (NMC, 2018e). The main aspects and requirements of these documents will be explored, as well as their application to practice.

The NMC standards

The *Future Nurse: Standards of Proficiency for Registered Nurses* (NMC, 2018b) sets out exactly the outcomes required for those wishing to enter the nursing register as a qualified nurse. The platforms forming the basis for this have been described above. Responsibilities related to the learning and teaching of others is articulated in 'Annexe A' under Section 4, suggesting that qualified nurses should be using evidence-based, best practice communication skills for working with people in professional teams, including demonstrating effective supervision, teaching and performance appraisal (NMC, 2018b: 30). This includes providing clear instructions, checking understanding, providing feedback, promoting reflection and maintaining related accurate records.

In the NMC (2018d: 5) *Standards Framework for Nursing and Midwifery Education* five headings are set out as principles to be followed in the educating of nurses:

1 Learning culture.
   o Ethical.
   o Open and honest.
   o Conducive to safe and effective learning that respects the principles of equality and diversity.
   o Innovation.
   o Inter-professional learning.
   o Teamworking.
2 Educational governance and quality.
   o Comply with all legal and regulatory requirements.
3 Student empowerment.
   o Empowered.
   o Learning opportunities.
   o Achieve desired proficiencies and programme outcomes.
4 Educators and assessors.
   o Suitably qualified.
   o Prepared and skilled.
   o Supported for their role.

5   Curricula and assessment.
- o   Students achieve the outcomes required to practise safely.
- o   Assess the safety and effectiveness of all learning environments.

(NMC, 2018d: 5)

As you can see from the above statements the NMC rate safety, ethical and legal principles, diversity and inclusion, teamworking and empowerment as necessary in developing the nursing workforce. The NMC (2018e) document *Standards for Student Supervision and Assessment* emphasizes three headings that underpin supporting students in practice, which is a role you will find yourself involved in at some level as soon as you are practicing as a qualified nurse. The headings are:

1   Effective practice learning.
- o   Deliver safe and effective learning experiences for nursing and midwifery students in practice.
2   Supervision of students.
- o   Principles of student supervision in the practice environment.
- o   Role of the practice supervisor.
3   Assessment of students and confirmation of proficiency.
- o   Assessing and confirming students' practice and academic achievement.
- o   Role and responsibilities of the practice assessor and the academic assessor.

Therefore, you can see that the NMC are promoting the close partnership between accredited education providers (AEI) and practitioners delivering healthcare to educate and develop nurses that can practise with the safety of service users and patients as a primary responsibility. In order to do this, there are three main roles between the academic providers and practitioners involved in healthcare delivery, the academic educators and assessors, practice supervisors and practice assessors, and each have differing responsibilities in relation to education, support, supervision and development.

Practice supervisors must be safe and effective role models, up to date with current evidence-based practice methods. They should work closely with students in the practice area commensurate with their scope of practice and level to facilitate the appropriate learning required for their stage of programme, providing feedback on needs, progression and development of students to their practice assessors. Student nurses in a practice area must always be supervised in practice settings. They must be provided support for continuing professional development and be aware of current appropriate standards (NMC, 2018e).

Practice assessors must conduct assessments to ensure that students are meeting the desired outcomes and progression relative to their stage of training. They must plan appropriate time to gather feedback, observe and assess the students in relation to their required outcomes, record such confirmation on progress and provide feedback as to strengths and needs in relation to such progression. This needs to be conducted by liaising with the student's practice supervisor for feedback and discussion with an academic assessor. A practice assessor should not be the person acting as practice supervisor or academic assessor. These roles should not be held simultaneously. Practice assessors need to be adequately prepared for the role via adequate continuing professional development with a high level of interpersonal skills and understanding of assessment processes. They must be up to date with the relevant proficiencies required from students on their nursing programmes (NMC, 2018e).

Academic assessors also collate feedback and make assessments as to how the students operate in the academic environment. They must liaise closely with practice assessors in order to make recommendations as to whether students have met required proficiencies in relation to their stage of programme and whether they can progress to the next stage. They must also be prepared to fulfil the role according to the requirements of the academic institution they work for. Similar to practice assessors they must be excellent role models, communicators and with good knowledge related to the proficiencies required of nurses and their own particular programmes. They too cannot act as practice supervisor or practice assessor simultaneously (NMC, 2018e).

It can be seen from all these applicable NMC standards that whatever level of nursing you are at you may find yourself supervising or assessing students in your practice area. This requires you to liaise with the students' academic institutions to ensure you are up to date with the current nursing programme, its proficiencies and requirements aligned to the NMC proficiencies, whilst acting as a role model and providing effective supervision and assessment for progression.

There is a clinical aspect to this in relation to your own performance, yet you will have to develop these wider responsibilities within the transition to your role. According to Stevens and Duffy (2017) nurses must make the transition from their clinical roles to also providing instruction to others. Their study suggests that this involves familiarization to the clinical environment, familiarization to the programme students on placement are undertaking there, and the proficiencies that it entails. They require development in facilitation and clinical instruction, learning, teaching and assessing. They also need excellent communication and collaboration skills.

Establishing effective working relationships in practice supervision

As a practice supervisor your role will be to ensure the satisfactory support and guidance of junior staff and student nurses, ensuring they are welcomed into the interprofessional approaches to care and ensuring they become a valued member of the healthcare team, even if supernumerary. The subject of teamwork is discussed in detail elsewhere in this book, so here we will look at how team relationships are used to facilitate and support the learning of junior staff (and in some cases senior staff), students and other team members.

The NMC (2018g) point out the importance of working with and communicating with other healthcare professionals in healthcare services; importance is placed on the development of interprofessional relationships. Hughes and Quinn (2013) highlight that interprofessional working is a cooperative exercise where traditional distinctions between professions are maintained whilst demonstrating a willingness to share specialized knowledge to meet patient needs more efficiently. Much can be learned in an interprofessional context, and as a practice supervisor you would need to provide opportunities for such learning to those students entrusted to you. There is a developing culture of 'lifelong learning' for all professionals working in the healthcare services, so there can often be a wide range of professionals considered to be students or learners, from those on pre-registration courses to those on post-registration courses (Hughes and Quinn, 2013). The needs of all these professionals will need to be addressed in such environments. A nurse may find themselves acting as a practice supervisor, practice assessor or academic assessor to a more junior student while being supervised, taught or practice assessed by others in their own environment. It also means that, in the context of this chapter, the term 'student' will normally mean a pre-registration nursing student but can also refer to those whom newly qualified nurses will often teach, including a new member of staff, a junior member of staff, or a student of any healthcare profession. Speakman (2020) suggests that teamworking and interprofessional approaches to healthcare are now a primary focus for providers, that healthcare education needs to have an emphasis on partnerships with other professionals and interprofessional education (IPE), and that collaborative practice (CP) depends on different professionals effectively communicating and engaging in teamwork. Therefore, the care environment needs to be one in which all groups of staff can be educated together.

Muijs and Reynolds (2018) suggest that the 'climate' of the environment is a very important aspect in developing working relationships between those considered as teachers and their students. This does not mean 'climate' in the sense of temperature and physical environment (although this is important, as will be discussed later), but relates to the climate of the relationships formed within it, such as how 'warm' or 'cool' the relationship between the parties is. This can be observed in the formality or informality placed on the learning/teaching relationship, the nature of support that is fostered, and the nature of trust in the person's knowledge, skills, authority and approach. Billings and Halstead (2020) highlight that revision of nursing programmes and experiences are inevitable due to vastly changing aspects in society and a need to ensure nurses are prepared with knowledge and skills to provide optimum care. Young and Maxwell (2007) suggested a shift in professional education away from a style where expert knowledge is passed to students in a distant manner and the student is a passive recipient, towards more student-centred approaches where they are more actively engaged. This approach helps to develop their confidence and skills in lifelong learning, problem-solving and critical thinking. Traditional modes of educating nurses meant the passing on of knowledge from the expert to the student. However, this can be overwhelming for both the teacher and the student, with students not always being able to transfer knowledge across contexts (Ignatavicius, 2018). In order to engage students in identifying their own learning needs (while maintaining standards), an important basis will be the nature of the relationship developed between the two parties involved: the educator and the learner.

ACTIVITY 7.1

Consider your experience as a student thus far. Identify your most positive experiences of learning in practice and how your practice supervisors or assessors established a positive working relationship.

1   What steps did they take to develop and maintain this?

Race (2015) proposes that successful learning comprises wanting, needing, doing, feedback and digesting. Therefore, to facilitate this process, the practice supervisor should take steps to find out the learning needs of the student and what they want and need in relation to their experience and requirements. This includes knowing the curriculum of the course they are on, their level of experience, their learning styles and specific requirements related to their placement. A carefully planned programme of activities is then needed, in which they can be involved, with regular opportunities for learning formally and informally, and an opportunity for regular feedback on their performance.

One of the key approaches to effective relationships is ensuring that **rapport** occurs. 'Rapport' derives from the French verb *porter*, which means *to carry*, and rapport means *to carry back*. Therefore, in the sense of building relationships, rapport occurs when information is carried back to the original person, or, more accurately, *matched*. This includes the matching of non-verbal, vocal/tonality and verbal content. On a basic level, the words that are understood by the student should be used to create the basis of the relationship, which should be developed from there. In such an encounter the supervisor and learner develop shared meaning by concurrent sending and receiving of non-verbal, tonal and verbal messages (Arnold and Underman Boggs, 2016). This principle also fits with the notion of **advanced**

organizers, as suggested by Ausubel et al. (1978): that the best starting point is to begin from where and what the student already knows. This requires the practice assessor/supervisor to listen carefully and observe, and have conversations with the student, to ascertain this.

Stein-Parbury (2018) emphasizes the importance of interpersonal skills between professionals and ultimately patients/service users. It is essential to establish atmospheres in which trust, confidence, participation and the opportunity to respond freely are created. To do this, a student should find their practice supervisor approachable, therefore early contact and intervention is essential, at which point ground rules are negotiated and a plan of action set out so that outcomes can be met.

It is important to consider that interprofessional learning (IPL) may be an approach taken in the learning, teaching and assessment of students. Wilkes et al. (2013) suggest that IPL is increasingly utilized in health professional education so that best practice and support are shared with a view to providing optimum care for the patient by exploring health professional practice concepts and gaining perspectives of other's roles. Therefore, throughout the remaining sections, although the focus is on student nurses, this should be considered within a wider IPL framework. Ensuring these relationships are facilitated is an important part of the practice supervisor role.

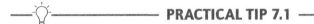

——————————————— **PRACTICAL TIP 7.1** ———————————————

Ground rules can be set as follows:

- Provide a clear induction to the practice environment including its physical layout, team members and the policies and procedures that guide it.
- An induction pack should be made available including helpful information about the practice environment and its purpose.
- Introduce the student to all members of the care team.
- The initial conversation should include questions to ascertain the student's previous experiences, knowledge and requirements for their placement with you.
- Highlight opportunities to observe and be involved in working with nursing staff and other healthcare professional team members.

Finally, it is important to ensure equity for students with diverse needs and recognize their differing learning needs.

Once you have developed a relationship with the student and oriented them to the working environment, to fully perform the roles of supervisor and assessor you will need a good understanding of the theory and practice of learning, teaching and assessing. These concepts will now be further explored.

Learning

As a practice supervisor you will be responsible for facilitating the students' experiences. The word 'facilitation' derives from the French *facile*, which means 'easy'. Therefore, a straightforward translation in this context is: making it easy for the student to learn. In order to do this, there is a need for the facilitator to understand the nature and theories of learning, which can be a complex issue. Although there are several different schools of thought and theories related to learning, and there are many overlapping principles, there are similar concepts with differing names and different concepts with similar names. Learning is often considered a permanent change in behaviour. In our case a change in the behaviour of nurses. Illeris (2018: 2) states that learning can be defined as 'any process that leads to permanent capacity change and which is not solely due to biological maturation or ageing'.

Three main schools will be considered here:

- The behavioural school of learning theory.
- The cognitive school of learning theory.
- The humanistic school of learning theory.

The subcategories and terminologies used to explain the concepts are so wide, deep and broad that they will not be discussed in fine detail for the purposes of this book. Instead, we will give you a whistle-stop tour of the main ideas behind these learning theories. The notion of experiential learning (learning by reflecting on experience) and different learning styles will also be considered to give you essential background knowledge before we outline some guidance for organizing teaching.

Behavioural learning theory

Merriam and Bierema (2013) argue that the behavioural learning theory (or behaviourism) is so embedded in our lives that we cannot perceive its actual presence, yet it has been the most influential approach to learning in the past century and forms a strong basis for education. Here, the aim is to reduce knowledge and skills into small measurable outcomes which are then rewarded in order to strengthen them. Behavioural theorists align with the earlier definitions of learning as being more or less any permanent change of behaviour resulting from experience, with demonstrable behaviours being a major focus.

The behavioural theory tends to refer mainly to the stimulus-response relationship of a human or animal with their environment. Behavioural approaches concentrate mainly on the development of behaviours (usually observable and therefore outward) as opposed to internal thought processes. This is the strength of behaviourism, but it is also its weakness, as it tends to reduce human learning to sets of behaviour without much thinking. The theory is based on the stimulus-response principle, whereby the resulting response is reinforced (strengthened) by reward or punished (weakened) by aversive methods. Jensen (2008) described behaviourism as a rule-based approach that manipulates learners and the environment to such an extent that they have no voice or choice in the process. This may be correct, but such rewards and punishments do help to shape responses and can lead to ways of motivating students. For example, consider Maslow's (1954) hierarchy of needs (Figure 7.1) which you should know well from your nursing studies: once one stage is satisfied, we can move to

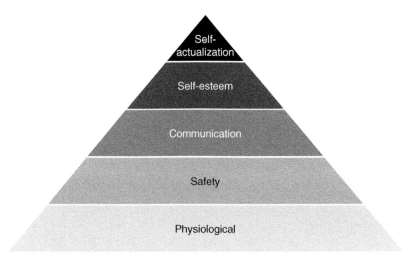

Figure 7.1 Maslow's hierarchy of needs (Maslow, 1943)

the next stage. This need to move to the next stage is a motivating factor for the learner and the rewards and punishments help to shape the way in which the learner gets there. Hughes and Quinn (2013) offer some criticisms of Maslow's hierarchy of needs, such as that there is evidence of people reaching the higher stages while having deficits in the lower stages and that it does not quite explain why people engage in activities that might not be related to any biological or intellectual deficits. However, it is important to note that, in assisting learners, the practice supervisor needs to be aware of how to maintain motivation by increasing rewards and reducing punishments. In this way, the student is accepting of the methods chosen to learn. If a student is punished or sanctioned, then they are less likely to take the same risk in learning again.

Classical conditioning

The first aspect of behavioural theory that we consider here is classical conditioning. According to Bates (2016), classical conditioning arose from the work of Pavlov, famous for his work in noticing the changes in how dogs salivated in response to differing stimuli with or without the presence of food, and later work by John B. Watson applying similar mechanisms (associating aversive experiences to specific stimuli) to human subjects, particularly the infamous 'Little Albert' experiments. In these experiments, a young child (Albert) was given a cuddly toy and subjected to a loud, startling noise at the same time, which eventually led to the child becoming fearful of the cuddly toy alone. Pavlov and Watson could be deemed to be credited as the founders of the behaviourist movement. To conduct such experiments in the modern age would be ethically very questionable, but from these research studies it has become understood and accepted that the basic element of learning is association – that is, association between the stimulus and the response (Figure 7.2). The response of the subject is the behaviour to which the whole theory relates. In nursing terms, the stimulus is the trigger or situation with which the student is presented, and the response is their resulting

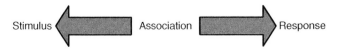

Figure 7.2   Association between stimulus and response

behaviour. So, as a practice supervisor you need to understand the necessary stimuli and expected behaviours in specific nursing situations: for example, a student may need to learn the correct response when presented with stimuli such as a chart highlighting a rise in a patient's temperature.

Operant conditioning

Operant conditioning (so-called because it relates to 'operations' in the environment) was developed by B. F. Skinner and built on the work of the classical conditioning researchers and on the work of Thorndike (Aubrey and Riley, 2016). Thorndike noticed that behaviours of animals that were, at first, random (law of effect) became strengthened when repeated and rewarded with food (law of exercise). Skinner's work introduced similar aspects but recognized the power of the reward or the punishment in shaping behaviour. The rewards act as a *reinforcer* and therefore strengthen certain behaviours. For example, if a reward is given to a person immediately after a desired behaviour is demonstrated, the person is more likely to exhibit that behaviour again. The reward therefore acts as a positive reinforcer of the behaviour. If it is desired to reduce or extinguish certain behaviour, then instead of a reward, an aversive experience, or a *punisher*, would be given immediately after the behaviour, with a view to weakening, decreasing the frequency, intensity or severity of the behaviour.

Behaviours can also be strengthened or reinforced by other means: for example, if a person is experiencing something that is aversive to them, they may develop a behaviour to avoid the experience. Therefore, removing this aversive experience should strengthen certain escaping/avoidance-type behaviours. Nothing is being given after the behaviour to reward it; instead what *is* happening is the punishment is given before the actual behaviour and the behaviour is intended to stop this: for example, if we are too hot, then we would remove a layer of clothing to cool down. This is known as 'negative reinforcement' because the stimulus is removed and the behaviour is still strengthened. So, we learn to remove layers of clothing if we are too hot in future. The removal of the aversive stimulus (in this case, heat) is rewarding and the behaviour is strengthened.

Basically, the association now occurs not only between the stimulus and the response, but by the association between the response and the

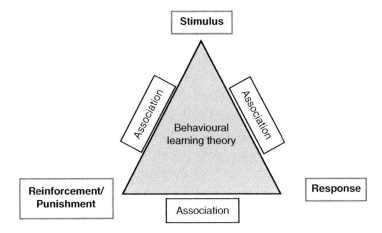

Figure 7.3 Operant conditioning

wider external response that provides reward or punishment. This is illustrated in Figure 7.3 and Table 7.1.

It has been suggested above that reward or punishment is totally controlled by external means, but this is not entirely accurate. Rewards or reinforcers can be either **intrinsic** or **extrinsic**, and many things in life can be used as reinforcers. Intrinsic reinforcers come from within the person, such as feelings of satisfaction and self-competence, and extrinsic factors come from the environment, such as praise, pay, privileges and good grades.

Applying operant conditioning in practice

To apply operant conditioning to your practice as a newly qualified nurse, you need to consider how to provide reinforcement to the learners with whom you may be involved, which should be appropriate to the level they are at in Maslow's hierarchy of needs. As far as possible, the reinforcers should be positive and rewarding to provide encouragement. It could be safely assumed that the students'

Table 7.1 Operant conditioning

	Rewarding experience	Aversive experience
Presented	Positive reinforcement (strengthens behaviour it follows)	Punishment (weakens behaviour it follows)
Removed	Punishment (response cost: weakens behaviour it follows)	Negative reinforcement (strengthens behaviour of escaping)

physiological and safety needs are met, so they are more likely to be motivated by social praise, which should reward their need for communication and self-esteem, thus encouraging them to develop the skills and outcomes further. Reprimands for doing the wrong thing are punishers, and although effective in the short term, can be damaging to relationships and reduce the students' willingness to participate in learning experiences. They are likely to limit further communication and damage self-esteem unless communicated in a professional, constructive and kind manner. Rather than telling a student that they are doing something wrong (an example would be saying something like 'No, No, that is totally wrong!'), phrase your response in a constructive way by saying something like 'You need to do it this way', or 'You need to improve that technique', and then tell them how to do it. Once they do something approximating what you want, give them the reward.

ACTIVITY 7.2

Think of the learning experiences that you have had during your nurse education.

1   What kinds of rewards were you given by those teaching you in practice?
2   How did you feel when you were rewarded or punished?
3   Consider the positive rewards that you could give to a student under your supervision in your workplace.

Shaping

As well as setting up stimuli, expected behavioural outcomes and rewards, an important aspect in behavioural approaches is to reduce expected knowledge, skills and behaviours into smaller components that can be achieved easily, then subtly developed into more complex skills. This is known as 'shaping' – whereby understanding and skill are developed in a gradual process. By reinforcing the student on completion of the skill or being able to demonstrate some knowledge, they can then be moved on to the next level. Shaping is important when a student is not able to meet a learning outcome. The skill should be broken down so that they can therefore achieve an easier step (leading them to be able to be reinforced), which is then developed into more complex stages, step by step (Aubrey and Riley, 2016).

Social learning theory

Another important learning theory applicable to learning in clinical areas is that of social learning theory or role modelling, based on the observations of Albert Bandura. The basic principle is that learners will imitate the behaviours of others. If these are rewarded and reinforced, then such behaviours will be strengthened. This theory is based around research that involved observations of how children responded after seeing others behave in certain ways before them, concluding that they were quite likely to copy or mimic behaviours of adults that they had witnessed. Therefore, it is important, as a nurse, to demonstrate exactly the types of skills and abilities that you wish your learners to develop, as they will imitate you. The more the approach is witnessed, the more likely this will then be repeated by the learner. It is important that these behaviours are not just modelled in a teaching/learning situation, but that they are also practised continually, because the more the learner witnesses a correct technique or practise, the more that will be modelled (Wlodkowski and Ginsberg, 2017). If the learner is only exposed to correct techniques while being taught, but then witnesses different behaviours occurring more frequently in the everyday world of practice, they will probably adopt the latter approach. This is the notion of taking 'short cuts', or not 'practising what is being preached', but copying what are the most prevalent observable approaches.

ACTIVITY 7.3

Think of some of the practice supervisors with whom you have worked.

1   What kinds of role models were they in relation to being consistent with what they taught you and how they practised?
2   Consider those you thought to be the best in teaching you and the methods they used to model the practices for you.

Cognitive learning theory

Cognitive learning theory is important to understand as it provides a deeper explanation of how people learn and understand. It includes the internal mental processes of the learner as a fundamental basis. According to Gopee (2018), it involves learning by internal purposive action involving thinking, perceiving, information processing and memory. Cognitivism answers the criticisms of behavioural learning theory of simply being programmed responses to external stimuli. Cognitive theory includes the learner's ability to discriminate, generalize and transfer skills, knowledge and understanding to new or different situations. The different situations are usually the real-world domain in which the skills are practised. Cognitive learning theory includes the notion of thinking between the stimulus and the response (Figure 7.4). To do this, perception, memory and information-processing as internal mechanisms are important factors. Therefore, to assist students, we need to understand the impact of these processes and how to develop them.

A main proponent of cognitive learning theory is Bloom, who developed a taxonomy (or classification) of educational objectives related to cognitive learning (Hughes and Quinn, 2013). Bloom (1956) suggested that a skill consists of three main domains:

- A psychomotor component (the actual hand-eye coordination and behavioural motor/physical dexterity necessary).
- An affective component (the attitude and application required to carry it out effectively).
- A cognitive component (the level of understanding about the task that is required).

For example, if you consider learning a clinical skill such as taking blood pressure, there is first the 'hands on' element of learning how to operate the equipment; second, one learns how and when the skill is relevant and appropriate to carry out on a patient; and third, a student must understand the anatomy and physiology of the cardiovascular system. Bloom developed this taxonomy to represent the sequential and deepening levels of the cognitive domain.

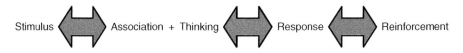

Figure 7.4 Cognitive learning theory (unlike that shown in Figure 7.2, this theory includes the notion of thinking between the stimulus and the response)

1 **Knowledge.**
This is knowing straightforward facts about the subject/issue being considered.

2 **Understanding/comprehension.**
This is knowing how the subject/issue works or what its utility is.

3 **Application.**
This is the ability to put the subject/issue into practice in the real world or to be able to explain its uses.

4 **Analysis.**
This is the ability to break the subject/issue down into its component parts.

5 **Synthesis.**
This is the ability to transfer the understanding about the issue and come up with new ideas of how it can be used.

6 **Evaluation.**
This is the ability to place a value on all aspects involved in the issue as they are applied to different situations. Evaluation utilizes judgement based on the evidence provided in previous levels.

(Hughes and Quinn, 2013)

The lower levels (1 and 2) suggest that the learning is achieved by reception or rote (when we learn something by repetition, 'parrot fashion' such as learning 'times tables' by heart in mathematics). This may be an important way to learn but is very superficial. The methods employed can be used to convey information itself, but the learner may have very little understanding about it.

The latter stages in the taxonomy (3, 4, 5, and 6) show how the individual can develop higher-order thinking skills so that the knowledge provided now has meaning. At these stages, the learner is more likely to be discovering the knowledge, understanding, application and value from the learning themselves, and involves a move from superficial understanding to deeper understanding. This notion of 'surface learning' (superficial repetition of knowledge) to 'deep learning' (advanced critical evaluation of the concepts) was highlighted by Marton and Saljo (1976).

ACTIVITY 7.4

Consider a topic or skill that you have recently learnt at university or on placement. If you had to teach this skill to someone else:

1   How would you break the teaching session into sections applying Bloom's taxonomy above?

The concept of 'meaningful learning' as opposed to 'rote learning' was discussed by Ausubel et al. (1978), who suggested that understanding the students' previous knowledge as a starting point is important, as otherwise they will not be able to make the links between new knowledge being presented and what they already know and understand. According to Hughes and Quinn (2013), Jerome Bruner (1960) suggested the notion of 'discovery learning' as being the polar opposite to reception learning. This concept suggests that the nature of learning is more valuable to the individual if they find things out for themselves, which leads to deeper learning (Figure 7.5).

The notion of moving to deeper levels of learning by making associations with the student's prior knowledge and experiences, and building on this cognitive learning, requires several considerations. Bates (2016) suggests that Bruner's theories require students to be actively involved in a process rather than being spoon fed. This is very important in clinical settings. Therefore, your role is to do more than provide information, you also need to design sessions so that students can discover and

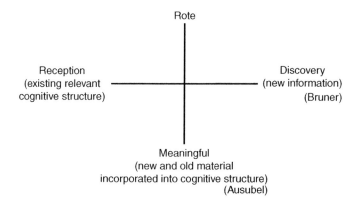

Figure 7.5   Methods of learning

Adapted from Quinn, S. and Hughes, F. (© 2013) *Principles and Practice of Nurse Education* (6th edn). Cengage Publishing. Reproduced by permission of Cengage Learning EMEA Ltd

identify the relationship between information and knowledge in specific contexts. Feedback at each stage is very important.

These aspects relate very closely to cognitive development theories proposed by Piaget, that a learner 'assimilates' information by processing it against prior held knowledge and that prior beliefs can 'accommodate' the new knowledge into a whole new set of understandings and behaviours. Jean Piaget had an influential role in the sphere of theory related to children's cognitive development, as did Lev Vygotsky, who suggested that it is not only the individual child's potential that is important in learning, but also the opportunities, environments and socialization that can enrich their learning. This he called the 'zone of proximal development' (ZPD) which means that an individual can have a certain potential capacity for learning, but that this can be hindered in poor or lacking social and learning environments. The tools that help to widen the ZPD include language, stories, art and role models. This became known as 'Cultural Historical Activity Theory' (CHAT) (Aubrey and Riley, 2016). These aspects lead to the concept of 'Scaffolding'. According to Bates (2016) this relates to the teacher's role in engaging and supporting development by developing incremental steps in understanding and then making them more complex as the learner understands and applies these further.

Bates (2016) outlines that Jack Mezirow's 'Transformational Learning Theory' can be considered within the cognitive domain. Mezirow suggests that experiences are the basis of learning. It involves the individual's view of the world (**meaning perspective**) and knowledge and values relating to their experiences (**meaning schemes**).

- **Experience of life** – This is the starting point in any learning event.
- **Critical reflection** – This is a fundamental aspect of adult learning where the individual questions the validity of their values and beliefs.
- **Rational discourse** – Exploring the meaning of their beliefs and values and sharing these views with others.

This approach depends on the aspect of reflection which is a crucial aspect in nurse education.

Transformative learning is defined as the process by which we transform problematic frames of reference (mindsets, habits of mind, meaning perspectives) – sets of assumptions and expectations – to make them more inclusive, discriminating, open, reflective and emotionally able to change. (Mezirow, 2018: 115)

This is achieved by considering 'instrumental learning' (task-oriented) or 'communicative learning' (critical self-reflection). As a practice supervisor you will need to balance these aspects in your support of the student (i.e. exposing them to clinical situations whilst creating space for discussion and reflection).

———————————————— **ACTIVITY 7.5** ————————————————

Think of some of the aspects that you have learned throughout your nurse education.

1   How were these knowledge and skills developed?
2   What kinds of explanations were you given that helped your understanding?
3   What approaches hindered your understanding?

Brain-based learning

Another factor related to improving the cognitive abilities of individuals is brain-based learning. This means that to facilitate learning, we should not only look at the nature of learning, but also incorporate the physical and physiological understanding of how the brain works.
   Brain-based learning/teaching is based on three aspects:

- **E** – active *ENGAGEMENT*
- **S** – purposeful *STRATEGIES*
- **P** – based on *PRINCIPLES* derived from neuroscience

Jensen (2008: 4)

Jensen (2008) highlights that the brain is designed for selection and survival. It is actually poorly designed for formal instruction and efficiency or order. This is the most important aspect as it explains a wide range of behaviours, even negative ones which are designed in some way to assist the individual to have their needs met and to survive. Basically, brain-based learning requires us to ensure that all physical needs are met, such as those in Maslow's hierarchy of needs (water, food, air, safety and shelter), or these will interfere with effective learning. So, it is a matter of creating optimal physical conditions to ensure optimal cognitive functioning. There is a need to ensure that there is a balance between the amount of stimulation and relaxation offered to provide good learning experiences. Too much stimulation causes stress and a feeling of threat, so learning is reduced. Too much relaxation means there is very little change in environmental stimuli, which provides little opportunity to learn new things (Jensen, 2008). Therefore, in supervising a student you need to consider a variety of activities and the time scale in which they are employed.

As human beings, we gather in information about the world around us through our senses. We also process our experiences of the world internally in a sensory way. So, for example, when remembering or imagining, we create sensory experiences internally. We process information in the following ways:

- Visually.
- Auditorily.
- Kinaesthetically.
- Olfactorily.
- Gustatorily.

In other words, we see, hear, feel, smell and taste, then process this internally to form our understanding of the world (Freeth, 2016). The activities that we provide for a learner to develop understanding of the situation need to incorporate differing aspects of these sensory processes. Individuals have preferences for certain sensory modes in differing situations. Therefore, you might match your instructional approach with a student's preferred method of processing information – that is, visually, auditorily, kinaesthetically, and to a lesser extent olfactorily and gustatorily. However, as you cannot always easily find out individual preference in instructional situations, we must consider varying our activities to ensure that we do match them at least on some level.

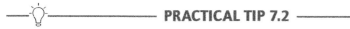 **PRACTICAL TIP 7.2**

The use of pictures, drawings, diagrams or objects might satisfy those with a visual preference. Discussion, questions and answers or reading some narrative about the topic might satisfy those with an auditory preference. Getting hands-on experience and being involved in completing tasks might satisfy those with a kinaesthetic preference, and so on. The use of all these types of activity might produce a sensory-rich learning approach in which the learner can develop in relation to the aspect that they are learning.

It is important to consider these different sensory modes and preferences as they play a large part in learning and instruction.

———————————————— **ACTIVITY 7.6** ————————————————

Think of the sensory mode from which you most prefer to learn: visual, auditory or kinaesthetic.

1   What kinds of activities appeal to that preference?
2   For example, do you prefer to be shown things such as diagrams or pictures?
3   Do you prefer discussions or questions and answers about topics?
4   Do you prefer hands-on practical experiences?
5   If you like all these approaches, which one do you have the strongest preference for?

Multiple intelligences

Howard Gardner (1993) developed the concept of people demonstrating preferences for different modes in different situations and challenged the previously accepted concept that intelligence could only be measured by using Intelligent Quotient (IQ) tests. He suggested that, because of these preferences for different sensory processes, individuals expressed their intelligence in different ways and therefore could be disadvantaged by the former established ways of assessing intelligence. He named these 'multiple intelligences'. Basically, someone might not be able to solve problems using one processing approach but may be able to do so if they use the approach that they prefer. These multiple intelligences or processing preferences are as follows.

- Visual/spatial.
- Verbal/linguistic.
- Logical/mathematical.
- Bodily/kinaesthetic.
- Musical/rhythmical.
- Interpersonal.
- Intrapersonal.

The notion here is that you can assist a student to learn, by either matching their preferred 'intelligence' or by using a variety of approaches to ensure that their preference is at least not missed.

⌾ ─────────── **PRACTICAL TIP 7.3** ───────────

Following the above approach may not always be easy in busy clinical areas, so the aspect of getting to know the learner well is important. Then you can involve them in activities and situations in which they can best learn.

Experiential learning

An approach considered within the cognitive school that assists in the process of multiple intelligences mentioned above is experiential learning. This is a bridge between the theory of learning and the concept of preferences for learning styles. It is an approach proposed by Kolb (1984) based on the previous work of Lewin and includes the concepts of assimilation and accommodation purported by Piaget (Aubrey and Riley, 2016). In the experiential learning cycle, the student goes through several stages in order to optimize the learning potential.

Kolb argued the importance of the person–environment interaction, and therefore the experiences that the learner has and the way in which they process the information. According to Hughes and Quinn (2013), Kolb sees learning as a core process of human development and not merely a readjustment to change. Learning is recognized as being 'gained through experience'. This gave rise to the concept of the experiential learning cycle.

- **Concrete experience (CE).**
  This is the actual event or activity. Being involved enables individuals to become immersed in actual clinical learning situations.
- **Reflective observation (RO).**
  This occurs after the event, allowing the learner to reflect on their experiences from different perspectives.
- **Abstract conceptualization (AC).**
  This stage is used to develop explanations of what has happened, come up with new ideas, and begin to understand logical theoretical approaches to be applied in the situation in future.
- **Active experimentation (AE).**
  This is then used to test developing hypotheses as a problem-solving approach in practice.

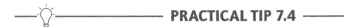

PRACTICAL TIP 7.4

When instructing a student in the clinical area, these phases following the experiential learning cycle are important.

1   Provide the student with the experience.
2   Follow this up with some time for discussion and reflection on the situation and gather information about it.
3   The next stage is to include some problem-solving exercises or question and answer sessions based on the theoretical knowledge necessary for the situation.
4   Finally, the student needs more supervised practice in the situation to establish the knowledge and skills needed in the specific context. In doing so, learning from experience should take place.

Let's reflect on this a little more.

ACTIVITY 7.7

Think of a skill that you learned in the clinical area. Reflect on this and identify the parts of the skill development that linked to the stages above.

1   What forms did this take?
2   Did you always go through the whole experiential learning cycle or only parts of it?
3   Which parts of the cycle did you prefer?

It is important to note in this theory that the concepts of concrete experience and abstract conceptualization are opposites. The same is true of reflective observation and active experimentation. Both have, on one side, some involvement in the practical arena and, on the other side, more internal or information-gathering and problem-solving processes. According to Hughes and Quinn (2013), this relates to preference of perception (how information is taken in by the individual, such as a preference for concrete experience or abstract conceptualization) or a preference for processing (how information is internalized, either by active experimentation or reflective observation). However, it must be noted that although it is popular as a tool in health professional education and curricula it is not necessarily supported by empirical evidence.

The theories of brain-based learning – multiple intelligences and experiential learning – provide an opportunity to further discuss the concept of learning style preferences. This is because they allude to individual preferences in cognitive style, sensory modality and instructional approach.

Learning styles

As mentioned earlier, learning styles are preferences of students for an approach towards the subject matter to be learned. McKenna et al. (2018: 280) suggest that:

> learning styles refer to the way in which individuals approach learning situations to process information.

In 1983 Curry proposed that learning styles fell into different categories (see Figure 7.6).

- The inner circle, **personality traits**, refers to aspects of an individual's personality. These are considered fairly fixed and unchangeable.
- The middle circle, **information processing style**, refers to the ways that the students cognitively deal with their learning experience and how they prefer to process the required information for learning. These are fairly stable but can be adapted.
- The outer circle, **instructional preferences**, refers to the methods of instruction most liked by individuals. This is fairly changeable.

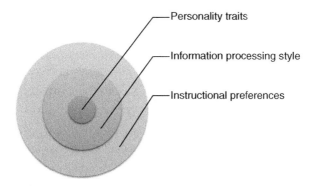

Figure 7.6 Onion model (adapted from Curry, 1983)

McKenna et al. (2018) go on to state that the association between learning styles and learning achievements remains contentious, so some caution needs to be applied. In a systematic review by Coffield et al. (2004), several issues were raised regarding the use of learning styles; the authors pointed out that care must be taken before you apply the use of learning styles without carefully considering their validity and usefulness. The review showed that validity and reliability was questionable in several learning style theories and tools. The authors do point out, however, that it is accepted that the main value in understanding the concept of learning styles is for students/learners to be able to raise their awareness of their own and others' learning styles as a self-awareness activity. It is beyond the remit of this chapter to discuss all learning-style theories and tools; instead, the learning styles proposed by Kolb (1984) and Honey and Mumford (1992) and the VARK tool developed by Neil Fleming in 1987 (Fleming, 2014) will be discussed here, as they are very commonly used in nursing education.

Kolb

Kolb (1984) suggests that if individuals prefer certain types of learning at specific points of the experiential learning cycle, then they may prefer that particular style of learning more broadly (see Figure 7.7). Therefore, at various points within the cycle various styles are developed.

- Between concrete experience and reflective observation, the learning style is known as being a '**Diverger**'. This means that you may be imaginative and aware of meaning and values and prefer observation to action.
- Between reflective observation and abstract conceptualization, the learning style is known as being an '**Assimilator**'. This style suggests a preference for reasoning, having ideas and logical problem-solving.
- Between abstract conceptualization and active experimentation, the learning style is known as being a '**Converger**'. This style suggests being good at solving practical problems and making decisions.
- Between active experimentation and concrete experience, the learning style is known as being an '**Accommodator**'. This style means that you are intuitive and can adapt to changing situations using trial and error.

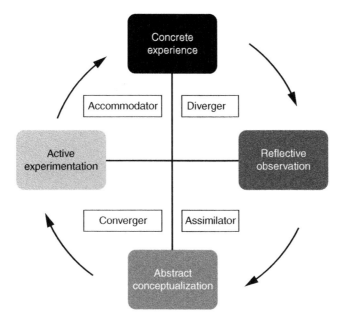

Figure 7.7 Learning styles (Kolb, 1984)

Kolb, D.A. (© 2015) *Experiential Learning: Experience as the Source of Learning and Development* (2nd edn). Reprinted by permission of Pearson Education, Inc., New York

By identifying students' preferences and matching the sensory mode, cognitive or instructional approach, optimal learning should be achieved. Kolb suggested that students tend to fall into one of the learning style classifications due to their past experiences and then develop preferences for that approach. Therefore, developing (matching) instruction methods towards those preferences should benefit the learner. Kolb developed the 'Learning Style Inventory' (LSI) which was a questionnaire designed with behavioural statements that represented each learning style, which when analysed suggested which style was preferred. However, Coffield et al. (2004) suggested there was little validity to the instrument. Despite this it still appears to be one of the most popular considerations in education.

Honey and Mumford

Honey and Mumford (1992) accepted and built upon Kolb's model, but disagree with the polar nature of the preferences and argue that each individual style has strengths of its own. This means that an individual can be an 'all-rounder', meaning they can learn in differing situations, or maybe just have a preference of one learning style, suggesting that that approach will provide the best learning experience for them. They accept the main premise of Kolb's styles, but have a different perspective from him.

Honey and Mumford's styles (1992) are as follows:

- **Activists.**
  This style relates to Kolb's concrete experience preference. Someone with this preference would prefer here-and-now activities and like to get involved in lots of new activities. However, they often get bored once into a project and look for new experiences.
- **Reflectors.**
  This is similar to Kolb's reflective observation preference. Individuals with this preference like to gather information and ponder all perspectives before making decisions. They are likely to keep diaries and listen to all sides of a debate.
- **Theorists.**
  This is similar to Kolb's abstract conceptualization preference. People with this preference like problem-solving and logical approaches based on evidence and knowledge.
- **Pragmatists.**
  This is similar to Kolb's active experimentation. This is applying what is learned in practice. People with a preference for this style like to try things out in practice and experiment with new techniques and approaches.

According to Bates (2016) the style preferences relate to:

1 How the person takes in information: through **doing** (activists) or **thinking** (theorists).
2 How the person internalizes information: through **observing** (reflectors) or **experimenting** (pragmatists).

Honey and Mumford suggested that different, less-established preferences of the individual can be developed by widening the repertoire of the types of learning activity to which they are exposed. In a similar way to Kolb, they also designed a 'Learning Style

Questionnaire' (LSQ) to be used to ascertain the individual strength of preference for each style.

VARK

More recently the **Visual – Aural – Read/Write – Kinaesthetic (VARK)** learning styles tool developed by Fleming (Fleming, 2014) has become popular in the education and health professional education fields (Stirling, 2017). This is very similar to the concept of 'multiple intelligence'. Stirling (2017) suggests the tool has been well tested and is a simple, straightforward tool to use. It is easy for students to complete and for staff to interpret.

* **Visual** – Students learn best from visual aids and demonstrations.
* **Aural** – Students learn best from verbal explanations.
* **Read/Write** – Students learn best from text-based materials.
* **Kinaesthetic** – Students learn best from interactive, hands on experiences.

Abbott and Shaw (2018) suggest these classifications help in identifying students' preferred style for learning and aid the instructor in designing activities to match these.

McKenna et al. (2018) found that nursing students were multimodal learners suggesting that more than one mode is preferred and that students can learn from a variety of approaches.

In considering learning styles, the main premise is to understand that individuals all learn differently, so if only one approach is used, then some learning will not appear accessible to some students. Ideally, some form of assessment (or, indeed, the use of a formal tool such as the LSQ, LSI or VARK) to ascertain individual preferred styles should be completed so that the most appropriate type of instructional method that matches the style of the individual learner can be employed for effective learning to take place. Alternatively, in the absence of such knowledge or in dealing with larger groups of individuals, a variety of techniques need to be employed for learners to be able to take best advantage of the learning opportunities available. However, caution should be taken due to the criticisms that have been highlighted about the validity of the concept of learning styles.

ACTIVITY 7.8

Having read the descriptions of learning styles given above (Kolb, Honey and Mumford or VARK):

1   Which would you prefer, and why?
2   What kinds of learning activities do you engage with most and which ones provide you with the most effective means of learning?
3   How would you apply these with the learners you may supervise?

Humanistic learning theories

The final topic related to learning theories to be discussed is humanistic learning theory, sometimes referred to as adult learning theory (Hughes and Quinn, 2013). In behavioural learning theory, the locus of control is external to the student as the instructor manipulates the environment and the reinforcers or punishers; in cognitive learning theory, the locus of control could be considered as shared between the instructor and the learner, as some more explorative approaches are used rather than straightforward stimulus–responses. Humanistic theory places the locus of control firmly with the learner. It differs in that the principle suggests that the learner is the one that brings with them the motivation to learn; therefore, the supervisor needs to act as a facilitator rather than instructor, or as is commonly stated in the anecdote, 'a guide on the side as opposed to a sage on the stage'. Candela (2020) suggests this main difference is because humanistic learning theory deals with the value, worth, dignity and integrity of individuals. It has as a fundamental principle consideration of the capacity for human growth and development and an individualistic approach. Race (2015) suggests that maximizing potential for the learner is paramount in the humanistic theory. It is now much more accepted that teaching skills for personal success is about creating access and opportunity for all regardless of status.

The main theorists to consider within this field are Maslow (1954), Malcolm Knowles (1980) and Carl Rogers (Rogers and Freiburg, 1994). As mentioned earlier, Maslow's hierarchy of needs does form a basis for how individuals' learning can be reinforced by having their needs met. In the humanistic learning theory, the higher-level needs of communication, self-esteem, and self-actualization are the internal drivers and motivators for the individual to pursue learning, therefore suggesting that the individual comes with a desire and a preparedness to learn. Maslow's concept of self-actualization is a major motivator and driver for individuals wishing to experience new or further learning opportunities. Hughes and Quinn (2013) suggest that Maslow basically referred to self-actualization as the person becoming the best that they can be and is related to discovering their identity and purpose or destiny. However, they point out that there are criticisms due to the cases on which the theory was based and that there are exceptions to the rules suggested.

Merriam (2018: 84) describes the humanistic perspective as 'focussed more on how adulthood could be distinguished from childhood learning'. The formal type of education (which is usually applied to children) is known as 'pedagogy', which basically means the art and science of teaching children (note that the term 'pedagogy' is also a term used to describe teaching methods or strategies). According to Candela (2020), Malcolm Knowles introduced the term 'andragogy' as a concept relating to the teaching of adults. Knowles believed the art and science of teaching adults is different from strategies required with children.

In this philosophy it is suggested that adults come with their own motivating factors, individual preferences and aspirations. They can make their own decisions, so therefore, in respecting this, adult learners may enter into some form of agreement with the teacher as to how best to meet their own individual needs. Obviously, in nursing, some of these outcomes are set, for example, in the NMC (2018b) standards of proficiency and the various learning outcomes incorporated into nursing courses. However, processes should be in place whereby the individual identifies and negotiates what and how they need to learn to achieve the outcomes. This is a basic tenet of adult learning and humanistic approaches.

Facilitating in adult learning

According to Hughes and Quinn (2013), Carl Rogers suggested that the instructional role is being a facilitator. Negotiations take place with the individual and a 'learning contract' is developed. A learning contract should include aspects such as the learning outcomes to be achieved, some sort of personal development plan that might identify the strengths, needs and goals, a description of learning actions and the activities to be undertaken, and an agreement of the product and evidence to be produced to demonstrate achievement of the outcomes. In doing so, each individual learner may have very different approaches to achieving the outcomes, but the outcomes and the standards still remain, and quality is maintained. So, as a practice supervisor you may take up a coaching role, giving advice, suggestions and acting as a support mechanism for the student when they are undertaking their learning journey.

In order to be successful in such a facilitator/coaching role, Carl Rogers suggested that there is a fundamental requirement for the facilitator to embody unconditional positive regard incorporating trust, empathy and genuineness. Unconditional positive regard is the polar opposite to the conditional aspects of behavioural learning theory, whereby conditions are firmly put in place before rewards and reinforcements, sanctions or punishments are provided. It means that there is a sense of acceptance and respect about the learner with no conditions on that acceptance. However, it is a form of mutual responsibility and the student should also therefore show respect to the facilitator. Race (2015) states that Rogers' principle of facilitation is not a didactic role, rather it means that the facilitator should enter a professional relationship with the learner, thereby embodying the personhood of both, and breaking down barriers so that learning will not be affected by power or authority. The basis of ensuring good facilitation is the art of communicating well on an adult level with the learner. Outcomes need to be identified and, in nurse education, these outcomes are givens and are basically non-negotiable in order to meet NMC requirements; however, how you meet them is negotiable. In teaching junior nurses, you quickly need to establish trust. This means that you need to act as a role model without expecting them to do things that you would not be prepared to do yourself. It is important that you are aware of current evidence-based practices to deliver appropriate, relevant and best advice to the students.

ACTIVITY 7.9

Think of the practice supervisors/assessors with whom you have worked.

1   What steps did they take to gain your trust?
2   How did they negotiate your planned learning experiences to meet your course requirements?
3   How did you recognize when unconditional positive regard was being employed with you?

Teaching

In this section teaching approaches that can be utilized in practice by newly qualified nurses will be discussed. Teaching methods, as mentioned earlier in the chapter, are sometimes referred to as 'pedagogy', which Muijs and Reynolds (2018) describe as effective teaching. Pedagogy is a term originally used interchangeably to refer to teaching children, which was also later applied to all teaching strategies including those related to adults, before Knowles' concept of 'Andragogy' was introduced (Merriam and Bierema, 2013).

Constructive alignment prompts the health professional to consider the following questions:

1 **What do I want the learner to know?** (Intended learning outcomes.)
2 **How will the learners optimally learn this?** (Type and sequence of teaching and learning activities.)
3 **How will I know the learners have learnt this?** (Assessment.)

Croy (2018) outlines that taking these factors into account, as well as the attributes expected of the graduating student, should lead to deep learning and the ability to make sense of the larger picture. Therefore careful planning is required to structure teaching approaches that suit the needs of the student and their requirements.

Setting a learning outcome is the first stage in ensuring alignment in learning. According to Race (2015), learning outcomes should be more than official statements in course documents – they should underpin all teaching and learning situations. Setting clearly identifiable learning outcomes can be done in a discussion with the student or more formally written into their assessment documentation. The outcomes should include the person completing the outcome (the learner, the student, you, etc.) and what they need to do ('will administer an intramuscular injection', 'will record a clients' history', 'will complete a behavioural assessment'), when they will do it ('at the end of the session', 'by the end of today', 'by the end of the placement'), and the degree of success needed to complete it ('successfully', 'independently', 'under supervision', etc.).

The following are some examples of learning outcomes.

- 'You will administer an intramuscular injection by the end of today under supervision'.

- 'The learner will record a client's history by the end of this week independently'.
- 'The student will complete a behavioural assessment of a client by [specific date (e.g. 1 January)] independently'.

Sometimes, more formal learning outcomes are written, with a stem statement such as:

- 'By the end of this teaching session [module, course, etc.], the student will be able to demonstrate ...'

Following the stem statement, the actual required behaviour/activity/skill of the student is included, using such verbs as described in Bloom's taxonomy earlier.

1 'By the end of this teaching session [module, course, etc.], the student will be able to demonstrate **knowledge** of the principles of anatomy and physiology'.
2 'By the end of this teaching session [module, course, etc.], the student will be able to demonstrate an **understanding** of the principles of anatomy and physiology'.
3 'By the end of this teaching session [module, course, etc.], the student will be able to demonstrate **application** of the principles of anatomy and physiology'.
4 'By the end of this teaching session [module, course, etc.], the student will be able to demonstrate **evaluation** of the principles of anatomy and physiology'.

In each of the above cases, deeper levels of learning need to be demonstrated. Therefore, the way in which these outcomes are tested would need to be different.

1 A simple multiple-choice test might be used to examine their knowledge.
2 A deeper question requiring some explanation in the answer (written or verbal) might be used.
3 An observed structured clinical examination (OSCE), which involves the direct observation of clinical skills assessed using a checklist, might be used to ascertain how skilled they are at applying their knowledge by working with a patient (usually simulated in exam conditions but can be in real-world context).

4   Some problem-solving or research answering a specific assign-
    ment might be used to probe the depth of their knowledge of how
    principles are transferable across different fields, perhaps even
    followed up by some oral questioning or 'viva voce' (live voice)
    examination.

Plan

The starting point in teaching is planning. As a practice supervisor
some situations may be spontaneous and opportunistic, as they occur
in practice, so there may not be enough time to plan thoroughly. For
all other situations, time must be spent on thinking about the instruction or formally planning it. This would usually include some consideration of detail of the students involved, the aim of the teaching and
learning outcomes to be achieved, teacher activity, student activity,
times and venues, methods of assessment, and methods of evaluation
(Hughes and Quinn, 2013). In order to do this, it is useful to be aware
of how learning theories are applied and the level of Bloom's taxonomy at which outcomes are expected to be demonstrated. Jakeman
et al. (2017) suggest undertaking a survey of learners' expectations
prior to any learning and teaching session. For example, dependent
on the maturity of the student, you may use Kolb's (1984) experiential
learning theory to scaffold new information with what they already
know. In relation to clinical teaching in practice, Bandura's social
learning theory where they learn from others through role modelling
may be appropriate. You may need to understand the principle of positive reinforcement theory, applying Skinner and Thorndike's work
where people learn when they are motivated by reward, i.e. passing
the programme or receiving praise from the patient, practice supervisor, practice assessor or academic assessor.

Learning environments

One of the major factors you would need to consider within your plan
is the environment in which the learning and teaching takes place.
This includes the venue, equipment, resources, reducing potential
distractions and ensuring it is appropriate for the teaching method
employed. It also means ensuring that you create a climate for learning where physical, psychological and social factors are addressed
adequately for the student, and are rewarding for them (Muijs and

Reynolds, 2018). You must consider similar environmental aspects within the clinical area, ensuring they are appropriate for the function of the aspect to be practised and, like all nursing resources and equipment, should be well-maintained. These principles should also be transferred into ensuring the learning environment is appropriate for the function of teaching the student(s).

Resources should be prepared and available before the instruction is given. Scheduled or timetabled use of rooms is advisable, but sometimes the learning experience may present itself spontaneously. Communication with other members of staff is important as they also will need to know when the instruction is occurring.

A clinical environment is an authentic learning environment for learning many aspects of nursing. However, sometimes it may be necessary to deliver the teaching in an area away from the clinical environment. Hughes and Quinn (2013) highlight that environments where learning is facilitated should be non-threatening so the learning itself is valued and can be reflected upon, more than focusing on the impact any negative environmental factors may have had. This requires careful planning and preparation. It is important to remember how Maslow's hierarchy of needs can influence a learner's experience of the event. So, for example, temperature and ventilation can affect physiological needs, the state and upkeep of the environment can affect safety, noise and other distractions can affect communication, and so on.

Structure

In whatever environment or situation you may find yourself in when teaching, such as informal or formal clinical settings, or in formal teaching environments, you need to ensure you create and follow a structured approach to achieve optimum outcomes. According to Scheckel (2020) a structured approach consisting of identified clear goals, precise content and processes allows students to function with a great deal of independence whilst adhering to the rules and focusing on outcomes. Therefore, the structure of the session needs careful thought, but can follow a simple format, as suggested in the adage of 'tell, tell and tell'. This basically means you should tell them what you will tell them (expected outcomes), tell them (provide content), and then tell them what you have told them (recap and evaluate). In other words, provide an 'introduction' outlining what will occur in the session and stating the learning objectives. The next aspect is 'development', in which these aspects are fully explored. Finally, there is the 'conclusion', in which the content discussed is summarized as a review. This structure should be used in any form of teaching approach whether formal, informal or opportunistic.

Muijs and Reynolds (2018) suggest that teaching approaches fall into three distinct types, into which most strategies can be classified.

- **Direct instruction.**
  This is where the authority lies with the teacher and includes information giving and demonstrations.
- **Interactive teaching.**
  Here, students are encouraged to participate and provide answers or raise questions in more discursive forums, seminars or coaching approaches.
- **Constructivist teaching.**
  This relates to problem-based approaches, in which there is some responsibility on behalf of the student to undertake some exploration and information-gathering to solve a 'real-world' problem.

Some sessions with students will incorporate one or more, if not all, of these aspects. Whilst there is a growing emphasis on technology, Sinclair et al. (2017) argue that teaching approaches should not necessarily be sacrificed for 'edutainment' style instructional design. It is important that authentic strategies are used for learners to make connections from their learning to clinical practice.

Methods

Gopee (2018) rightly points out that as a healthcare provider your main priority is in attending to the needs of your service users. Teaching activities may be more sporadic and opportune, as well as timetabled teaching activities with specific learners. In working as a practice supervisor, you may take a student-centred approach whereby you recognize the needs, learning styles and placement requirements for the students and plan a programme of events for them, as well as taking advantage of learning opportunities that arise whilst providing care in the clinical environment. Although opportune, it may be useful to work with the student in such incidences by using Kolb's (1984) experiential learning cycle as a basis for ensuring that concrete practice experiences are reflected upon, critically analysed and ideas that the students can then try out in practice can be developed under your supervision.

In direct instruction, you may be utilizing more didactic approaches as a teaching method. If taking place in the practice setting, this may be along the lines of a short presentation to a small group of individuals. A mini-lecture (in similar ways to a large-scale lecture) is an efficient way of sharing information quickly (Hughes and Quinn, 2013). Care must be taken in using technology to present the information, such as 'PowerPoint' or other presentation platforms. Just as with learning environments, visual aids should be neat, tidy, uncluttered and spacious. The information should be kept to a minimum and the points explained. Further detail can be developed through questioning or by providing supporting materials such as handouts. Non-verbal and verbal aspects need to be carefully orchestrated to create engagement with you as a presenter and to emphasize relevant or important points. It is also important for managing the students and any disruptions that may occur (Race, 2015).

Another form of direct instruction is by providing a demonstration. This might be in the practice area or in a lab or simulation area. Simulated learning involves imitating some facet of life, such as the use of equipment, including mannequins or actors who take on roles of patients (Hughes and Quinn, 2013).

Demonstration

A demonstration is described by Hughes and Quinn (2013) as a visualized explanation of facts or principles. The number of students observing such a demonstration needs to be carefully considered, as the presence of too many students will restrict the effectiveness of what can be observed, or what can be asked about the procedure. Once again, all equipment should be prepared and be in working order, and all needed resources should be at hand. Demonstrations should be broken down into clear steps with a clear step-by-step commentary. Feedback following opportunity to practise the skills should be delivered quickly (Gopee, 2018).

Simulated learning

Simulated learning (SL) is a popular educational technique that allows interactive and immersive activity by recreating all, or part, of a clinical experience. Real patients are therefore not exposed to risks as these activities take place in simulation laboratories using equipment and models that recreate authentic clinical situations (Unsworth et al., 2016). These models vary from very simple replicas of parts of the body to very high-fidelity computerized mannequins. Presado et al. (2018) point out that SL replicates real-life situations and the nature and proximity normally found in them which can be imitated in differing modalities (i.e. the further away learning is from the actual reality of a situation, the lower the fidelity). To attain high fidelity, technology and situations that aim to closely mimic real-life incidents should be used in a secure and safe setting. Wiseman and Horton (2011) suggest that simulation-based education (SBE) requires scenarios that create visual, tactile and auditory situations that replicate as closely as possible the situations found in daily clinical practice. According to Nystrom et al. (2016), there are three main phases when implementing SL. These are briefing, simulation and de-briefing. When briefing, the context of the scenario or problem is presented to the students. From this they would problem-solve and demonstrate how the solution might be applied in the situation. Finally, the students would be debriefed about what was correct or not, and what changes would help improve the situation. As this takes place on mannequins or other technological devices there is no risk of any real person being harmed.

Small group interactive teaching

Using demonstrations could be considered as interactive teaching. However, interactive teaching can also be small individual or group sessions, such as seminars or tutorials. These methods align with the student-centred humanistic approaches that have developed over the past 30 years. According to Race (2015) as education systems either utilize large lectures for economic rationalization due to growing numbers, or more digital methods, small group teaching is more important than we think. This is due to the fact that it is about getting people to work together and producing a collaborative environment where people learn together and can develop a range of transferable interactive skills not available in large lectures or online. Small group teaching might include role play, discussions, setting up of debates or microteaching (Hughes and Quinn, 2013). The skills of questioning need developing as well as the ability to 'scaffold' learning, which means developing a basic understanding of the topic, then discussing increasingly complex aspects of the area under study. Things to consider are forming of groups, group size and group activities which all need to be carefully managed to avoid dominance of individuals or some participants acting as passengers (Race, 2015).

Problem-based learning (PBL)

Constructivist teaching basically means providing the student with problems, or exercises, in which they need to seek out information to answer them. Sullivan (2020) highlights that problem-solving such as PBL improves outcomes, peer working, interpersonal skills, critical thinking and confidence. It is based on the delivery of a trigger or scenario reflecting real-world problems. There is a period of group facilitation to highlight information inherent in the situation, to develop hypotheses, and to identify gaps in knowledge. Following this, there is a period of self-directed study during which students appraise evidence and return to the group to provide answers or solutions to the problem at hand (Phillips, 2020).

Simply put, PBL is an approach that reflects a structure whereby students are directed around a problem and need some self-discipline to find the solution. Muijs and Reynolds (2018) suggest that any such approach follows a basis of a start phase in which the problem is given, an exploration phase in which the problem is analysed and information gathered, a reflection phase in which the information is shared and reconstructed in light of the problem, and finally an application and discussion phase, in which the problem is solved and the learning gained is extrapolated and identified.

Assessment

As a qualified nurse, you may find yourself involved informally or formally in the assessment of student nurses. The role of practice assessor is one that you may find appealing once you have settled into your role as a qualified nurse. A nurse can become a practice assessor when registered and with 'appropriate equivalent experience for the student's field of practice' (NMC, 2018e: 8). They must demonstrate preparation or prior evidence of learning relevant to the role and receive ongoing training as well as being appraised of the proficiencies and outcomes for the courses their students undertake. A practice assessor should not be the same person acting as a student's practice supervisor. As a nurse you may find yourself in both roles but not with the same student.

As a newly qualified nurse, although not a practice assessor, you may be expected to participate in assessments in the practice area by observing and giving feedback on a student's progress to the practice assessor.

Lidster and Wakefield (2019) in reviewing the NMC (2018e) standards suggest that assessment has the following main aims:

- To provide a basis for job selection.
- To contribute to the development of effective practice learning environments.
- To maintain standards through governance and accountability.
- To motivate learners and inform them of their progress.
- To escalate concerns regarding failing students.
- To inform academic assessors (and, in this case, practice assessors/supervisors) about students' fitness to practise and confirmation of proficiency.

As a newly qualified nurse, you may get the opportunity to be involved in some selection interviews, but it is the last four aims of assessment that are most important for you. The practice assessor/supervisor's responsibilities are related to assisting in the development and progress of the learner and in making sure that standards are met. Race (2015) suggests that the purpose of assessment is for students to set their sights high and be able to achieve their intended outcomes. It is the final analysis which determines their qualifications and future careers. Therefore, the practice assessor should communicate what the 'goalposts' are and provide instruction on the nature of how they will be assessed and on what they will be assessed.

Hughes and Quinn (2013) suggest that assessment serves the purpose of providing valuable feedback to the student on their performance, development and progress, and whether learning has taken place. Ultimately, it leads to a judgement as to whether they are worthy of a publicly recognized award and right to practice.

Types of assessment

Muijs and Reynolds (2018) suggest that assessment takes up one-third of a teacher/practice assessor's time. This shows how interlinked teaching and assessment are: they could be considered within the same continuum of learning, and there could not be learning without both instruction and assessment. There are two important types of assessment.

- **Formative:** this is where information is gathered in an ongoing manner and the student is provided with feedback about how they are performing. It can still be a formal process. This type of assessment has being found to have a positive effect on achievement.
- **Summative:** this is where final judgements on the student's performance against specified criteria are made. This type of assessment is used as the quality control mechanism and to ensure that appropriate standards are met.

————————————————— ACTIVITY 7.10 —————————————————

Reflect on your nursing course and your experiences of assessment in practice.

1   What types of assessment have been used in order for competencies to be passed in your portfolio?
2   From the methods used by the practice assessors whom you had, what were the most beneficial approaches used to provide formative feedback?

How to provide feedback

When providing feedback on students, it is important that the mechanisms of judgement-making are understood. Assessment can be judged by the performance of the learner compared with others, known as 'norm referencing', or they can be judged by their performance against given criteria, known as 'criterion referencing'. The latter is often used as a basis in nursing and higher education in order that the learners demonstrate that they meet the minimum standards required (knowledge of content and demonstration of skills).

Norm and criterion referencing

Gopee (2018) suggests that norm referencing is where the individual can have their performance compared with their peers; any deficiencies are highlighted, providing an opportunity to identify needs and actions to be taken to improve performance. Norm referencing can often highlight the expectations related to levels of performance: for example, more would be expected of a third-year nurse than a first-year nurse in relation to certain activities (this may also be reflected in the expectations within the criteria). By comparing results on a group level adjustments can be made in order to reflect the performance of the individual against the group as a whole.

Criterion referencing is an evaluation of performance decided against pre-determined criteria (Gopee, 2018). This is because the knowledge, skills and competence of the learner must be accounted for against statutory requirements. The development of assessment criteria is important to create reliability in the assessment process. This is almost the same as producing a checklist of aspects that can be ticked off on completion, or a set of behaviours describing how well someone has completed the task. The criteria are important, as ideally what is wanted is that at least two or more assessors can arrive at the same decision considering the facts observed. This is known as inter-rater reliability.

An example of criterion referencing taken from the NMC (2018b: 18) standards of proficiency is:

> demonstrate the knowledge, skills and confidence to provide
> first aid procedures and basic life support.

This is a set standard, but problems with interpretation may still arise, as criteria will still need to be established for determining terms such as 'skills and confidence', and there is a need for a clearer definition of what 'first aid procedures' are and how they can be identified and measured. A good assessor will explore such criteria with the learner, identifying, negotiating and agreeing on the terms and how they are demonstrated in the real-world context. For example, while working with people with learning disabilities in the community, you might discuss with a student specialist approaches to communicating, such as using sign language or a communication board, for those with limited communication abilities.

Hence, getting to know the student, identifying clear outcomes, providing supportive instruction, stating the method of assessment, and then making unambiguous decisions on the performance of the outcome is an important and continuous process.

ACTIVITY 7.11

Look back over your nursing practice portfolio. Identify the factors involved that were related to formative assessment.

1   How were these structured and what processes occurred?
2   In what way were the summative elements approached differently?
3   Identify aspects that were norm-referenced and those that were criterion-referenced.

In your portfolio, there will be some proficiencies or competencies that you are required to pass. These might be considered as criterion assessments. Feedback where you are compared with your peers or others, perhaps with feedback such as 'you performed at a higher standard than expected for your stage of training', might be considered norm referencing.

Assessment in practice

Throughout a nursing course, students will have been exposed to a variety of assessment methods in their formal educational setting. These may include seen and unseen timed examinations, production of assignments and essays, OSCEs and individual or group presentations. Students will come into the clinical area with specific sets of competencies that are expected to be demonstrated in order to satisfy the NMC (2018b) proficiencies. Hughes and Quinn (2013) suggest that assessment in the workplace may revolve around how the student constructs their personal practice portfolio, which may include reflective diaries as well as the competencies needed to be achieved. The main method of assessing a student's progress is by observing them in practice as they complete their required skills and tasks.

Observation

It is important that an effort is made in the relationship-building aspect, as being observed can be quite unnerving for the student.

The observations may be rated against a checklist developed to identify the stages of the task and the criteria against which the student is being judged. Observations could be made in close proximity or in a more 'long-arm' fashion. However, a practice assessor cannot sign off a competence for a student if they have not actually observed it themselves or have not been provided with reliable testimony of observations from other recognized practice supervisors.

A checklist for assessment

Overall, it is important that assessment:

- Is valid, reliable, consistent, fair and honest.
- Has closely aligned learning outcomes, teaching activities and methods of assessment.
- Includes the student being given appropriate feedback that is commensurate to their performance and supportive of their further development.

ACTIVITY 7.12

Think of how you have been assessed in practice.

1   How were the assessments set up?
2   How were the observations conducted?
3   How were you provided with feedback?
4   What techniques were used to put you at ease?

Evaluation of learning

The NMC (2018d) outline that evaluation of learning is an important factor as it is linked to educational governance and quality.

By evaluating students' experiences, further lessons may be learned and changes incorporated to improve future learning situations (Hughes and Quinn, 2013).

Evaluation can be:

- Formal or informal.
- Systemic or episodic.
- Formative or summative.

Howard (2009) suggested that evaluation is important to improve outcomes, teaching processes, learning achievement and ultimately patient/client care. They argue there are two major components of evaluation, as follows:

- To evaluate factual/physical aspects linked to learning outcomes, all of which are easily measurable. (Has learning occurred?)
- To evaluate systems and processes that support and contribute to the fixed components of the course. (Are the mechanisms working in an appropriately supportive way?)

Most nursing courses have formal ways of evaluating students' experiences throughout their education. These might be on a modular level or at course level. There are also mechanisms to explore their learning experiences while in practice. There might be tripartite meetings between the student, their personal tutor, and their practice assessor/supervisor in the clinical area. Evaluation may be required as a part of their formal portfolio documentation, and they may need to complete this as part of their mandatory requirements.

If an evaluation is completed formally, then there is usually some sort of questionnaire or instrument designed for the purpose. Most of these are answered anonymously, but it can also be transparent by identifying who filled in a questionnaire, if necessary. Race (2015) suggests that involving students in self-assessment and peer assessment can help them to build confidence in their own abilities and in providing evaluative information. This increases their confidence and they can draw up the agendas for what is to be evaluated. As a newly qualified nurse, you may not be called on very early in your career to be involved in devising formal evaluations. However, you may work with learners for whom there is a need for informal evaluation.

As discussed above, the main evaluative questions quite simply are as follows.

- **What have you learned?**
  This can be expanded to assess whether or not the student has learned aspects that reflect their intended learning outcomes and wider learning opportunities.

- **What has helped/hindered your learning experience(s)?**
  This can be expanded to include the student's thoughts and feelings related to environmental factors, the teaching and learning activities, and supportive mechanisms that they have experienced.
- **What could be done to further improve the learning experience for future students?**
  It is important to let the person know that their views are valid and that they are being listened to. However, it is also important not to change approaches immediately (unless there is something remarkably obvious that needs to be changed), as evaluations tell you how an individual perceives a situation, and because individuals perceive situations differently, change should only be considered if there are consistent evaluative comments requiring some need for change or improvement.

Summary

Newly qualified nurses have a crucial role to play in the practice-based education of student nurses, junior staff and often other health professionals. It is important that, alongside being a good role model, practice-based teaching and assessment follows these golden rules:

- Get to know your students and their course requirements.
- Understand the principles of learning and teaching.
- Set appropriate learning outcomes.
- Create environments that are physically, psychologically, and socially conducive for learning.
- Design relevant teaching and learning activities to optimize students' learning experiences.
- Use a range of assessment methods to ensure that students meet the learning outcomes.
- Provide constructive feedback on performance, including clarity on how to improve.
- Evaluate all aspects of the practice assessing/supervising/teaching experiences.

This chapter has looked at the NMC (2018e) standards in relation to supporting learning and assessment in practice. We have discussed learning theories and how these should shape our approaches to facilitating learning for students. The nature of assessment was discussed, as well as how to develop effective learning environments and teaching methods in a practice setting.

In this chapter, we have also looked at several learning, teaching, practice supervising and assessment approaches.

8

GETTING THE JOB THAT YOU WANT

Graham Ormrod and Rob Burton

THE AIMS OF THIS CHAPTER ARE TO:

- Offer strategies to assist you in finding and getting the job you want.
- Help you to reflect on your strengths and areas of development.
- Explore how best to prepare for interview.
- Assist you to match your strengths with the person specification.
- Offer insight into the interview procedures.
- Promote strategies on coping with disappointment and how to get the next job.

Introduction

You have come to an absolutely crucial time in your career not only as a student, but also with regards to your future career generally. No doubt you will have thought about this moment since you started your nursing course and probably even further back than that. Starting and successfully completing your course will have been the first few steps in what will hopefully be a long, exciting and fulfilling career.

You will probably have also been talking about job opportunities to your friends and colleagues more and more as the time for decision-making became closer and closer. Discussing your thoughts, plans and aspirations with those whom you trust can be very positive; however, this can also occasionally lead to *more* misunderstandings and confusion, and thereby raise, rather than reduce, anxiety at this already highly pressured time. Therefore, be cautious!

In this chapter, we will explore various ways of ensuring that you show yourself in the best light, help to increase the likelihood of getting your ideal job, and generally do yourself justice. It is important to remember, however, that despite what you might now think, there will always be more than one job out there for you. You might presently think:

> This job on the paediatric intensive care at the local trust is the only job for me.

Or

> Working in the team with that community psychiatric nurse who was so supportive when I had my placement there is an absolute must!

Considering very specifically the job that you would like is clearly an important step in actually getting it. However, the crucial stage here is consideration of *why* this particular job is so attractive. It is essential that, as far as is possible, the reality of the job is clear to you and that the reality meets both your current skills and expertise, and also your aspirations.

It is important to reduce the risk of becoming disheartened by putting 'all of your eggs in one basket'. One of the great things about nursing as a career is its variety – a variety that brings many different options and opportunities. Being able to recognize and grasp these opportunities, while matching them to your skills, experience and ambitions is a key part of finding a suitable and rewarding job.

So where might you start your career?

According to Hood (2017), every nurse has an established set of values – that is, values that they see as being important in their life. No two nurses share an identical set of values and selecting the ones that are the most important can be a difficult task. Nurses learn professional values as part of their socialization as a student, but some of these values can change over time. Hood (2017) suggests that certain areas of nursing generally cater to different sets of values. So, nurses who value technologically complex skills tend to pursue what might be broadly viewed as critical care environments. Depending on the field the nurse is in, this environment can be found in intensive peri-operative areas, accident and emergency, or some areas caring for individuals with particularly complex challenging behaviours. Nurses who place greater value on long-term relationships may choose to explore career options in other areas, such as in caring for those with long-term conditions, school nursing, or caring for clients with learning disabilities in their own homes. While not claiming to fully capture the complexities of the personal and professional context, this type of initial approach and consideration might help to work out where you see yourself heading in your career – not least because, as Hood (2017) further asserts, unlike most other professions, nursing offers many career opportunities that fit with a nurse's *personal* values and allows them to develop a personal vision of their future.

So, once you have identified your future vision and identified your career direction, what strategies might you use to make this happen? If you speak to your practice supervisor, practice assessor, mentor, personal tutor or other colleagues, they may tell you that they didn't arrive at their current job along a carefully crafted and meticulously planned career path, but that they took advantage of interesting opportunities as their insight and particular interests became clearer. While it may be true that most careers don't necessarily follow exact and predictable paths, it is also true that opportunities don't simply appear out of thin air and there is a need to be proactive in exploring any possibilities.

A structured 'linear' career path, if such a thing exists, would follow a sequential series of carefully judged steps and may best suit the nurse who enjoys structure and meeting designated deadlines.

> In three years, I will be a mentor or practice supervisor for students, by five I will be a charge nurse and by ten years I will be working as a nurse specialist in palliative care.

However, a lot of nurses have a fulfilling and enjoyable career following a far less 'linear' career path, relying more on unpredictable circumstances and key critical career incidents. Such paths are not totally random, however, and can still be formulated by considering particular and specific interests and relevant outside experiences, and then seizing the opportunities as they arise.

Nursing, and healthcare generally, takes place in a context of continual change, shifting demographics, innovation, rapidly evolving technologies and often challenging environments (NHS England, 2017a). This is probably truer now than ever before. Exploring and recognizing the possibility of a less linear path in your career *may* increase the likelihood of taking opportunities creatively as they arise and encourage a more flexible approach in times of such rapid change. However, it might conversely encourage a less focused approach to career development, leading to inertia and feelings of being 'left behind' *if* the individual nurse is not continually reflective of their current position and proactive in their exploration of career possibilities.

The term 'career mapping' can be used to denote the continuous process of career development. This is when any career changes unfold as the nurse engages in professional practice and lifelong learning, having identified their individual values, coupled with what Hood (2017: 552) calls an 'envisioning' of their nursing career. This overall vision, essentially picturing yourself in the future, creates a *blueprint* for personal action to make that envisioned future become reality.

Getting your ideal job can be very complicated. Some considerations are often called internal – that is, essentially about *you* – whereas others might be viewed as more external – for example, the current job market or the competition for the job that you want and so on.

One of the tools that can help clarify your thinking in relation to both internal and external issues of career planning is the **SWOT analysis** (Table 8.1). Much of the development of the SWOT analysis came from the area of sales and marketing, and in this context phrases such as internal (meaning the strengths and weaknesses of a particular organization) and external (the opportunities and threats from outside of the organization) might appear more appropriate and fitting. However, the process can also be very useful for an individual wishing to clarify their career planning.

Table 8.1 A partly completed example of a SWOT analysis

	Strengths	Weaknesses
I N T E R N A L	Current knowledge of specific clinical area from my placement	Newly qualified – therefore lack of experience
	Good teamworker	Need to stay in particular local area
	Enthusiastic and well motivated	First time had to apply for a job
	Chose the area for 'elective placement' so face is known	Nervous of 'blowing own trumpet'
	Opportunities	**Threats**
E X T E R N A L	Recent investment in the service – so opportunities are available	Whole cohort looking for a job at same time
	Department are looking for newly qualified staff	More experienced competition
	Job is at local trust	Possibility of trust merger so may need to work cross-site

---
ACTIVITY 8.1
---

1 Complete a SWOT analysis similar to the example above. Be honest and realistic, but also as creative as you can, and avoid false modesty. Remember this is only an initial guide to where you might concentrate your thinking.

It is important to consider weaknesses as 'areas that could be further developed'; therefore this analysis will be not only a reflection of your current self, but also a record of your potential.

2 Try to put yourself inside a prospective employer's head, particularly as you consider your strong points. What might they be looking for?

If this is the first time that you have undertaken such an analysis, you may find it easier to start by simply listing key words. This can be developed further if necessary.

So, what are you going to do with this information? You are going to use it to 'market' yourself! This can be a three-step process.

Determining your objectives

Your objectives might include:

- Your ideal job.
- Other jobs that you might consider.

- How you intend to make the transition from student to registered nurse.
- Your two-/five-/ten-year career goal.

Developing a 'marketing' strategy

Think about the following:

- Which organizations or trusts might you 'target' to achieve your objectives?
- How will you discover what opportunities are available there?
- How will you then communicate your wishes to them?
- What help can I get to do this? What support network have I got? Could the university help? Could my practice supervisor, mentor or other colleagues help?

Putting together an action plan

It is essential that the strategies are turned into actions:

- What do I need to do?
- When do I need to do it?
- What are the goals that I want to achieve?
- What are the specific timetables and deadlines?

Short-term career planning

The above processes allow you to focus more clearly on your realistic goals and objectives, which make it more likely that you will accomplish them. Your SWOT analysis may have highlighted barriers to your achieving these goals, such as lack of motivation or procrastination, or perhaps fewer personal barriers, such as family and peer pressure, or even financial considerations.

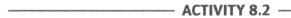

ACTIVITY 8.2

Consider your current situation.

1   What is it with which you are happiest?

Now consider what would improve this situation in the future.

(Continued)

(Continued)

2   What kind of activities do you particularly like?
3   What kind of activities do you avoid?

Write your thoughts in Table 8.2.

Table 8.2   Activities I enjoy and activities I avoid

Key activities	
Activities I particularly enjoy	**Activities I try to avoid**

   Once you have made this list as comprehensively as possible, take a close look at your proposed career path and the job for which you thought you might apply.

1   How does your list match the key characteristics of your ideal job?
2   Are there any surprises?
3   Does your proposed job have more likes or dislikes?

Preparation: What type of job do you want and why?

If you allow it to be, finding a job can be quite a traumatic and disheartening experience. To help to keep you focused and motivated during what can be quite a long and arduous process, it is important to consider who might be your support network. Who might be able to offer you advice and support?

──────────────── **ACTIVITY 8.3** ────────────────

Write down who you might include in your support network. How, specifically, might they be able to help?

──

   As your nursing career progresses, you will undoubtedly develop a supportive professional network of colleagues and friends. This can facilitate learning by sharing best practice, discussing differences in practice, exploring current and future priorities and initiatives, and generally helping and encouraging you. Your support network may be less structured and less obvious at this stage in your career; however, there are still people who might support and advise you. One obvious person who might help you during this time is your personal tutor, who hopefully will be a trusted adviser who has seen you grow and develop professionally during the time on the course. Similarly, you will have practice colleagues who have contributed to your growth and development as they have been supporting and assessing your practice.

Support networks outside of nursing, such as friends and family, appropriately utilized, might also be able to assist you in clarifying your thinking. Such 'critical friends' can often put into words more precisely the skills that you have but might be quite reluctant to acknowledge as you generally struggle to 'blow your own trumpet'.

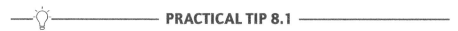

PRACTICAL TIP 8.1

It is fair to say that just as nursing equips us with many transferable skills in other areas of life, the converse is also true: other areas of life equip us with transferable skills for nursing. This is important to remember when you are trying to sell yourself. So why include aspects of your 'personal' life in your application, curriculum vitae (CV) or even at interview?

- What might being involved in the local parent–teacher association say about your abilities and skills?
- What does the fact that you have completed the Duke of Edinburgh's Award say about your ability?
- Similarly, why might the fact that you like to go hill climbing in your spare time be of any interest to a prospective employer?

The above examples can be included in your application or discussed at interview as they offer evidence of skills that may be valuable to an employer. They may show that you are reliable, trustworthy and committed. *Or* they may show you are self-reliant, a good time manager and able to complete difficult tasks. *Or* they may even indicate that you have a well-rounded personality and have strategies outside of work that may help you to handle pressure and stress. *Or* all of the above!

Although you should include only *relevant* information, it is still possible to be quite creative by including information that makes you stand out from the crowd.

Finding the job

By now, you would have confirmed the type of work that you prefer and clarified the skills that you have to match the requirements of this role. So how can you find the jobs that are presently open to applications? It is important that you know about the many resources available to locate employment opportunities.

- Each trust or employer will have an area accessible to employees and others where internal job openings are advertised. Do you know where this is in your current placement area? Ask your practice colleagues for advice.
- Similarly, current vacancies will be available on the employer's website.
- There are also many websites available that allow you to search f or specific jobs appropriate to newly qualified nurses. For example, in the UK:
  - **www.jobs.nhs.uk**
  - **www.rcnbulletinjobs.co.uk**
  - **www.jobmedic.co.uk**

- Some nursing journals also contain classified advertisements with available opportunities, such as *Nursing Times* (www.nursingtimesjobs.com).
  This website also offers an email service, through which you can receive email updates on all the suitable jobs.

- You may also find some jobs in your local paper.

The next difficult question: 'When should I apply?'

There is no absolutely correct answer to this, unfortunately – especially for student nurses coming to the end of their nursing course. The variables involved here are as follows:

- Is there a job available?
- Is it appropriate for a newly qualified staff nurse?
- When does the vacancy need filling?
- When can I start?

Because of all of these different and uniquely personal considerations, it is important not to be too disappointed if you do choose to apply and you don't get invited for interview, or if you do receive an invitation for interview, but do not subsequently get appointed. Obviously, this may simply be because they need someone to start *now*. If you are unable to take up the opportunity for a few months, then you may be unsuccessful simply due to that fact.

Therefore, although it is true to say that there may never be agreement on when is best to apply in these circumstances, it seems logical to say that more than a couple of months prior to the time at which you can officially start may inevitably lead to disappointment. Although *all* interview experience may be seen as useful in some way and part of a useful and ongoing learning process, even if, in real terms, you have no chance of being ultimately appointed, it is likely to irritate the interviewer if you have not been open and transparent about your position and ability to take up the opportunity. Discussing your specific situation openly and honestly with the contact person on the job advertisement may reduce your potential for disappointment and the likelihood of wasting their valuable time.

Remember that you may want the next job in that particular area and you don't want to be remembered as a time-waster.

So, how can you increase your chances of getting an interview?

It is important to think of the interview as a wonderful opportunity and recognize that you are largely in control of the impression that the interviewer will form of you. Although many people might be critical of the whole interview process generally as a means of matching the right person with the right job, it is not purely chance if someone is successful at interview.

You will probably have heard people say, and may have also said yourself:

How can they really know about me in such a short time?

Or

It is just whether your face fits or not, it isn't really about the individual person that's why it's so unfair.

Or

It is just about being in the right place at the right time.

There may be some truth in these comments, however, it is important to realize that the interview process is not simply determined by chance, and that you can have significant control and influence over the way in which the interview is conducted and more importantly over the outcome. We can be critical all we like, but interviews are not going to go away; indeed, employers spend a significant amount of time, effort and money trying to ensure that they pick the right person for the job.

Before going any further, it is appropriate to reflect on Graham's own experiences of searching for a job, and later being on an interview panel.

No doubt everyone will have their own unique, sometimes less than perfect, recollections of their experiences of getting a job. The preparation, the selection process, interview, feedback, disappointment or elation and even the subsequent nervousness as reality hits home. Often the most memorable incidents are not necessarily the most positive, and perhaps that is human nature. You may look at a qualified nurse and think, 'I would love a career just like theirs', however it is almost certain that they have a back catalogue of unsuccessful job applications, setbacks and apparently career-defining disappointments. Disappointments that in hindsight generated other exciting and surprising opportunities that became career-defining for them.

I can still vividly remember 'coming second in a one-horse race' for a job opportunity that everyone appeared to assume was mine. I was the only person shortlisted and felt nervous but well-prepared, only for it to turn into a disaster! In retrospect I was over-prepared but at the same time fundamentally ill-prepared, attempting to cover every possible question that might conceivably be asked and thereby forgetting the essentials in the process. The pre-interview presentation, something I did virtually every day in my job, was a catastrophe, well over the time allotted, over complicated and dense with information. The rest of the interview continued on pretty much the same, unfortunate course as by the end of the presentation I was in such a state that the initial and inevitable 'easy' question, 'Why do you want this job?', totally threw me. If I had been asked an incredibly complicated question about the minutiae of current government health policy I may have been ok. Despite the significant time and effort I had devoted to the interview my experience was, unfortunately, quite brutal evidence of my inappropriate planning and incorrect preparedness.

...and breathe....

As is probably evident from reading this reflection, at the time it felt devastating and left me in a state of shock for what appeared to be a considerable length of time, not least as my interviewers were colleagues who I saw and worked with on a regular basis. A comment from one of the panel was 'What happened? That wasn't the Graham I know'. However, this painful event taught me so much and ultimately led to career-defining decisions that subsequently resulted in a career full of many exciting and fulfilling experiences. This one interview fundamentally challenged my previously held career beliefs and aspirations, and ultimately led me to a change in direction and the decision to apply to work at a university. The particulars of this story have been relayed to many students to highlight how wonderful opportunities can often come from circumstances that can initially feel devastating. This is hopefully both helpful to them and wonderful therapy for me!

No one finds the process of getting a job easy and occasional setbacks and disappointments are inevitable. However, although very difficult and challenging, these setbacks **must not** *be taken personally or used as overwhelming evidence that your career is pretty much over already. It may well sound trite when a friend or loved one says 'there are other jobs you know', but it is essentially true and will always be so.*

Looking for, and applying for, a job needs to be given the priority it deserves. Whilst undoubtedly very important, it is only one part of a rewarding life and one specific, idealized job should never be viewed as critical or urgently life-confirming. Often the job that seemed like it was going to be 'just ok' turns out to be the best and most rewarding job you have ever had. Conversely it can take merely a couple of minutes on the first day of a new job to realize, or at least believe, that an error has been made. In one job I very quickly recognized that my decision to apply for the post had been based purely on the opportunity to work with staff who had been so supportive to me as a student, only to find that most of them had moved on by the time I arrived.

It is crucial, therefore, that the whole context of the decision-making process is clear in your mind and appropriate preparation and planning are made to increase the probability of you doing yourself justice. This will continue to be the case throughout your career and it is, therefore, advisable to regularly reflect and thereby be in a position to make positive decisions early. Being 'fed up' and desperate to change jobs before you start to look is not the most helpful position, not least as finding another job can sometimes take considerable time.

Having been on many interview panels over the years, my perspective on interviews has changed considerably. Always remember that the panel is simply made up of people who are looking for a potential future colleague, someone who can offer them a solution to a problem they currently have. Some members of the panel may be very experienced, whereas others may be less so and may be almost as nervous as you, which can sometimes explain any less-than-perfectly expressed or unclear questions. Always feel free to ask for clarification, it is unlikely that a question has been presented in a way to purposefully confuse or trip you up. As an interviewer I once asked a candidate the same question twice. Despite what the candidate thought this was not some fiendish plot or mind game designed to produce some deep psychological reaction. It was simply an error by a relatively inexperienced interviewer. An error that I only discovered, with growing realization, when reading my notes as I offered feedback and then rather sheepishly offered the candidate the job. Thankfully, despite my apparent lack of proficiency, the candidate still accepted the opportunity and became a very valued colleague. This anecdote also indicates the genuine control and influence that the interviewee ultimately has. A good interview panel will recognize this and endeavour to provide a supportive experience that puts the organization in a good light. As an interviewee, you can make a decision on whether you want to work with them in the future by your perception of the general atmosphere of the interview, the panel's attitude and the respect shown to you during the whole recruitment process.

Good luck!

How can you improve your chances of success?

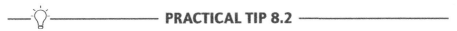 **PRACTICAL TIP 8.2**

Remember that the best students don't necessarily get the job; the best prepared do.

The three main ways in which you can improve your chances are preparation, preparation and preparation! For example, it is essential to keep up to date with what is happening in healthcare generally and especially in the specific area in which you are interested. If you don't, you could quite easily come unstuck at an interview when a question is asked that relates to current practice, policies or new initiatives in that particular area. Knowledge and understanding of the current major issues will allow you to impress the interviewer with your insight and also your enthusiasm. It is undeniably impressive to an interviewer if a candidate is able to relate their knowledge of current issues to the specific job for which they are being interviewed.

Application form and/or CV

You never get a second chance to make a first impression. The unique personal profile on an application form or curriculum vitae (CV) tends to be the first thing the potential employer will read apart from the routine matters of name and contact details. Therefore, it is vital that you use this opportunity to work for you. The point of this section is to summarize, in no more than a few words, your major qualities and 'selling points'. The person reading this is not interested in what a wonderful person you are. They are, however, very interested in whether:

- You can do the job on offer.
- You have a real understanding of what the job entails.
- You have the appropriate experience and history.
- You will be able to do the job well.
- You will get on with the rest of the present team.

So it is important to concentrate on the benefits that you can bring and keep to the facts, avoiding overblown exaggeration and hype.

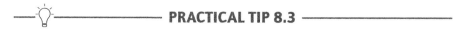

PRACTICAL TIP 8.3

If you write your application form or CV as a 'solution to someone else's problem', it should make a favourable impression on the reader – that is, the person who needs that solution.

Unfortunately, this approach does mean that each job application is deserving of a very specific and individual approach, which can feel onerous and time-consuming. However, this time is definitely worth it: not only does it improve the impression that you are giving and the impact your application will make, but it also concentrates your mind on precisely why you are the right person for this particular job. There is no more certain way to lose a job than to speak of caring for patients undergoing surgery when the prospective employer is a charge nurse on a medical ward, for example.

Hopefully your preparation, reflection and the exercises that you have undertaken to clarify your thinking and understanding will have made you confident about what makes you stand out and right for the job. Let's be honest: if you don't know this by now, you cannot expect those reading your application form to invest significant effort into exploring and spotting it for you.

CV template

There are many different types of CV template available. Avoid gimmicks and unfamiliar formats as these can detract from, rather than enhance, the information included. The important thing is to make it easy for the reader to pick out the content that they are looking for so that the CV shows you in your best light as a prospective candidate (see Figure 8.1 on p. 262).

Application form, job description and person specification

Each job advertisement will include both a job description and a person specification. It may sound obvious, but these are very important documents! The job description will include details such as job title, job location and who the job holder is accountable for and to, and so on. It will also include a job summary or job purpose. For example, this section may include a paragraph similar to this:

> The post holder will participate in the delivery of high standards of care to children and their families. They will assess the care needs and develop, implement, and evaluate programmes of individualized nursing care within a multiprofessional setting, and work collaboratively and cooperatively with others to meet the needs of children and their families/carers.

The job description should then give more specific and crucial aspects of the job and the role, including areas such as:

- Clinical duties.
- Management.
- Professional/education.
- Health and safety.

Studying the job description thoroughly will enable you to confirm both your interest in this particular job and also the appropriateness of your application.

While no two job descriptions will be identical, they generally tend to include certain information. Figure 8.2 shows a fictitious example that could help you to assess your current position and focus your preparation.

Curriculum vitae	
Name	**Work experience** (most recent first)
Address (home and term)	Date Trust, hospital or company name, Job title Main responsibilities
	Skills gained (communication, teamwork, interpersonal, problem-solving)
Telephone (home and mobile)	Skills
Email	For example, IT skills
Personal profile	Other relevant skills
A succinct, approximately three-line summary of your unique selling points which will make you stand out from the crowd	Interests and activities
	Only include these if they are focused and relevant to the specific job for which you are applying
Education and qualifications	
	References
Date University, Course, Qualification Subject	Usually at least two appropriate references are required
Dissertation (if relevant to job)	
Date School/college	
A levels (grades if good)	
Other qualifications	
Date School	
GCSEs – number of subjects, including Maths and English	

Figure 8.1   CV template

Title: Qualified Nurse

Grade: Band 5

Reports to: Charge Nurse

Accountable to: Charge Nurse

Job summary: To be responsible for the assessment, planning, implementation and evaluation of evidence-based individualized programmes of care. The post-holder will also assist in the management and organization of nursing work in the ward/department.

Key responsibilities:

1 **Clinical/professional**

   1.1 To work within the code of professional standards of practice and behaviour, and within the policies, procedures, and guidelines of the department.

   1.2 To ensure that high standards of nursing care are maintained and act when standards are not being maintained.

   1.3 To participate in the assessing, planning, implementation, and evaluation of individualized programmes of care.

   1.4 To recognize changes in clients' conditions that require the intervention of others and refer on as appropriate.

2 **Management/operational**

   2.1 To support the Charge Nurse in risk assessment and minimization.

   2.2 To manage verbal complaints, inform the Charge Nurse, and refer on when unable to resolve.

   2.3 To participate in the investigation of incidents/complaints as required.

   2.4 To establish and maintain effective communication within the multidisciplinary team.

   2.5 Have an awareness of team members' skills/capabilities and be able to delegate tasks appropriately.

   2.6 Act as an innovative and enthusiastic role model, providing leadership, guidance, and advice to staff on operational and professional issues.

3 **Education/training**

   3.1 To support the Charge Nurse in providing a suitable and effective learning environment for students.

   3.2 To take responsibility for own continuing professional development and performance.

   3.3 To support the development of other team members.

4 **Quality/research**

   4.1 Monitor and ensure that standards of care are maintained and that policies/procedures and protocols are adhered to.

   4.2 Ensure own practice is evidence-based.

   4.3 Contribute to and participate in programmes of audit, including utilization of results in practice.

   4.4 Support the Charge Nurse in aspects of patient and public involvement.

   4.5 Actively participate in benchmarking clinical practice along with other areas.

Figure 8.2 A sample job description

The person specification

The other key document is the person specification. Again, it is essential that you study this carefully to see what characteristics are either essential for the job or merely desirable. Table 8.3 shows a specimen person specification that includes some of the generic points often included in such documents. The main thing to recognize is the fundamental rationale behind such documents. They exist to help to ensure that the *right* candidates are placed in the *right* jobs. They are also incredibly helpful for you to clarify the role you are applying for, prepare appropriately, ensure that you meet the essential requirements, and ultimately ensure that you stand a good chance of being successful in your application.

Table 8.3 Example of an NHS foundation trust person specification for a qualified nurse – Band 5

Requirements	Essential	Desirable	How identified
Qualifications	First-level registration		Application form Portfolio/profile
Experience		Experience working in specialty	Application form Portfolio/profile
Training	Willingness to take responsibility for own continuing professional development	Insight into issues of recruitment and selection	Interview
Special knowledge/ expertise	Knowledge of nursing conditions and treatments relating to specialty Knowledge of local and national initiatives	Venepuncture Knowledge of specific drug therapy related to specialty	Portfolio/profile Interview
Disposition: adjustment, attitude, commitment	Approachable and supportive to support staff Positive attitude Ability to prioritize workload of self and others Flexible and adaptable Good interpersonal and communication skills		Interview
Practical/ intellectual skills	Ability to motivate staff Excellent written and verbal communication skills	IT skills	Application Interview
Attendance record	Ability to maintain a satisfactory level of attendance		References

The person specification has four main aspects, as follows:

1   The specific requirements of the post.
2   The qualities, experience and skills that the candidate *must* have to be even considered for further discussion at interview.
3   The qualities, experience and skills that the employer would *prefer* the candidate to have before they invite them for further discussion at interview.
4   The way in which these qualities and skills are to be identified: application form, portfolio/profile, reference or interview?

─────────────────────── **ACTIVITY 8.4** ───────────────────────

By using the example in Table 8.3 or a real person specification, work through each of the items in it, and note down a personal example that shows that your experience, skills or personality fit closely with what is required.

1   Consider and write down how you would provide appropriate evidence that you fit these requirements.
2   Write your answers in proper sentences and say them out loud.
3   How comfortable does it feel to say the words?

   Imagine saying them for the first time in the stressful environment of an interview. The more you are able to rehearse, the more comfortable you should feel at the real interview.

───

Clearly, you must provide proof that you have all of the characteristics marked as essential if you are to be successful in the interview. If this proof is to be identified at the point of application, it is essential that you include such evidence/proof in your application form. If you do not include it, you will most likely fall at the first shortlisting hurdle. If you are not experienced enough for a job, then you might think 'fair enough', but imagine the greater disappointment of not being invited for interview simply because you omitted to highlight your experience comprehensively, perhaps on the assumption that you might be offered the opportunity to further explore this at interview.

The person specification helps you either to confirm or discover what is really wanted for the role, allowing you to match your experience and skills to indicate to your prospective employer that you could do the job. So, if you lack some *essential* experience or skill, then considering that job application may be a waste of time; however, one area of weakness in the *desirable* column may not be devastating if you can 'wow' them on all of the others. Including examples of how quickly you have learned things in the past may offer reassurance that although you might not be as experienced as other applicants, you would be worth investing in (or taking a risk on!) because of all of the other excellent attributes that you would bring to the team.

If the job is not for a newly qualified staff nurse, there is little that you can do about that: this is simply not the job for you at this particular time. However, the effort you put in, and the preparation and thought invested in the application procedure, will certainly help when the right opportunity does come along. It is important not to *waste* valuable time, mindful of the effort and commitment that it takes to get a job – but continually considering your strong points and areas that you might need to develop may mean that you are ready when the next job comes along.

And, of course, the next job could always just be your ideal job!

Professional portfolios/profiles

As you can see from the above person specification, evidence of suitability is often provided by means of your professional portfolio or profile. A key requirement of professional practice according to the UK's Nursing and Midwifery Council *Code* (NMC, 2018a) is the continued development of specialist knowledge and competence to address the new and ever-changing demands of the complexities of modern professional practice.

Since April 2016 to renew professional registration with the NMC all nurses have been required to follow a revalidation process that demands evidence to demonstrate that they practice safely and effectively. This includes production of evidence of 35 hours of continuing professional development relevant to their scope of practice, examples of practice-related feedback, several written reflective accounts and reflective discussion (NMC, 2016a). This requires you to demonstrate responsibility for your own learning through the development of a portfolio of learning and practice, and to be able to recognize when further learning and development may be required. Your professional portfolio or profile is an opportunity to showcase the professional skills and accomplishments that have been generated as part of the completion of your nursing course. Maintaining a professional portfolio/profile is in the spirit of lifelong learning and reflective practice, and it is also habit-forming.

Even though an impressive and appropriately focused portfolio/profile may not get you the job, it may well be the 'casting vote' if you are competing with other students for a particular job. There are no hard-and-fast rules as regards what a good portfolio/profile should contain, but do make sure that the priority of the portfolio/profile – that is, the key documents included – are related to the specific job for which you have applied and emphasize your suitability to take on this new exciting role.

Some other application tips

- Increasingly, applications are completed online and if they do not offer the provision of spellcheck, take special care to verify that all of the information that you are providing has no spelling or punctuation errors.
- Consider sending a cover letter if possible. This can not only provide a general introduction and shed positive light on your personality, but also give you an opportunity to include positive aspects about yourself that might not be appropriate to put in the job application itself.
- Always ensure that you give appropriate references. It will probably be expected that one reference/final summary be from your university. If you choose not to utilize your university reference, this will inevitably raise questions in the mind of the employer.
- Any further referees need to be chosen carefully. You need to know that they will be supportive and positive, and have insight into the requirements of the job being applied for to enable them to tailor their reference accordingly.

- Remember that you are applying for a professional post and the references need to reflect that. Your choice of referee may be a 'friend', but be aware that they are offering the reference in their professional capacity and not in their capacity as a friend, and that this professional insight must be the main thrust of the reference.
- Remember also that it is common courtesy to inform a person before you use their name as a reference. You are risking the possibility of a less favourable reference if the request for a reference is a surprise to the referee!

Pre-interview

Consider ringing the contact person to confirm receipt of your application and discuss the key aspects of the job, as this shows interest and commitment. Imagine the scene during the shortlisting process: 'Well, this person never even bothered to contact me'. Obviously, not a good start! It is, however, essential to treat this step as an integral part of the application process and therefore to rehearse it carefully. It is also important to ring at the most appropriate time to catch the person at their best time, when they are most able to speak to you. This also indicates an appreciation of the circumstances of the ward, department or work environment generally.

Your phone call may lead to an informal visit. If it does, again treat this as seriously as any part of the recruitment process. If the person interviewing is unable to speak to you, they may ask a trusted colleague to do so. However, rest assured that the interviewer is very likely to subsequently ask them their opinion and first impressions of you as a potential colleague. You may also want to consider a 'ghost visit' to the area. This means visiting unannounced as perhaps a member of the public would. What are your impressions of the place? Does it feel like somewhere that you might be happy to work? If there are staff there, do they look professional and supportive? If there are clients there, do they look content and supported? Although it would be rash to make a decision based solely on such a visit, it might be part of your overall decision-making process.

A word of warning: you are visiting an environment in which confidentiality is paramount and you are simply visiting the open access and public areas to gain a flavour of the environment. This is not a covert spying mission, and if you treat it as such, be prepared to be escorted from the premises by security and wave goodbye to any chance of employment.

ACTIVITY 8.5

Many universities and placement providers give final-year students the opportunity to undertake practice job interviews. These can be very helpful, because you can receive some objective feedback in advance of a real interview.

If you do not have an opportunity to participate in these, do practise answering interview questions with a friend or by yourself so that you have rehearsed what you are going to say.

The interview

So, the letter arrives inviting you for interview. How do you feel? Elated or full of trepidation? Enthusiastic or terrified? These emotions are totally understandable, but wasn't this why you applied for the job in the first place? It is perfectly normal to worry that you may go through all of the stress and anxiety of preparation for nothing. Coping with this anxiety is important, as interviewers can often detect it – and it inevitably affects your performance in a negative way. Try to think of your application as doing someone a favour by being the person that they need to do the job.

The people who interview you are likely to be complete strangers, unless you are applying for a job in an organization in which you have already worked or have been a student. Interviews are just a common-sense way for people to find out about each other and ask each other questions. So, as well as the employer interviewing you, you also have the chance to make your own decisions about the employer, the job on offer, and the type of work environment, ward or department, and so on.

Interviews are like examinations at the end of a course of study. You know that you have done well so far on the course and you know in advance roughly what areas the questions are going to cover. In the same way, you know that you have done well in the selection process up to this point or you would not have been invited for the interview. You also know in advance roughly what will be covered in the questions to be asked, because you have studied the details relating to the job. Similarly, most of the talking in the interview will be done by you and therefore you can have a fair measure of control over where the interview is going.

Of course, you cannot set the questions yourself, but you can calculate fairly accurately what subject areas will be covered and plan your answers accordingly. The only reason why you have been invited for interview is because the employer wants to find out more about you. You are not invited to be tricked, but to find out exactly who you are and how you would deal with certain situations likely to crop up in your job.

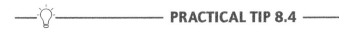

PRACTICAL TIP 8.4

Remember, employers are interested in three main areas:

- Your qualifications and skills.
- Your experience and work background.
- Your personality and character.

The most important of these is personality and character, because skills can be taught and experience gained on the job.

Ten questions you might be asked

Note: these are in no particular order.

1 Why do you want this particular job?
2 What do you think your key strengths are?
3 What do you see as the major difference between your role as a student and as a qualified nurse?
4 What would you do if you were asked to do something that was beyond your level of competence?
5 What do you like least about nursing?
6 What would you expect from me as your charge nurse?

7 What would you do if you were to witness poor practice by a colleague?

8 What part of being a student did you find most difficult?

9 Caring for patients can be quite stressful. How do you manage stress?

10 What are you most proud of in your career so far?

11 How would you redesign a teddy bear?

Question 11 is a rogue! However, it indicates that you need to always be prepared for a question totally out of the blue. This might appear a little underhand but may be used to see how you react. Remember that the employer wants a person to fill the post, so being purposefully obtuse and confusing is not the norm. Frightening tales of mind games being played by interviewers are usually simply rumours or urban myths ... although you never know!

Creating the best impression

It cannot be emphasized enough that first impressions are very important and that even though you will not get the job on image alone, it definitely helps. The impression that we give is based on so much more than just the words we speak. This first impression is based on appearance and behaviour generally, including clothing, posture, body language and facial expressions.

Evidence seems to indicate that, with regards to first impressions, there is a '93 percent rule'. What this means is:

- 55 percent of the impression that we get is from appearance and body language.
- 38 percent is from the way in which a person speaks, including the way in which the voice is used, clarity of speech and accent.
- Only 7 percent is from the actual words that we say.

This powerful realization is compounded by the fact that we are also highly affected by our visual impressions of others, particularly where quick decisions have to be made. Decisions with regards to a person's aptitude, friendliness, social status, education, politics and even religion or sexuality have been shown to be made within the first one to two minutes of initial meeting. Some evidence indicates that these impressions are made even more quickly, in some respects even within seconds, and we underestimate this at our peril. The secret of success is in understanding how other people perceive you and using this information to your advantage by making sure that the impression you create works in your favour.

Some people may view the above observation cynically as another example of the inappropriateness of interviews as a fair and equal process. However, this is not about pretending to be someone else or putting on an act, but more about enhancing your strong points and minimizing your weaker ones. Your appearance is the most important aspect of the first impression that you create.

- A smart appearance shows that you have taken trouble over the way in which you want to come across and your choice of clothes indicates your attitude to yourself and to other people.
- Therefore, it is probably best not to go to an interview in your uniform, as you may have thought of doing.
- Similarly, it is advisable to avoid wearing too much perfume and smoking, as this may trigger some allergies in the interviewer, and the smell of smoke not only emphasizes the habit, but also creates a very negative impression for some people – something that you most definitely do not want to do.
- It is advisable to arrive five to ten minutes before the scheduled time, as this gives time to relax and calmly consider your thoughts. Hopefully you have also been able to visit the venue for the interview previously to give you one less thing to worry about and to work out the practicalities of getting there on the day. This preparation, along with arriving in good time, reduces anxiety. Arriving just prior to the scheduled time indicates appropriate self-confidence without putting undue extra pressure on the interviewer if you arrive too early.
- Whilst you are waiting, try to look relaxed, but 'busy': read a professional journal, or your set of potential questions, or your CV. If the interviewer accompanies the previous candidate to the waiting area, they will therefore be given a positive first impression.

- It is imperative that you bring all of your certificates and records as asked for in your interview confirmation letter. These may need to be photocopied, and if you fail to bring them as requested, it gives a less-than-favourable impression with regards to your organization, preparedness and even your ability to follow instructions. All of this might lose you crucial 'points' in the inevitably competitive job hunt.

When it is your turn, start off on a positive note by greeting the interviewer with direct eye contact and a firm handshake, and enter the interview room smiling naturally at all of the interviewers present. This approach indicates not only confidence and assertiveness, but also a friendly and interested approach.

Sit well back in the chair (when invited to do so) and lean forward slightly giving the impression of just the right amount of keenness and interest. This position should also be comfortable, thus avoiding having to change your position too frequently, thereby distracting the listener from what you are saying. Equally distracting can be lots of hand movements, so you may want to consider clasping your hands lightly in your lap or resting them on the arms of the chair. While gestures undoubtedly add variety to speech, too much gesturing can also imply anxiety and tension.

Practising interview techniques definitely brings rewards and instils confidence, so even though it might sound slightly bizarre to say 'practise sitting in a chair properly', give it a go. Hopefully, you will reap the rewards and you can then recount your funny and slightly embarrassing story to your new colleagues once you have been offered the job!

As mentioned above, you will be doing most of the talking in the interview and therefore you might consider rehearsing some answers as well. It is very likely, for example, that you will be asked what you consider to be your strengths. Remember that you may not be asked in *exactly* those terms, but it is probably safe to assume that the underpinning reason for asking at least one question will be to further explore your strengths and qualities. Therefore, as you already can take a good guess that this is going to be asked in some guise or other, it is a good idea to rehearse the aspects that will inevitably be included in your answer.

According to the person specification above, for example, you 'know' that you are going to be asked a question that is related to your 'ability to prioritize the workload of self and others'. Therefore, an answer to such a question can, to an extent, be considered and rehearsed. It is also effective to rehearse your answer aloud. Your answer may include comments with specific examples such as:

> In my final placement I was lucky enough to be given the responsibility for the holistic care of a group of clients, supported by my mentor. This included the appropriate delegation of aspects of care to a support worker. I found this experience very rewarding and confirmed to myself that I was able to ensure high-quality care by prioritizing not only my own workload but also the workloads of others.

While this in no way attempts to be an ideal answer, it indicates certain areas that you might consider. If so, literally saying those or similar words for the very first time to complete strangers (or some might argue more stressfully to the charge nurse from the very placement you are describing!) when you are anxious, 'on show', and your mouth is a little dry, is not ideal. Therefore, some level of rehearsal may well help.

The STAR approach (Situation –Task –Action –Result)

The **STAR approach** is a technique that is sometimes used by interviewers to gather information about your capabilities and thereby your suitability for the job. It attempts to predict your future performance based on the past. An insight into this technique may help you to prepare prior to the interview.

Situation

You will be expected to present a recent challenge and situation in which you found yourself. This may be explicitly asked for, such as: 'Have you ever been in a clinical situation in which you were asked to do something you were unsure about? What did you do?' Or they may be less explicit and start: 'What would you do if …?'

Both of these examples offer you a chance to show evidence of how you would deal with situations you may come across in the job.

Task

What did you have to achieve in this situation? If, in all of your answers, the task as you broadly describe it was the maintenance of safe and quality care, you will not go far wrong. The interviewer wants someone *appropriately* confident, but not *overly* so. They want you to be an integral part of a functioning and supportive team, able to safety deliver high-quality care, but also to be mindful of your accountability and relative inexperience.

Action

What did you do and why? Were there alternatives and if so why did you reject them? If you are being interviewed by the charge nurse, for example, they will want to be reassured that you would be safe and competent, working in the best interests of the client at all times, especially in the charge nurse's absence.

Result

What was the outcome? What did you learn from this experience and how might you use this learning in the future?

How to answer: Some golden rules

- Always be honest. Perceptions of dishonesty or 'being economical with the truth' are bound to worry the interviewer, not least as it casts a doubt on all of your answers. Remember also that the NMC *Code* (2018a: 20.2) says: 'act with honesty and integrity at all times'.
- Always describe things in positive terms. If you are asked about a difficult or negative experience in your training, discuss this in terms of how you used the situation to learn and develop, and how you turned it into a more positive experience. If you speak of

previous situations negatively, the interviewer will inevitably think that you will be likely to speak negatively of them or their team in the future. Anyone who creates a negative attitude will always be overlooked in preference to the positive and keen candidate. Moreover, nothing attracts people like enthusiasm, and working with someone who is positive and keen is exactly what an employer wants.

- Some experts advise that you should generally limit your answers to three statements, with each aspect sharing something about yourself. Such targeted and focused answers show that you are able to be thorough, succinct and clear in your communication – an important part of your role as a qualified nurse.

- If you have been unable to show your knowledge during the course of the interview, this could be offered at the end of the interview. For example, 'I am aware of the importance of X new policy, and if I were successful, I would be very keen to contribute to the team implementing that change', or 'I would be very excited by the opportunity to being part of this thrilling new initiative'.

At the end of the interview

It is advisable to have a couple of questions ready, as you will invariably be asked if you have any. This can cause anxiety in students applying for their first job, not least with regards to which questions to ask. The main rule is: only ask a question if it is necessary and appropriate rather than simply because you feel you ought to ask one.

Questions about training opportunities or the chance to take on greater responsibilities in the future show keenness and may indicate plans to stay in the job, whereas purposefully difficult, 'smart', or obtuse questions are a sure way not to get the job. It is interesting to consider that some interviewers may be slightly anxious themselves when conducting interviews, and an interviewee who increases that anxiety is likely to be looked on unfavourably.

Avoid questions about holidays, uniforms, or any such practical questions. You can discuss those issues thoroughly after you have been offered the job. However, like many other aspects of the recruitment process, there are no absolute rights and wrongs in this. While admittedly you do not want to ask a question that might be difficult for your interviewer to answer and make them feel foolish, an insightful, articulate question may help you to stand out and indicates an interest and focus on the job. So, the advice here is to go prepared with a question, but do not feel that you need to ask it if the circumstances do not feel necessary.

Finally, always thank the interviewers for their time and attention, and smile again before you leave on the same positive note. You may also consider writing a thank you letter as soon as possible after the interview, as this shows appreciation and highlights courtesy as a personal strength. You never know what the future might hold, and if you are not successful this time, you may be keen to be in a good position the next time an opportunity arises – especially if this was your 'dream job'.

Post-interview: What do I do now? How can I get the next one?

You need to develop strategies to support you through the potential ups and downs of the job-hunting rollercoaster. It is quite easy, and to an extent inevitable, to feel that all of the hard work and commitment you have put in to achieving your qualification and registration is in itself deserving of a suitable job in the area in which you really want to work. Unfortunately, unless you are very lucky, it is likely that you are going to have to learn to cope with rejections.

This is why a personal support network is so important to help you to deal with and learn from the experience.

First of all, it is important not to take this rejection personally. Any job opportunity is likely to have attracted a number of applications and this is especially true at the end of your course, as many students are in exactly the same boat. Requesting post-interview feedback from the interviewers is not unacceptable. It really helps in identifying what you could have improved, which is useful for future references and interviews. You can even ask for this if you got the job too. You can improve your odds of getting a job by:

- Getting feedback as soon as possible.
- Reflecting on the feedback as objectively as possible (not easy especially immediately after the event).

- Being very selective and applying only for jobs for which you are a very good match.
- Using the techniques highlighted in the chapter that will give you that hidden advantage.
- Being professional at each stage in the process.
- Avoiding getting into a vicious spiral of an 'all or nothing' mentality whereby this feels as if the only appropriate job has now gone.
- Getting the disappointment out of your system as soon as possible to ensure that you are in the best frame of mind to make the most of the next opportunity that comes along.

Summary

Being successful in applying for a job is far from simply good luck. There are genuine and *relatively* easy steps than can be taken to improve your chances. Some of the steps, both positive and negative, are reiterated in Table 8.4.

Table 8.4 Improving your chances for getting a job: Common mistakes and reasons why applicants are successful

Some common mistakes	Some reasons for success
Lack of specific and focused preparation	Flexibility and caring and helpful attitude
Not answering the question fully or properly, e.g. answers too short or full of waffle	Positive attitude, especially in the face of challenges
Not showing any enthusiasm for the job	Enjoying working in a team
Not being clear about skills and abilities, i.e. too vague or too modest	Looking smart
Using jargon	Evidence of continual learning
Not showing full consideration of all aspects of the job, e.g. indicating a dislike for some key aspect of the role	Ability to handle change
Having an untidy appearance or too relaxed an attitude	Punctuality
Panicking	Ability to offer examples to highlight claims
	Use of endorsement of others, e.g. 'My practice supervisor said …'
	Giving specific examples to show competence, adaptability and expertise

Planning your career and making career decisions is clearly an important aspect of your life, but it is essential that this is put into true perspective. Do not put so much pressure on yourself that it stops you from making any real choices, decisions or plans, and *never* turn down an interview just because you are scared. Like someone once famously said: feel the fear and do it anyway.

9

PREPARATION FOR PERSONAL AND PROFESSIONAL DEVELOPMENT

Val Ely, Rob Burton and Graham Ormrod

THE AIMS OF THIS CHAPTER ARE TO:

- Define and explore the concept of preceptorship to provide you with strategies to both seek and undertake preceptorship successfully following your qualification and registration as a nurse.
- Define preceptorship and continuing professional development (CPD) in terms of determining their relationship to your professional role.
- Define and explore the concept of CPD to ensure that you become a successful lifelong learner, in both your personal and professional practice, capable of planning your future career development.
- Identify how CPD will form part of your Nursing and Midwifery Council (NMC) revalidation requirements.
- Explain how credit gained from formally accredited CPD activity can contribute to your future academic qualifications.

- Illustrate throughout how preceptorship and CPD are related to the NMC *Standards for Nurses* (2018b; 2018c; 2018d; and 2018e).
- Highlight some strategies useful for your personal and professional development planning and life coaching.

Introduction

This chapter will examine the issues of personal and professional development from the point of qualification and beyond. It will focus on personal and professional development from the point of initial registration and **preceptorship**. This chapter will then proceed to examine **continuing professional development** and how this is key to Nursing and Midwifery Council re-registration and **revalidation** requirements. Finally, throughout this chapter the relationship between preceptorship and continuing professional development linked to the NMC *Standards* and *Code* (2018a; 2018b; 2018c; 2018d; and 2018e) will also be explored.

The Chief Nursing Officer for England recognized that the transition from student nurse to registered nurse is a 'challenging time for new nurses' (Department of Health, 2010). This view was echoed by NHS Employers (2018) too. In their view a quality preceptorship programme is essential to ensure the best possible start for newly qualified nurses. Preceptorship follows the practice supervision and practice assessment process, which was formerly referred to as the mentorship process (NMC, 2018e) in pre-registration nurse education. Practice supervision and practice assessment is experienced by all student nurses during their pre-registration nursing education at both undergraduate and postgraduate level. As will be seen in this chapter, the elements of preceptorship in registration as a nurse with the Nursing and Midwifery Council includes the individual newly registered nurse taking responsibility for their own personal and professional development and then embarking on a process of lifelong learning. This, from the outset, makes the connection from pre-registration nursing education and training to 'lifelong learning', which is referred to by regulatory bodies as continuing professional development (CPD), or as it can also be referred to in the nursing and health professional context, learning beyond registration (LBR). With the implementation of 'Revalidation' by the NMC (2019b), CPD is also key to individuals retaining their professional registration.

Therefore, to assist those nurses nearing registration or those who are newly registered, this chapter explores personal and professional development in the context of preceptorship, practice supervision, practice assessment, CPD and revalidation. We will also discuss some personal and professional development planning approaches related to coaching and goal-setting, which you may use during your career beyond initial registration.

Definition of preceptorship

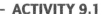
ACTIVITY 9.1

As you approach qualification as a nurse, note down how you would define the term 'preceptorship'.

The Department of Health (DH, 2010) reviewed many definitions of the term 'preceptorship' when developing its preceptorship framework. Key definitions include:

> A foundation period ⌈of preceptorship⌉ for nurses at the start of their careers which will help them begin the journey from novice to expert. (DH, 2008b)

> A period ⌈of preceptorship⌉ to guide and support all newly qualified nurses to make the transition from student to develop their practice further. (NMC, 2006)

> A period of transition for the newly registered nurse during which time he or she will be supported by a preceptor, to develop their confidence as an autonomous professional, refine skills, values and behaviours and to continue on their journey of life-long learning. (DH, 2010)

However, for the purposes of this chapter, our preferred definition of preceptorship is:

> Preceptorship is a term used for a consolidation period following Registration with the NMC. It will help ease your transition back into and develop your clinical practice. (HEE, 2017)

ACTIVITY 9.2

Now that you have read some of the available definitions, which definition do you prefer in terms of your aspirations for your impending period of preceptorship?

It will be useful to write down your own definition of this term so that you can negotiate your learning needs and styles when your period of preceptorship begins.

Preceptorship in nursing

The NMC originally published preceptorship guidelines in 2006 as part of their Post Registration Education and Practice (PREP) standards. These guidelines were the only non-statutory requirements contained within PREP. However, they strongly recommended a period of preceptorship on entering registered practice for the first time, entering a new part of the NMC register, or for those trained as nurses abroad. This guidance addressed the role of the newly registered nurse, often referred to as the **preceptee**, and the member of staff who supports them during this period, the **preceptor**. These NMC guidelines also outlined the one-year suggested length for the period of preceptorship and the preparation requirements for preceptors.

Health Education England (2015) in *Raising the Bar* further endorsed the relevance of preceptorship in nursing. They asserted that high-quality preceptorship is related to 'Assuring predictable and sustainable access to ongoing learning and development for registered nurses' (Theme Six). Plans were put in place to develop and implement preceptorship standards by April 2018, and they have already implemented their *Preceptorship and Return to Practice* programme (HEE, 2017).

Therefore, preceptorship is confirmed as an important activity in which you will be involved immediately following your qualification and registration as a nurse. In addition, as a 'preceptor' of the future, you are likely to provide preceptorship for many other newly registered nurse colleagues.

Benefits of preceptorship in nursing

The current *Preceptorship Framework for Newly Registered Nurses, Midwives and Allied Health Professionals* (DH, 2010) outlines the benefits of preceptorship to the newly registered nurse (preceptee), the preceptor, their employer and the nursing profession. However, ultimately, the goal of preceptorship is the provision of safe and effective nursing care to patients/clients by the newly registered, but still accountable, nurse. In keeping with the purpose of this book, it is worth taking this opportunity to focus on its key benefits for the newly registered nurse.

ACTIVITY 9.3

Thinking ahead to your role as a qualified nurse, how would preceptorship benefit you both personally and professionally?

Threaded through the list of benefits identified by the Department (DH, 2010) are issues important for both personal and professional development. The newly registered nurse can expect preceptorship to:

- Develop their confidence.
- Provide professional socialization into their working environment.
- Increase their job satisfaction leading to improved patient/client/ service user satisfaction.
- Provide them with the feeling that they are valued and respected by their employing organization and that this organization will invest in them and their future career aspirations.
- Commit them to the organization's corporate strategy and objectives.
- Develop an understanding of the commitment to working within the profession and regulatory body requirements.
- Encourage personal responsibility for maintaining up-to-date knowledge and skills.

ACTIVITY 9.4

Refer to your list above.
   Are there any similarities or differences to the benefits of preceptorship identified by the Department of Health (2010)?
   If so, it might be helpful to amend your list so that you can share with your preceptor from the outset how you hope preceptorship can benefit you.

Elements of preceptorship

The Department of Health (2010) outline some elements to preceptorship for the newly registered nurse, preceptor and the employer, which in turn could be used to produce learning outcomes for a preceptorship programme or for newly registered nurses undergoing this process with their preceptor. The elements of preceptorship for the newly registered nurse are summarized below. Preceptorship provides the opportunity to:

- Apply and develop the knowledge, skills and values already learned.
- Develop specific competences that relate to the preceptee's role.
- Access support in embedding the values and expectations of the profession.
- Produce a personalized programme of development that includes post-registration learning, e.g. leadership, management and effectively working within a multidisciplinary team.
- Reflect on practice and receive constructive feedback.
- Take responsibility for individual learning and development by learning how to 'manage self'.
- Commence lifelong learning.
- Enable the embracement of the principles of the NHS Constitution (DH, 2015).

―――――――――――――――――― **ACTIVITY 9.5** ――――――――――――――――――

Review these elements of preceptorship to determine your learning outcomes for your role as a newly registered nurse and your requirements from preceptorship.

Implementing preceptorship

The Department of Health (2010) believes that good preceptorship comprises two key learning strategies to fulfil their suggested elements of preceptorship – namely:

- Core theoretically based learning activities, whether taught, blended or distance learning.
- Supervision/guided reflection on practice.

The Department of Health (2010) further suggests that these **core theoretically based learning activities** provided should be between four and six days in length, with the **supervised/guided reflection of practice** taking around 18 hours. They recommend too that the preceptorship programme should take place over a period of six to twelve months and be linked to appraisal.

─────────────────────── **ACTIVITY 9.6** ───────────────────────

Does four/six days of core theoretically based learning activities and 18 hours of supervised/guided reflection of practice seem appropriate for you to meet your preceptorship needs?

If not, consider how you will justify needing more or less than these suggested time periods.

───

Furthermore, according to the Department of Health (2010), the suggested learning methods for a quality preceptorship programme include:

- Organizationally based preceptorship, for example:
  o Action learning sets.
  o Self-directed learning.
  o Clinical practice focus days.
  o Reflective practice.
  o Shadowing.
  o One-to-one support (in person or remotely/electronically).
- Preceptorship facilitated in partnership with universities that is delivered through an academically accredited programme.
- Work-based learning, e.g. portfolio-building.
- Web-based/blended learning programmes such as the Edward Jenner Programme offered by the NHS Leadership Academy.
- Attitudinal and behavioural-based learning, e.g. through role modelling.

─────────────────────── **ACTIVITY 9.7** ───────────────────────

1 What learning methods would you prefer to use?
2 Does this help you to identify the learning activities and time that you will need for your period of preceptorship?

───

More recently the NHS Employers (2018) have moved away from stipulating the explicit nature of preceptorship learning strategies and methods and instead have recommended that a:

> preceptorship programme should be a structured period of transition for the newly qualified nurse, midwife or allied health professional when they start employment in the NHS. During this time, he or she should be supported by an experienced practitioner (a preceptor), to develop their confidence as an independent professional, and to refine their skills, values and behaviours. Having expert support, and learning from best practice in dedicated time gives a foundation for lifelong learning and allows nurses to provide effective patient-centred care confidently.

Irwin et al. (2018) also identify that team preceptorship can be a valuable way of providing this process to the newly registered nurse as reported by preceptees. However, Currie and Watts (2012) assert that, whatever learning strategies and methods are deployed within preceptorship programmes, what will be pivotal to their success is how employers provide commitment to the programmes in their organizations, and undertake monitoring, evaluation and further development of such programmes.

─────────────── **ACTIVITY 9.8** ───────────────

Think ahead to your first post as a newly registered nurse.

1   Are you familiar with the preceptorship process in your new employing organization?
2   Have you read any policies, etc., on preceptorship by your new employer?
3   Also, how would you prefer to receive preceptorship? Would you prefer an individual or team approach?

As we move from examining preceptorship towards exploring CPD and revalidation, we will see how similar learning strategies and methods are available for personal and professional development. Thus, good preceptorship is vital for establishing a pattern of successful lifelong learning and CPD which will enable the newly registered nurse to re-register annually and revalidate tri-annually.

Preceptorship in the future

Following consultation in 2017, the NMC launched their new:

- *Standards of Proficiency for Registered Nurses* (NMC, 2018b).
- *Standards Framework for Nursing and Midwifery Education* (NMC, 2018d).
- *Standards for Student Supervision and Assessment* (NMC, 2018e).
- *Standards for Pre-Registration Nursing Programmes* (NMC, 2018f).

These new standards will present new challenges for the preceptorship process and the preceptors supporting the future newly registered nurse. In turn the Nursing and Midwifery Council may seek to provide further preceptorship guidelines, meaning that preceptorship will remain a dynamic process. It will be important for all registered nurses to keep up to date with any changes relating to their regulatory body. Indeed, keeping up to date as a registered nurse leads us into our next part of this chapter which will now focus on **CPD** and **revalidation**.

The relationship between preceptorship, practice supervision and practice assessment, CPD and revalidation

As a newly qualified and registered nurse prior to the implementation of the new NMC standards listed above, you will have probably experienced **mentorship** throughout your pre-registration nursing education. The NMC (2008b) stipulated that:

> Students on NMC approved pre-registration nursing education programmes, leading to registration on the nurses' part of the register must be supported and assessed by mentors.

Furthermore, if you had undertaken your pre-registration nursing education after September 2007, you would have had a **sign-off mentor**. The NMC (2008b) stated that the sign-off mentor, who had fulfilled additional criteria in their mentor training, made the final assessment of a student's practice to ensure that the required proficiencies for entry to the NMC register had been achieved. Some of you could have provided the role of a mentor and/or sign-off mentor to student nurses already. However, the NMC (2018e) *Standards* have now replaced the terms '**mentor**' and '**sign-off mentor**' with the terms '**practice supervisor**' and '**practice assessor**'. All registered health and social care professionals can provide supervision to a student nurse but in terms of NMC registrants providing this role the NMC (2018e) Section 3 states that the role and responsibilities of the **practice supervisor** include:

- Serving as a role model for safe and effective practice in line with their code of conduct (NMC, 2018e: 6).
- Supporting learning in line with their scope of practice to enable the student to meet their proficiencies and programme outcomes.
- Supporting and supervising students, providing feedback on their progress towards, and achievement of, proficiencies and skills.
- Possessing current knowledge and experience of the area in which they are providing support, supervision and feedback.
- Receiving ongoing support to participate in the practice learning of students.

ACTIVITY 9.9

Read the NMC (2018e) *Standards for Student Supervision and Assessment* related to the supervision of students (Sections 2–5).

Whether you have already provided mentorship and/or sign-off mentorship previously or not, consider whether you are able to become a practice supervisor. If you need any further CPD to undertake this role, what will your development needs include?

In terms of the NMC registrants undertaking the new **practice assessor** role, NMC (2018e) Section 7 states that their responsibilities include:

- Conducting assessments to confirm student achievement of proficiencies and programme outcomes for practice learning.
- Seeking feedback from practice supervisors to inform assessment decisions.
- Undertaking and recording practice assessments based on conduct, proficiency and achievement which also draw upon student records, direct observations, student self-reflection and other resources.

- Maintaining their current knowledge and expertise relevant for the proficiencies and programme outcomes they are assessing.
- Working in partnership with the nominated academic assessor to evaluate and recommend the student for progression for each part of the programme, in line with programme standards and local/ national policies.
- Ensuring there are sufficient opportunities for the practice assessor to periodically observe the student across environments to inform decisions for assessment and progression.
- Ensuring there are sufficient opportunities for the practice assessor to gather and coordinate feedback from practice supervisors, any other practice assessors and relevant people to be assured about their decisions for assessment and progression.
- Understanding the student's learning and achievement in theory.
- Communicating and collaborating between practice and academic assessors at scheduled points in the programme structure and student progression.
- Ensuring that they do not act as a practice assessor, academic assessor and practice supervisor for the same student.

ACTIVITY 9.10

Continue to read the NMC (2018e) *Standards for Student Supervision and Assessment* related to the assessment of students (Sections 6–10).

Whether you have provided mentorship and/or sign-off mentorship previously or not, consider if you are able to become a practice assessor. If you need any further CPD to undertake this role, what will your development needs include?

By now an immediate difference between preceptorship, practice supervision and practice assessment seems to be clearly visible. As we have read in this chapter so far, preceptorship is only 'strongly recommended' by the NMC but it is not compulsory. Practice supervision and assessment, on the other hand, are compulsory NMC requirements within pre-registration nursing education programmes (NMC, 2018e). However, NHS Employers (2018) assert that all employers should require their newly registered and appointed staff to undergo the preceptorship process despite it not being made compulsory by the NMC. Indeed, the NMC (2016c) have also recommended that employers should provide a period of preceptorship for newly registered nurses but have currently fallen short on mandating this process. Therefore preceptorship, practice supervision, practice assessment, CPD and revalidation are further closely linked. There are no mandatory or statutory requirements involved in becoming a preceptor or providing preceptorship, although it is recognized that individual employers may require preceptors to undergo training as part of their related organizational policy.

However, in complete contrast, to become a practice supervisor the NMC (2018e) requires that nurses must be prepared for this role and have:

- Ongoing support to prepare, reflect and develop for effective supervision of and contribution to student learning and assessment.
- Understanding of the proficiencies and programme outcomes they are supporting students to achieve.

Likewise, to become a practice assessor the NMC (2018e) requires that nurses:

- Undertake preparation or provide evidence via prior learning and experience that demonstrates achievement of the following minimum outcomes:
  - Interpersonal communication skills, relevant to student learning and assessment.
  - Conducting objective, evidence-based assessments of students.
  - Providing constructive feedback to facilitate professional development in others, and knowledge of the assessment process and their role within it.
- Receive ongoing support and training to reflect and develop in their role.
- Continue to proactively develop their professional practice and knowledge in order to fulfil their role.
- Have an understanding of the proficiencies and programme outcomes that the student they are assessing is aiming to achieve.

The vehicle for achieving this knowledge and skill set will begin with preceptorship and then CPD. Equally, to become a preceptor, practice supervisor and/or practice assessor, you may undertake a course to prepare you for this role. This will be part of your CPD, so again a link is established between preceptorship, practice supervision, practice assessment and CPD. These courses may be accredited if provided by a university, so you may be able to count this towards a higher academic award too. More discussion with examples will be provided on CPD and academic accreditation later in this chapter. Finally, as preceptors, practice supervisors, practice assessors and indeed NMC registrants, nurses must keep their knowledge and competence up to date; providing evidence of this is mandated by revalidation. This is required by the NMC (2018a) *Code*, thus establishing once again the relationship between preceptorship, practice supervision, practice assessment, CPD and revalidation.

Definition of the term 'continuing professional development' in nursing

As with preceptorship, there are a number of ways of defining CPD within the differing professional contexts to which the term applies. In healthcare the Health and Care Professions Council regard CPD as:

> the way in which registrants continue to learn and develop throughout their careers so they keep their skills and knowledge up-to-date and are able to practise safely and effectively. (HCPC, 2019)

However, this is the term used by the RCN (2016) to define CPD which is the one we prefer to use within this chapter:

> Continuing professional development (CPD) is described internationally by a variety of terms. These include: continuing nursing education, lifelong learning and professional skills development (among others). While there is no universally agreed term for CPD, there is a generally accepted understanding of its purpose – to help nurses maintain an updated skills set so that they are able to care for patients safely and competently.

CPD requirements in nursing

The NMC have stipulated CPD requirements for nurses since 2008 in their PREP standards. However, the latest standards on CPD from the NMC are contained within their revalidation requirements, which we will review below.

———————————————— **ACTIVITY 9.11** ————————————————

Visit http://revalidation.nmc.org.uk/ and read the 'Revalidation' microsite. Consider how you will manage your revalidation from the point of initial registration to your re-registration every three years.

CPD and revalidation

CPD is a key element of most international nursing boards and councils' requirements for continuing registration and definitely is a key component for NMC revalidation. Revalidation was first formalized by the Department of Health (2007b). The Department noted that previous and traditional systems of professional regulation saw individual health professionals, such as nurses, being deemed fit to practise for life following their initial professional qualification. Such individuals were registered with a professional or statutory body and remained on that register without having to demonstrate ongoing **fitness to practise** through CPD. Their place on the register was held on trust by society throughout their careers. This trust largely had its origins in social deference from the public and patients towards healthcare professionals and authority. However, the Department (2007b) also noted that, since the Second World War, a much greater informed and assertive public now increasingly rejects passive acceptance of authority and unquestioning obedience to establishments such as hospitals and healthcare professions such as medicine and nursing.

One of the reasons that the public is likely to challenge authority in healthcare is greater access to information through the media, social media and the internet. High-profile cases nationally have challenged beliefs about the future of professional regulation for both the public and professions concerned. Such high-profile infamous UK cases include those centred on the professional behaviour and conduct of enrolled nurse Beverley Allitt, registered nurse Colin Norris and Doctors Harold Shipman, Richard Neale, Clifford Ayling, William Kerr, Michael Haslam and Ian Paterson.

The Bristol Royal Infirmary and Alder Hey inquiries, as well as the inquiries into Maidstone and Tunbridge Wells Hospitals and the Mid

Staffordshire Hospitals, revealed that many patients died due to both individual and organizational failings. In a more deferent age, such individual and collective failings might have escaped both public and media scrutiny. However, today, no such 'hiding place' exists, and the public therefore demanded that their politicians act.

The White Paper *Trust, Assurance and Safety: The Regulation of Health Professionals in the 21st Century* (DH, 2007b) presented before Parliament implemented new arrangements for professional regulation. For individual healthcare registrants, professional regulation introduced revalidation across all disciplines. Revalidation required that individuals demonstrated periodically their continuous fitness to practise. A key requisite of revalidation is CPD. To implement the White Paper, the Department of Health (2008c) set out principles for non-medical revalidation. CPD is included as principle 5. Here, the Department stipulates that CPD is:

> the process by which individual registrants keep themselves up to date with healthcare developments in order to maintain the highest standards of professional practice. It should be seen as an integral part of revalidation and may provide supporting evidence that a practitioner submits to the regulatory body for consideration at the time of revalidation judgement. CPD needs to be relevant to the practitioner's scope of practise, where such scope has been defined. (DH, 2008c)

The first health professional registrant group to undertake CPD were doctors who commenced this process in December 2012. All healthcare professions are now required to undertake revalidation to periodically re-register. For nurses the NMC implemented their revalidation requirements from April 2016 and are currently concluding their first three-yearly cycle of this new regulatory process. Once revalidation had been implemented the NMC then withdrew their Prep Standards from use. More will be discussed on CPD and revalidation in the next section where we look at the NMC revalidation requirements.

NMC revalidation requirements

Paragraph 6.2 of the NMC (2018a) *Code* requires you as a registered nurse to:

maintain the skills and knowledge necessary for safe and effective practice. As such, you will need to continue to develop your knowledge and skills after initial registration to enable you to work safely and effectively within your chosen nursing scope of practice. This means that you will continue to deepen your knowledge, skills and experience in any relevant areas outlined in these new standards of proficiency.

In order to fulfil the requirements of revalidation, nurses must demonstrate that they are reflecting on their practice and maintaining their CPD in relation to their scope of practice. If nurses occupy specialist roles which require particular knowledge or skills, the standard required in that scope of practice should reflect the standard of those who have traditionally occupied these role duties such as doctors. As Brazier and Cave (2016) point out this is both a legal and a professional requirement.

To plan for your revalidation nurses should ensure that their knowledge and skills remain current for safe and effective practice. They must also consider their own scope of practice and CPD needs in line with both the new NMC (2018b) proficiencies and the NMC (2018a) *Code*. Whilst revalidation is required tri-annually, nurses should have an annual appraisal with their manager. In this appraisal a review should take place with your manager as to the scope of your current practice and any future changes required. This will then identify your CPD needs to meet the new proficiencies required.

The NMC (2018b) proficiencies for registered nurses introduced examples of new proficiencies which nurses are expected to achieve prior to registration. These include:

- Intravenous administration.
- Chest auscultation.
- Pharmokinetics.
- Pharmacodynamics.
- Pharmacology.
- Whole systems assessment.
- Prescribing practice. However, should nurses be required to undertake a prescribing role within their scope of practice they would first need to successfully undertake an NMC recognized prescribing course and abide by the NMC (2019d) *Standards for Prescribers*.

ACTIVITY 9.12

Consider how your current and future practice addresses the new NMC (2018b) proficiencies for registered nurses.

Can you identify any CPD needs? If so, addressing and evidencing these will be useful for your revalidation.

To help you with revalidation all the NMC requirements are helpfully laid out on their revalidation microsite at: http://revalidation.nmc.org.uk/

Registered nurses need to be really familiar with this microsite and also have an NMC online account as revalidation evidence needs to be submitted by this means. In short, revalidation was designed to be straightforward to enable registered nurses and midwives to demonstrate that they practise safely and effectively. The requirements of revalidation are that registrants submit to the NMC evidence of undertaking:

- 450 practice hours, or 900 if renewing as both a nurse and midwife.
- 35 hours of CPD including 20 hours of participatory learning.
- Five pieces of practice-related feedback.
- Five written reflective accounts.
- A reflective discussion.
- A health and character declaration.
- A professional indemnity arrangement.
- Confirmation of revalidation by another NMC registrant.

In terms of CPD requirements, registrants must have undertaken 35 hours of learning activities relevant to their scope of practice in the three-year period since their registration was last renewed or when a registrant first joined the NMC register. Registrants can check their revalidation date within their NMC online account. Of these 35 hours registrants must undertake at least 20 hours of participatory learning. Examples of participatory CPD learning include:

- Structured learning (direct or distance learning).
- Accredited college or university learning event.
- Workshops, conference.
- Peer review activities.
- Coaching and mentoring.

- Structured professional clinical supervision.
- Undertaking short supervised practice for specific skills development.
- Group or practice meetings outside everyday practice, e.g. to discuss a new way of working.
- Participation in clinical audits.
- Practice visits to different environments relevant to their scope of practice.
- Participation in online chats such as those provided by @WeNurses on Twitter.
- Training related to job rotation or secondment, shadowing, etc.

In terms of recording CPD to fulfil NMC revalidation requirements, the NMC provide a suggested template. However irrespective of which template is used, the NMC require that registrants record the following information regarding all their CPD activity:

- The CPD method/activity.
- A description of the topic and how it related to their practice.
- The dates on which the activity was undertaken.
- The number of hours (including the number of participatory hours).
- The identification of the part of the NMC (2018b) proficiencies and (NMC, 2018a) *Code* most relevant to the activity.
- Evidence that the CPD activity was undertaken.

CPD, clinical governance and revalidation

Earlier in this chapter we discussed how various infamous high-profile incidents involving various healthcare professionals and organizations have led to the government setting up inquiries and responding with various policy and legislative changes. A key government response to the recommendations from these inquiries has been the implementation of or strengthening of clinical governance arrangements through the publication of White Papers first produced in the 1990s (DH, 1997; 1998). The current clinical governance guidance (National Quality Board, 2011) is overseen by the Care Quality Commission, with NICE being responsible for setting clinical standards since 2008 (DH, 2008a). The boards of provider units, local clinical commissioning groups and NHS Improvement all too have a role in setting, monitoring and enhancing the clinical governance agenda both locally and nationally. This is further discussed in Chapter 3.

Clinical governance also has many definitions, but the original and most well-known definition came from the Department of Health (1998: 33). Clinical governance is:

> A framework through which organizations are accountable for continuously improving the quality of service and safeguarding high standards of care by creating an environment in which clinical care will flourish.

Gottwald and Lansdown (2014) assert that CPD is a vital component of clinical governance, adding that CPD can be derived from either formal or informal learning processes. As we saw earlier, both learning approaches are also valued within the NMC (2019b) revalidation requirements. However, Gottwald and Lansdown (2014) further conclude that CPD needs to be undertaken at individual, team and organization level for it to be most effective in terms of clinical governance, and that this process needs to be managed by appraisal or personal development review. Appraisal or personal development review is a structured process whereby individuals can review their personal and professional development needs to date with an appraiser. Individuals can then make future development plans based on their learning needs and available learning opportunities which link to their preferred learning styles. These future development plans must also be aligned with both team and organization development objectives. This may help ensure that the self-development needs of individuals are supported if they explicitly link to the team and organization development needs as well.

───────────────── ACTIVITY 9.13 ─────────────────

Examine the clinical governance policy in your employing organization and determine what it requires in terms of your CPD and whether it will be managed by your appraisal.

CPD and the interdisciplinary context

Other healthcare professional groups have also been required to undertake CPD as a means of demonstrating fitness for re-registration. For example, allied health professionals have been required to meet the Health and Care Professions Council CPD standards since 2006. The current Health and Care Professions Council (2019) CPD requirements are deemed to meet current health profession revalidation requirements. Pharmacists too have been required to meet CPD standards since 2009. More recently the General Pharmaceutical Council (2018) have also implemented revalidation requirements for all their registrants.

Undertaking CPD with other professional groups is extremely valuable. As patient/client care involves an interdisciplinary approach, then it follows that CPD should involve joint learning to further develop the practice provided by all team members to their patient/client group. Equally, sharing resources from professional, statutory, and regulatory bodies related to CPD will be very useful to any healthcare professional and assist in maximizing resources. Joint CPD is indeed a learning activity itself if the outcome is a greater understanding of roles in the teams by the different disciplines. Finally, current regulatory processes for health professionals require testimony from other registrant colleagues, so again undertaking CPD with colleagues from other professions provides opportunities for development and revalidation.

─────────────── **ACTIVITY 9.14** ───────────────

Consider how you could undertake CPD with other professional groups in your practice area. Highlight the advantages and disadvantages.

CPD and academic accreditation

Your pre-registration nursing qualification is likely to have been academically accredited. This means that, in addition to qualifying as a nurse, you have achieved an academic qualification from a higher education institution (HEI) or university. This qualification could be a diploma in higher education, but since 2010 it will have been a degree with honours. As discussed earlier, CPD can be undertaken in many forms and does not have to be associated with an academically accredited learning activity. This, as we have already seen, is particularly underlined by the NMC (2019b) revalidation CPD requirements.

However, if some of your CPD is undertaken as an academically accredited learning activity, you may wish to consider whether you can or wish to use any of the academic credit gained towards a higher academic qualification relevant to your practice.

To manage your academic development, it is important to have some understanding of the higher education qualification and credit infrastructure. The Quality Assurance Agency for Higher Education (the QAA) has a national framework for higher education qualifications (QAA, 2008). This qualifications framework with academic levels is summarized in Table 9.1. There are three undergraduate levels (levels 4–6) and two postgraduate levels (levels 7–8).

The crucial point to bear in mind with the National Qualifications Framework is that the QAA (2008) sets out descriptors for the achievement of qualifications at each of its levels. These descriptors are usually written as learning outcomes for each overall qualification. HEIs that deliver these qualifications may use credit points to organize the delivery of their qualifications, but the QAA (2008) does not insist on such a system. If credit points are used, then they are usually attached to modules, which then in turn form the overall academic

Table 9.1 The QAA (2008) National Framework for higher education qualifications

Typical higher education qualification	Level
Doctoral, e.g. PhD	8
Master's, e.g. MSc or MA Postgraduate diplomas Postgraduate certificates	7
Bachelor's degrees with honours, e.g. BA/BSc (Hons) Bachelor's degrees without honours, e.g. BA/BSc Graduate diplomas Graduate certificates	6
Foundation degrees, e.g. FdA, FdSc Diplomas of higher education (DipHE) Higher national diplomas (HND)	5
Higher national certificates (HNC) Certificates of higher education (CertHE)	4

Adapted from the QAA National Framework

qualification. Therefore, formal CPD learning activities that you undertake could provide, on successful completion, academic credits at a determined level. It may be useful to consider prior to undertaking such a learning activity whether the level of the credit enables you to complete a higher academic qualification.

Example

Referring to Table 9.1, if you already have a diploma in higher education (level 5), following the completion of your pre-registration nurse education, you may only choose to study academically accredited courses at the minimum of level 6 in order to progress towards a degree with honours. Likewise, if you have achieved a degree with honours (level 6) you may choose only to study academically accredited courses at level 7 to progress towards a master's degree. The UCAS website shows all currently available master's level programmes in the UK.

In terms of accumulating academic credits, you then may wish to consider how you could transfer these credits towards a higher academic qualification. This requires using the **Credit Accumulation Transfer Scheme (CATS)**. Therefore, you need to bear in mind how many credits you are accumulating and how many credits an academic award comprises in total. Another consideration is how the modules studied match the learning outcomes of a specific qualification towards which you may wish to transfer credit. The means of claiming credit using the CAT scheme is by the **accreditation of prior learning (APL)**. This allows relevant formal and experiential learning to be claimed.

In order to successfully manage your academic development, it is best to seek advice from appropriate academic staff. It may also be useful to plan your academic development within your appraisal. Any formal learning undertaken as part of academic study counts towards your 20 hours of participatory learning CPD stipulated by the NMC (2019) revalidation requirements.

Personal and professional development planning and coaching

So far in this chapter, we have explored formal requirements and mechanisms that you may face as a newly qualified nurse in relation to your preceptorship, continuing professional development and revalidation. It is now appropriate to look at more informal, yet nonetheless worthwhile, strategies for managing your own development, either independently or via facilitation from others. The following section discusses some approaches to assist you in identifying your needs and setting goals, so that, as you embark on your career as a qualified nurse, you have some idea of how to construct a pathway for your future. This might mean identifying how to survive and develop in the initial transition period or to make longer-term plans and identify the steps needed to get there. These will be useful as a basis for your discussions with your preceptor or supervisors in your workplace. It may also be helpful as a basis for the time when you might be the preceptor or coach for another newly qualified nurse.

Coaching

Henwood and Lister (2009) suggested that, in the world of healthcare, change is a constant, and initial education and pre-qualifying training plus CPD is not always enough to deal with this. Coventry et al. (2015) found that it was sometimes difficult for nurses to access continuing professional development due to culture and organizational workload issues, ultimately affecting competence and patient outcomes. Therefore, it is important to consider how you might access CPD yourself considering regulatory body requirements and the necessity for maintaining and enhancing knowledge, skills and attitudes in quickly changing health professional fields.

Nursing staff therefore need to develop the ability to care for themselves. Coaching helps an individual to prepare for other aspects related to healthcare professional development such as preceptorship, mentoring, CPD, clinical supervision and appraisal. According to Lawrence (2017), coaching by line managers or senior staff is one of the most effective learning, personal and professional development activities. An emphasis on relationship-building and providing feedback is an important factor in the coaching approach. Your preceptor may be able to assist you by using coaching techniques, which are being increasingly used in professional careers. Coaching is not necessarily about giving advice to others; it is more about facilitating and pointing the individual in the direction in which they desire to go.

Coaching is described by Mühlberger and Traut-Mattausch (2015) as a process based on goal-setting and devising solution-focused approaches to meet the goals, self-direction and growth of the individual. This involves the coach identifying the roles, responsibilities and boundaries between themselves and the person they are working with; providing flexible support; communicating effectively through active listening and questioning; facilitating learning and achievement of results via goal-setting and action plans and monitoring progress. However, the main emphasis is that the coach should only facilitate the individual to be able to coach themselves. Narayanasamy and Penney (2014) point out that a coach is a powerful resource when the process is conducted effectively by guiding individuals to solve issues and identify desired outcomes and strategies. It is not about directing, providing answers/solutions or solving problems for them.

Coaching can be considered as an intervention that arises from the field of positive psychology. Donaldson and Dollwet (2013) highlighted that although positive psychology is a relatively new discipline, it has burgeoned in the last twenty years or so and has entered the fabric of the workplace and organizational behaviour. They suggest that positive psychology focuses on how individuals thrive in the workplace and state that this requires working conditions where individuals gain new and meaningful knowledge and skills daily, which leads to higher levels of thriving at work. Employees find that they can achieve their goals, reduce stress and raise workplace well-being if they are included in a coaching process.

Coaching is a solution-focused approach which emphasizes strengths, resources and resilience to create purposeful, positive change (Grant et al., 2012). Solution-focused approaches concentrate on identifying the desired state/outcomes and creating strategies and pathways to achieve them. This approach increases the range of potential actions to achieve growth through reflection, creative strategy development and action planning, resulting in self-efficacy and well-being.

Barron and Sloan (2015) highlight that the coach is required to assist the individual in clarifying the purpose of the coaching relationship by exploring learning needs, expectations and goals. There is a need to be able to demonstrate compassion as a fundamental requirement in the coaching situation. Therefore, you need to be able to identify a coach that you can relate to but who is able to maintain professional boundaries.

ACTIVITY 9.15

Consider the people during your training that have assisted you most in your own development.

1 How did they foster the relationship?
2 What strategies did they use most effectively to facilitate your development?
3 What characteristics did they display in coaching you?

Self-awareness and goal-setting

Having another person act as a coach is very beneficial. However, as most of the approaches are facilitative, there are some of the aspects that you can initiate yourself. Self-awareness is an important factor recognized within the concept of emotional intelligence, a characteristic which is highly valued in nursing and one that is crucial in personal and professional development and relationships in the workplace. Kemp and Baker (2013) highlight the importance of reflection in CPD. The purpose of CPD is to ensure the increasing effectiveness and competence of the nurse whilst developing new ways of thinking. This is achieved by making changes to existing belief systems through examination and elaboration of them. They suggest that reflection can at times be uncomfortable, raising doubts and insecurity in the individual. However, it can foster critical awareness of practice and lead to enhanced learning experiences. Clancy (2014) suggests emotional intelligence is crucial for professionals in healthcare settings and that motivation and self-awareness are important factors in promoting improved healthcare outcomes. This is because it helps individuals to recognize what skills they have and provides opportunities for developing these further. This suggests some accountability lies with the developing nurse to cultivate their passion towards these ends. The first steps towards this involve setting clear developmental goals.

According to Cooper (2013) one technique which can be used to facilitate personal development is Neuro-Linguistic Programming (NLP). She suggests that as nurses we are all leaders, and lead others in learning the art and science of nursing. Part of this requirement is ensuring that people believe they are valued. Based on NLP, this requires you adopting a positive state which requires some self-awareness for recognizing how you are currently feeling and identifying strategies for changing this if necessary. There is a need for good rapport with others to understand their position and to create meaningful relationships in the workplace. Finally, the ability to demonstrate behavioural flexibility is important to find solutions to challenges. This is achieved by varying your own behaviour to elicit the desired responses in others to move towards the outcomes set.

NLP is not without its critics, particularly due to its lack of empirical studies; however, Pishghadam and Shayesteh (2014) highlight that even though there is not a body of evidence related to the theoretical aspects, the techniques and models in NLP are of use.

> Technically speaking, NLP could be taught to help improve memory, promote personal strength, adopt effective learning strategies, distinguish and reframe impeding educational beliefs, raise self-esteem, and optimize motivation. (Pishghadam and Shayesteh, 2014: 2096)

Therefore, although we should be cautious about some of the wider claims of NLP, Cassidy-Rice (2014) suggests that some NLP techniques can be beneficial in promoting personal and professional development. It has tools that help bring awareness into the ways we do things, to communicate elegantly with others identifying the way forward, and to develop actions leading to performing at higher levels. He argues that values underpin the pathways to change. These include:

- **Power values** – what we want.
- **Operational values** – how we get there.
- **Determination values** – how we evaluate.

This is very similar to the '**GROW**' model which is a recognized tool used by coaches (Law, 2013). Grow stands for **Goals**, **Reality**, **Options** and **Will**. A clear **G**oal is required. The **R**eality of whether it can be achieved needs to be evaluated. **O**ptions of steps and strategies to help you move toward the goal should be identified, including assessing how barriers can be removed. **W**ill is related to identifying motivating factors in getting started, which might include ensuring the steps are small enough to create quick and easy achievements, which builds up will and motivation to continue.

Identifying outcomes and goals in this process is the start of identifying what we want, before creating the strategy and methods of measurement to evaluate the achievement.

Lazarus (2015) outlines that there are three types of goals:

- **Outcomes** (Why). These are related to identifying the overall outcome and involve the rationale and motivating factors.
- **Performance goals** (What). These are related to what needs to be achieved and measured to demonstrate the outcome.
- **Process goals** (How). These are the steps that the overall aims are broken down into.

The simplest premise related to goal-setting is to state the goal in the positive – that is, to state what you want as opposed to what you don't want. For example, when searching on a website, we often quickly get to the pages we want by stating the aspect we are searching for in clear terms. The more refined and specific our terms are, the more successful the search is. Goal-setting needs to follow the exact same process.

Another aspect assisting in goal-setting is the concept of **logical levels** highlighted within NLP. Logical levels refer to the concept that individuals psychologically operate on a number of levels. In a similar way to Maslow's hierarchy of needs, the lower levels give rise to the higher levels (Alder, 2017). Goals can be set in relation to the level at which development is needed. The logical levels are shown in Figure 9.1.

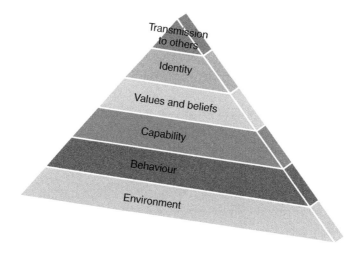

Figure 9.1 Logical levels

The logical levels are **environment, behaviours, capabilities, values and beliefs**, and **identity** (Alder, 2017). Each level feeds into the one above, so in relation to setting goals for your development, you can ask further questions such as the following:

- In what environment do I want/need to work?
- What behaviours do I need to develop?
- What capabilities would I need?
- What are my values?
- What would that say about me?
- What kind of a person/nurse do I want to be?

These questions could alternatively be considered as follows:

- Where do I want to be?
- What do I want to do?
- How do I want to do it?
- Why do I want to do it?
- Who will I become?

Your situation can be analysed at each level to identify goals that would impact upon them. This can be like a ripple effect: changes at one level can lead to changes at several levels. For example, if an environment becomes contaminated, behaviour must change as a result, and so on. Therefore, there is a need to understand what is happening at each level. Alder (2017) suggests that these levels define understanding, which influences our thoughts and solutions in the world around us. To develop pertinent personal development questions as nurses, then, we can simply frame them in relation to the levels. From these questions, we can set goals. This could be something as simple as: 'I want to work in intensive care environments'.

─────────────────── **ACTIVITY 9.16** ───────────────────

1 Identify a list of issues you would like to address within your preceptorship. Which of the logical levels do they fit in with: environment, behaviour, capability, values and beliefs, or identity?
2 Now set a positively stated goal (what you would want to achieve) for each level.

(Continued)

(Continued)

- Where do I want to be?
- What do I want to do?
- How do I want to do it?
- Why do I want to do it?
- Who will I become?
- How will I interact with others?

It is useful to note that if you get 'stuck' at one level, then you can look at the one below in order to set goals that will lead you to the higher level. For example, if it is a **capability** or skill that you feel you need to develop, then you might need to break the goal down into **behavioural** steps that build up the skill to master it.

According to Egan (2014), the basic premise of personal development planning or individual change goes through a process of understanding where you are now (**present state**) to where you want to be, or your goal (**desired state**), and how you intend to get there (**resources**). The goals that you set should be analysed and broken down into the various steps or stages that will take you through to the final process of achieving them. For example, if your desire is to become a nurse manager, then a smaller step might be to attend a management course. To get on a management course, your goal might be to seek out information on relevant management courses.

The discussion above has introduced the concept of setting outcomes that are relevant to your personal and professional development. By being able to create outcomes and identify resources, you can go into preceptorship, mentorship, clinical supervision or appraisal armed with clear goals to discuss with your superiors, or in some cases your peers, and in doing so identify your CPD requirements. Being forearmed in such a way sends a clear message that you have well-formed ideas about your career development.

Personal and professional development planning will be an important part of your career. It will be something that occurs constantly and can be useful to you in your career as a nurse.

Summary

This chapter has focused on the aspects that you will need to consider in relation to your own development once you have become a qualified nurse. We have looked at issues related to what you can expect from a period of preceptorship and how to be involved in, and manage, this for yourself.

We discussed the CPD and the requirements that you need to meet in order to continue to maintain your registration as a nurse with the NMC. The discussion has outlined some strategies and considerations that should assist you to do this.

Remember, becoming a qualified nurse is not the end of your educational journey throughout your nursing career. You could liken it to having completed your driving test. You have met the required standard and are considered safe to drive. However, once functioning in the real world as a practitioner in your own right, you continue to learn how to operate and get used to everyday or unusual circumstances, just as you must learn how to get used to driving without someone else providing you with instruction and supervision. So, really, it is just the beginning of a new phase. This means that you make lots of decisions. The difference from the driving analogy, however, as highlighted in this chapter, is that you can expect some guidance and supervision from a preceptor on qualifying. There should always be someone to whom you can turn for advice in these early transitional stages.

The need for CPD is a requirement to demonstrate that you are up to date with current practices and that you continue to be safe to practise, and therefore deserve the right to continue being a registered nurse through revalidation. The arenas in which nurses work are constantly changing, and you need to be able to change with the environments and approaches that are used in providing such a valuable public service.

Lastly, it is important to remember that this is your career. Therefore, personal development planning is important in that it assists you to align your CPD to the plans that you might make as your career develops and meet the requirements tri-annually for revalidation with the NMC. You may need to be able to set short-term goals to identify how you can develop in relation to the area in which you may work, or longer-term goals to assist you to move in a desired career direction of your choice.

Preceptorship is important in your transition to working as a qualified nurse.

- Preceptorship is required to ensure the provision of safe and effective care whilst you are in the transition from student nurse to registered nurse.

CPD is important in ensuring that you keep up to date with developing practice.

- CPD is essential to maintain your registration as required by NMC re-registration and revalidation requirements.
  Revalidation is a statutory requirement on healthcare professionals to ensure they are fit to remain on regulatory body registers.

- Nurses have undergone revalidation since 2016 and must fulfil all NMC requirements.

Personal and professional development planning and coaching:

- Assists in clarifying needs and goals.
- It helps to clarify your career direction and aspirations.

10

GLOBAL AND INTERNATIONAL NURSING

Rob Burton and Graham Ormrod

THE AIMS OF THIS CHAPTER ARE TO:

- Explore the concept of global nursing.
- Explore issues of nurse migration.
- Discuss requirements of registering as a nurse in other countries.

Introduction

According to the International Council of Nurses (ICN, 2019), their purpose is to represent nursing worldwide, to advance the profession and influence policy. It is well recognized that due to advances in technology and transport systems the world is a smaller place and is accessible to most who have access to these systems. According to Wong et al. (2015) globalization makes the world a smaller place with more people interconnected and interdependent with each other. Nurses aim to promote health regardless of borders and boundaries and are at the forefront of achieving this. There are around 19 million nurses worldwide that share these common principles. However, nursing on the world stage is not without its challenges.

Holmgren et al. (2018) outline that as international borders become unlocked on economic, social and cultural levels nurses are affected by the issues associated with globalization. Nurses make up the largest group of health professionals that need to cater for growing ageing and vulnerable populations, ill health, natural disasters, humanitarian crises and migration in times of global uncertainty and conflict. Wilson et al. (2016) highlight that nurses are fundamental in providing healthcare and access to it and make significant contributions to the global health agenda as advocates, care providers, managers and leaders, educators and researchers. In 2015 the United Nations (UN) released its agenda for building on the prior 'Millennium Development Goals' (MDGs) with its 'Sustainable Development Goals' (SDGs). There are 17 goals with targets for 2030, and as the World Health Organization (WHO) argue that health is a fundamental principle in all of these then nurses have a significant role to play globally.

The SDGs (UN, 2015) are:

1   No poverty.
2   Zero hunger.
3   Good health and well-being.
4   Quality education.
5   Gender equality.
6   Clean water and sanitation.
7   Affordable and clean energy.
8   Decent work and economic growth.
9   Industry, innovation and infrastructure.

10 Reduced inequalities.
11 Sustainable cities and communities.
12 Responsible consumption and production.
13 Climate action.
14 Life below water.
15 Life on land.
16 Peace, justice and strong institutions.
17 Partnerships for the goals.

www.un.org/sustainabledevelopment/
sustainable-development-goals

Figure 10.1 shows an infographic of the UN SDGs.

Benton and Shaffer (2016) conducted a review of the literature around these issues, and identified the following themes as key: child nutrition, education and women's health, food, Human Immuno-deficiency Virus (HIV) in Africa and elsewhere, methods and measures and midwifery capacity. They developed a matrix based on the SDGs and the ICN (2014) three pillars of 'professional practice, regulation and socio-economic welfare', in which nurses can contribute. They state that nursing should be a prime mover in achieving some of these goals, by direct action-oriented advocacy and aligning to the agendas in supportive coalitions. They highlight that there is a gap related to the nursing scholarship, which is required to produce nurses, leaders

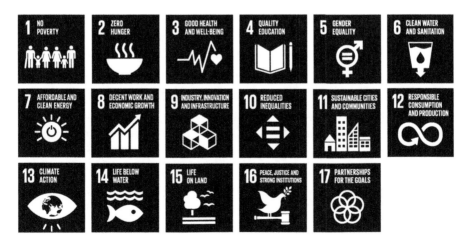

Figure 10.1 UN Sustainable Development Goals (2015) (www.un.org/sustainabledevelopment/)

Disclaimer: The content of this publication has not been approved by the United Nations and does not reflect the views of the United Nations or its officials or Member States.

and researchers that can influence future policy development. Griffiths (2019) outlines that research in nursing and midwifery in developing countries is a priority where nursing contributions are imperative due to poor health and healthcare workforce issues. A UK All-Party Parliamentary Group (APPG) on Global Health report discussing the 'triple impact' of nursing on 'better health, stronger economies and greater gender equality' emphasized the importance of nursing in these issues (Crisp and Watkins, 2018). A number of recommendations were made to highlight the contribution nursing should make in order to achieve these factors which echo the SDGs and the ICN pillars. These were to:

1   Raise the profile of nursing and make it central to health policy.
2   Support plans to increase the number of nurses being educated and employed globally.
3   Develop nurse leaders and nurse leadership.
4   Enable nurses to work to their full potential.
5   Collect and disseminate evidence of the impact of nursing on access, quality and costs, and ensure it is incorporated in policy and acted upon.
6   Develop nursing to have a triple impact on health, gender equality and economies.
7   Promote partnership and mutual learning between the UK and other countries.

(APPG, 2016: 6)

Figure 10.2 shows the triple impact of nursing themes.

The World Health Organization (WHO, 2016) point out that we are now in a period where the number of people aged over 60 years outnumber those aged under 5 years. The impact of this is vast. The changes in economic factors, urbanization and growth has led to the increase of unhealthy lifestyles, which in turn have led to the rise in the prevalence of non-communicable diseases such as diabetes and heart disease. Communicable diseases such as HIV/AIDS, tuberculosis, malaria and more recently the shocking ebola and zika viruses have also increased and of course the devastating and unprecedented coronavirus pandemic of 2020. Therefore, globalization is changing the nature of health, from maternal and child care to the burgeoning needs of older people. Nurses roles are crucial in responding to these health needs across the lifespan and in different settings across the world. It is important that nurses and midwives are prepared for

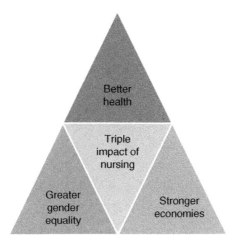

Figure 10.2 The triple impact of nursing

Reprinted from Crisp and Watkins (2018) The triple impact of nursing. *International Journal of Nursing Studies*, 78: A3–A4, with permission from Elsevier

these roles through their education, whereby knowledge and skills related to health promotion, disease prevention, treatment and rehabilitation are inherent.

As you complete your transition into nursing practice from being a student, you may soon come to recognize how these global factors could impact on your role as a nurse in a rapidly changing global environment. Therefore, it is necessary that you understand some of the issues related to globalization and the role nurses will have to play as these changes occur. The concept of 'Global Nursing' addresses these issues and so will be explored. As mentioned earlier, globalization leads to greater mobility and interconnectedness across international boundaries, which leads to issues related to migration. The impact of migration will therefore be explored further. As nurses do become mobile globally, you may find yourself in a position with opportunities to nurse in other countries, therefore some of the regulatory aspects of potential migration to some specific countries will be discussed in more detail.

Global nursing

In order to understand global nursing, it is important to understand the nature of globalization. Due to changes in technology, economic factors and travel accessibility the world is now figuratively a smaller place, with much more connectivity amongst populations.

> It encompasses a range of social, political and economic changes and is characterized by high mobility, economic inter-dependence and electronic interconnectedness ... to include two interrelated elements: the opening of international borders to increasingly fast flows of goods, services, finance, people and ideas; and the changes in institutions and policies at national and international levels that enable or promote such flows. (Bradbury-Jones and Clark, 2017: 54)

Wilson et al. (2016) reviewed the outcomes from a report looking at definitions of 'Global Health' and 'Global Nursing' developed by the global advisory panel on the future of nursing (GAPFON). These were as follows:

Global Health is:

> an area for practice, study and research that places a priority on improving health, achieving equity in health for all people and ensuring health-promoting and sustainable sociocultural, political and economic systems. Global health implies planetary health which equals human, animal, environmental and ecosystem health and it emphasizes transnational health issues, determinants and solutions; involves many disciplines within and beyond the health sciences and promotes interdependence and interdisciplinary collaboration; and is a synthesis of population-based prevention with individual holistic care.

Global Nursing is:

> the use of evidence-based nursing process to promote sustainable planetary health and equity for all people. Global nursing considers social determinants of health, includes individual and population-level care, research, education, leadership, advocacy and policy initiatives. Global nurses engage in ethical practice and demonstrate respect for human dignity, human rights and cultural diversity. Global nurses engage in a spirit of deliberation and reflection in interdependent

partnership with communities and other healthcare providers. (Wilson et al., 2016: 1530)

According to Nicholas and Breakey (2015), global health arose out
of the need to develop understanding of public health issues and communicable diseases, the need to gather data on populations, develop
social justice and equity, and focus on prevention rather than cure.
Health systems and global public health projects require leadership
for ensuring cost-effective, evidence-based approaches for integrated
health services that prioritize prevention, treatment and cure as a
continuum. Nurses are a fundamental part of the services required to
meet these aspects, working inter-professionally, across borders and
in situations with very different levels of technology available to support the approaches.

Wilson et al. (2016) highlight that the definition of global nursing arose from several identified themes from the relevant literature
on the subject. These themes included 'transnational', 'interdependent', 'glocal' (global and local health needs) and 'cultural competence'.
There are many interchangeable terms and some of these will be discussed further in this chapter.

These aspects arising from such global issues are integral within the
NMC standards of proficiency (NMC, 2018b) where the role of registered nurses in leading and coordinating care delivery for people of all
ages from different backgrounds, cultures and beliefs is identified as
paramount. The NMC code of conduct (NMC, 2018a) enshrines these
concepts within it across the themes of 'Prioritise people, Practise
effectively, Preserve safety, and Promote professionalism and trust'
(Bradbury-Jones and Clark, 2017). Therefore you should be able to
see that as a professional nurse your expertise should be able to cross
the boundaries of different countries and systems, as the principles
upon which you were trained are equally applicable across the world.

Global nursing is about developing knowledge about health, care,
persons, suffering and ecology in local and global contexts. This is
characterized by advocacy and activism from the nursing profession
with an aim towards sustainable development. This requires use of
knowledge and methods to reduce inequalities and social injustice.
Ultimately, knowledge in global nursing aims to alleviate suffering,
safeguard human dignity and contribute to health for present and
future generations (Holmgren, 2017: 172).

Arising from the above-mentioned triple impact report (Crisp, 2016), the ICN and WHO developed the project 'Nursing Now' which had 5 ambitious aims for nursing globally by 2020 – the 200-year anniversary of the birth of Florence Nightingale. These were:

1 **Greater investment in improving education, professional development, standards, regulation and employment conditions for nurses.**
    o   All countries have plans for developing nursing and midwifery.
    o   Increased investment in all aspects of nursing and midwifery.
    o   More nurses in training and employment, with clear progress in eliminating the global shortfall of 9 million nurses and midwives by 2030.

2 **Increased and improved dissemination of effective and innovative practice in nursing.**
    o   Nursing organizations collectively support a coordinated global portal of effective practice and innovation used by nurses and policy-makers around the world.

3 **Greater influence for nurses and midwives on global and national health policy, as part of broader efforts to ensure health workforces are more involved in decision-making.**
    o   All global and national policies on health and healthcare acknowledge the role of nursing in achieving their goals and include plans for the development of nursing.
    o   All national plans for delivering universal healthcare (UHC) make specific proposals to enhance and develop the role of nurses as the health professionals closest to the community.

4 **More nurses in leadership positions and more opportunities for development at all levels.**
    o   At least 75 percent of countries have a Chief Nursing Officer or Chief Government Nurse as part of their most senior management team in health.
    o   More senior leadership programmes for nurses.
    o   The establishment of a global nursing leadership network.

5 **More evidence for policy and decision-makers about: where nursing can have the greatest impact, what is stopping nurses from reaching their full potential and how to address these obstacles.**

    o A landmark study on the economic impact of nursing is published.

    o More articles on nursing's impact in peer-reviewed A* journals.

    o A coordinated global network on research on nursing is established.

(Nursing Now, 2018)

From this you may be able to understand that as nursing further develops itself professionally in wider regions of the world, and with the advancement of interconnectivity and ease of travel, you may find yourself working as a 'global nurse' at some point in your professional career. Jones and Sherwood (2014) describe professionally registered nurses, midwives and other health professionals as 'sources' suggesting they might be specifically prepared to work in other destinations or locales. Some countries may train nurses specifically for their own workforce as well as actively recruiting from other areas in order to ensure appropriate numbers to provide nursing services. As nurses are an important part of healthcare service provision in the global economy, several factors impact on their employment and deployment. These include the political system, the funding of health services, different legal and regulatory systems, and the cultural aspects of the population. As nursing becomes more mobile across the world, changes may occur within these differing systems.

As well as previous studies that have shown that more highly educated nurses and higher nurse staffing ratios improve patient outcomes, a review study by Coster et al. (2018) suggested that nurses improve the outcomes for their patients on international levels in low- and middle-income countries. This is due to their roles in working in acute settings, public health roles such as promoting health, vaccinations and hygiene, outreach and home visiting, nurse-led clinics and services, extended and specialist roles. They concluded that optimal deployment of healthcare professionals requires that care and treatment should be delivered at all stages of a patient's journey by a member of nursing staff who is:

> working to the maximum limit of their education, experience and competence who has the appropriate level of capabilities and skills to deliver safe care. (Coster et al., 2018: 81)

Watson (2019) argues that in modern times there are many challenges facing nurses in ensuring that the needs of populations living in dire situations throughout the world are shown compassionate and ethical approaches in meeting their health and well-being needs. She states that:

> Nursing has a global covenant with humanity, to sustain human caring, healing, health, and wholeness for humanity; in instances where human caring is threatened, be it biological or otherwise. (Watson, 2019: 1)

Due to the high value of nurses, their mobility across the globe is desirable, and movement is seen in the direction from lower economic situations to higher economic and more technical ones. Ortiga and Rivero (2019) highlight that this can be viewed as a 'brain drain' from those lower economic countries. However, they also suggest that the 'export value' of some nurses (from the Philippines in this instance) is their experience in dealing in more physical tasks with the patients, particularly when moving to countries where the developing professional status of nurses has resulted in moves to more technical-based and specialized roles for registered nurses. The implications of this for you is that you may choose to migrate to another country to practice, or you might find yourselves with nurses from overseas that have migrated to your country to work in your service. Either way, throughout your career you will find yourself working with many nurses that have trained, worked or both in differing healthcare service provisions and have experienced a range of differing levels of need for healthcare within their host countries.

According to an Organization for Economic Co-operation and Development (OECD) report (OECD, 2017), due to the mobility of overseas healthcare workers into other countries, there was a global code of practice on ethical recruitment developed by the World Health Assembly to respond to concerns of poorer countries losing their healthcare professionals and placing the healthcare systems under duress. However, according to the OECD, the overall average amount that foreign nurses constitute is five point nine percent of workforces, with six percent in the USA, 14.4 percent in the UK, 18.1 percent in Australia and the highest number in New Zealand with 25.4 percent across the OECD countries.

The ICN (2013) highlight that cultural competence is an important factor that today's nurses require if they are to operate in a global nursing profession. They suggest that nurses should demonstrate cultural competence by:

- Developing an awareness of one's own culture without letting it have an undue influence on those from other backgrounds.
- Demonstrating knowledge and understanding of different cultures.
- Accepting that there may be differences between the cultural beliefs and values of the healthcare provider and the client.
- Accepting and respecting cultural differences.
- Adapting care to be congruent with the client's culture and expectations.
- Providing culturally appropriate care so as to deliver the best possible client outcomes.

Johnson and Johnson (2015: 130) describe culture as 'traits that make up a particular group of people'. This includes customs, rites, social practices, food, dress, music and language.

Although there is not a clear definition, Harkess and Kaddoura (2015: 211) suggest that cultural competence is related to the complex integration of knowledge, attitudes and skills that enhances cross-cultural communication and appropriate effective interactions with others.

According to Bonello et al. (2018), awareness of cultural issues is important in understanding how interactions with others in professional settings can be affected if there are cultural misunderstandings. Their study into interprofessional education highlighted the cultural dimensions model of Hofstede which includes six aspects:

- Power distance.
- Individualism versus collectivism.
- Masculinity versus femininity.
- Uncertainty avoidance.
- Long-term orientation versus short-term orientation.
- Indulgence versus restraint.

(Hofstede et al., 2010)

These cultural dimensions can be either 'high-context' or 'low-context' depending on the historical development of the cultures they apply to and the complexity of the societies from which they developed

(Meyer, 2015). Meyer (2015) suggests that in relation to language/communication and cultural context, the USA is the lowest-context country, followed by the 'Anglo-Saxon' cluster of countries (Germany, Denmark, UK), next are the Latin-based language cultures (Italy, Spain, France and Latin America). African and Asian countries are seen as high-context, with Japan being considered the highest-context culture. High-context cultures tend to have long histories with relationship-oriented societies where networks of connections and traditions are passed from generation to generation. Japan is a society which is fairly homogenous, so these contextual elements are passed on and understood through each generation. As the USA has a relatively shorter history and is shaped by immigrants from around the world with varying languages, the need to pass on information quickly and flexibly applies and is therefore less based on tradition. A person from a low-context society may perceive someone from a high-context society as secretive, lacking communication skills and transparency as they will not be aware of the nuances and behaviours that support the interactions. Someone from a high-context situation may view someone from a low-context culture as condescending and patronising as they inappropriately state the obvious.

Cultural competence can be taught in nursing schools using various delivery methods including inviting speakers from certain cultural backgrounds. However, 'cultural immersion' seems to be a popular approach, including study abroad, exchange programmes and local cultural immersion. This may not always suit the actual purpose of cultural competence so nursing programmes need to ensure a considered approach to developing this, as opposed to tokenistic opportunities.

One of the ways that nurses can experience some of these aspects, cultural awareness, context, collaboration and communication skills is through mobility experiences. In some nursing courses there may be opportunity for students to access a mobility or exchange experience either as part of their academic programme or as part of a clinical elective placement. You may have had such an opportunity during your own pre-registration training. Such mobility experiences can sometimes be funded through projects such as the Erasmus programme in Europe, or the New Columbo Plan (NCP) projects across Asia and Australasia and other funding sources. Ortega et al. (2016) found that such mobility programmes or projects are useful experiences for students as they can develop their awareness of other cultures, the issues faced, and become global citizens as they are able to compare and contrast their own situation with those in the host country. This often leads to increased personal and professional development and offers some quid pro quo benefits to the hosting country. It must be recognized that this is not always the case and some risk assessment must be taken before embarking on such ventures, but there are positive outcomes to be found in the move towards global nursing. Hopefully, you may have had an opportunity for some form of exchange within your nursing programme. If not, and it is still available / feasible, it would be highly recommended to engage in such a project, as it helps with cultural competence and understanding of other healthcare systems and nursing. Johnson and Johnson (2015) provide some advice for nurses serving overseas or pursuing a career in a cultural context which is different to their own:

1   Be flexible.
2   Be open-minded.
3   Invest in language and cultural learning.
4   Seek out things you like in the new culture.
5   Make lasting friendships with locals.
6   Withdraw on bad days then quickly get back to work after a short break.
7   Regard each patient with unique value and dignity.
8   Think long-term.
9   Focus on disease prevention and health promotion over merely providing treatment.
10 Manage your expectations.
11 Take care of yourself physically.
12 Learn to disengage and ensure you have some downtime away from work.

(Johnson and Johnson, 2015: 132)

As the author has worked in a different cultural context within the nursing education system this advice is strongly recommended. Working and living in a different country and culture is not without its stressors and challenges but the experience can be very rewarding and enlightening.

Cultural competence does not only apply to nurses moving abroad to work or study, it also applies to patients travelling to access medical services in other countries. Lin (2016) highlights that the growth of medical tourism has led to an expansion of there being up to 18 percent of patients comprising people from many different racial and ethnic backgrounds accessing some countries specifically for medical procedures. This demonstrates that the issue of cultural competence in dealing with this trend is of high importance.

Therefore, education of nurses is an important consideration in order to develop professionals that can meet these attributes. Some nurse education courses will often contain students from culturally diverse and linguistically different backgrounds. A study by Fuller and Mott-Smith (2017) showed differences in perspectives of nurse educators from those of their culturally diverse students when identifying barriers. They found that the educators believed that the biggest barrier was language, whereas the students themselves suggested it was about the nature of forming relationships with their teachers and other students. They therefore recommended that nurse educators should make efforts to build and facilitate relationships for such students.

───────────────────────── ACTIVITY 10.1 ─────────────────────────

Think back to your nurse training.

1   What was the nature of relationships with students from culturally diverse and linguistically different backgrounds?
2   What barriers were faced by such students?

───

In a study analysing documents related to global nursing by Wong et al. (2015) they found that leadership and management of nurses within such global systems was of great concern. Buckner et al. (2014) investigated global nurse leadership concepts and identified there were six aspects that needed to be considered:

- **Creativity** (generating and recognizing ideas, alternatives or possibilities that may be useful in problem-solving and communicating with others).
- **Change** (improving the working conditions and safety of staff and patients).

- **Collaboration** (initiating new strategies, involving others and seeing opportunities for improvement).
- **Community** (developing support strategies, particularly in cultures based on collectivist values).
- **Context** (empowering those in the situation with knowledge and skills used to best solve the problems in that specific setting).
- **Courage** (being committed, presenting ideas and engaging peers).

In Wong et al.'s (2015) study, there were also issues of the quantity and quality of nurses that were involved in mobility situations. Nurses have contributed to health improvements in a global context. However, the importance of nurse education was also emphasized in relation to pre-registration preparation, post-registration and continuing professional development. Bittner et al. (2017) point out that this might be difficult as there is likely to be a shortage of nurse educators in the coming years relative to the required numbers to fulfil the aims of global nursing. Marć et al. (2019) highlight that there is an international shortage of nurses, which is likely to affect Europe, Asia and North America in the coming years. They argue that although there is no specific cause, as it is a multifaceted issue, this is mainly due to ineffective planning and use of available nursing resources, poor recruitment, an undersupply of a new staff, and global demographic conditions such as the ageing workforce. van den Broek and Groutsis (2017) also draw attention to the fact that for some nurses that move to work abroad there can be issues of vulnerability and safety, particularly in countries that are culturally quite difficult, and perhaps when they have entrusted such a move to be handled by intermediary agents that can turn out to be quite unscrupulous.

Nicholas and Breakey (2015) also suggest that as nurses are more able to transition to global contexts there is an important requirement to ensure interprofessional working is optimum. They suggest that ineffective interprofessional collaboration in poorer countries with less technological advances and economic status has led to poorer outcomes for patients who arguably are in the most need, therefore interprofessional learning is of the utmost importance in nurse education. However, they also found that poor interprofessional working also led to poor outcomes in resource-rich settings. Nicholas and Breakey (2015) recommend that this global agenda for nursing should challenge the nurse education systems worldwide.

There is growing competition for recruiting overseas nurses onto preregistration nursing courses and it is becoming a popular option for those wishing to study as an international student in other countries. However, there can be some issues with this in relation to acculturation and feeling a part of the wider population of nurses. Mitchell et al. (2017) found that international students on a pre-registration nursing programme faced some issues in relation to expressing themselves, mainly due to language barriers and lack of opportunities to overcome these (particularly within the clinical areas), and 'finding their place', as they often felt 'otherness' and in some cases directly discriminated against. These aspects would also be faced by qualified nurses that find themselves moving to work in other countries. According to Buscemi (2011), acculturation is the process in which individuals moving to a host country take on the characteristics of this, or a linear relationship between the individual's original culture and that of the host country not dissimilar to the stages of transition outlined in Chapter 2. In relation to such transitions as moving to another country, Vardaman and Mastel-Smith (2016) highlighted conditions faced during this process:

- **Meanings** (the reasons for moving, either for economic/status reasons or for contributing to the health of the host country).
- **Expectations** (related to the impressions they had on the potential lifestyle).
- **Level of knowledge and skills** (related to understanding of the host country, sometimes developed through movies or social media).
- **Environment** (related to interactions with others and principles of behaviour in nursing settings).
- **Planning** (related to economic factors and aspects such as language preparation).
- **Emotional/physical well-being** (related to factors such as absence from family and friends, change of diet and living conditions).

–––––––––––––––––––––––––––––– **ACTIVITY 10.2** ––––––––––––––––––––––––––––––

Reflect back on your nursing experience to date. Think of when you commenced your nurse training or a new nursing role.

How did the above transition factors related to acculturation apply to you?

––

Rosa (2017) highlights that nurses and other healthcare providers need to be aware of the global public health agendas and spark some global consciousness into their everyday work. This requires that you should empower yourself with knowledge related to planetary health and how that impacts both locally and globally. It also requires that these agendas are used to inform education and advocacy approaches at local levels whilst maintaining perspective on the implications of these globally. There is a need to integrate global agendas and strategies into policies and protocols in providing public health services. This suggests that you should reflect on global issues and the wisdom to be gained from transnational practices and how they can relate to whichever local population and community you serve in as a nurse.

Global nursing also occurs through the development of transnational teaching courses. As Ahmad and Buchanan (2016) highlight, the term 'glocal' demonstrates how some individuals espouse global intentions whilst preferring to stay in their own locations (due to reasons such as finances and family support), so access their 'global' education by studying with foreign institutions delivering on-site 'transnational' education in their own country. There has been a proliferation of these in recent years with many western universities providing professional and academic development opportunities for nurses trained in their own country. However, Arunasalam and Burton (2018) highlight that this is not without its difficulties, as there are sometimes barriers related to language, method of instruction, assessment approaches and different cultural and social expectations.

Naidoo and Sibiya (2019) point out that transnational education is a valuable commodity in the modern world, and that high academic standards can be fostered in furthering the development of nursing in host countries. Students are often exposed to educational circumstances different to those they are used to or have been exposed to. This may push them out of their comfort zones, which can be challenging, yet to some extent does help them in relation to experiencing and managing the 'culture shock' which is often recognized as a stage in transition theory and can be applied to moving to work within different cultures. Bonello et al's. (2018) study suggested that interprofessional education is welcomed and viewed as a positive approach, however, without careful consideration of cultural dimensions such as the low context-high context differences this may not always be well-received.

Nurse migration

Historically, Aiken et al. (2004) identified that the wave of large-scale migration of nurses was happening at a time when global health issues and targets were seemingly starting to be recognized and addressed. This migration of nurses from developing countries to developed countries creates risks that the source countries would be depleted of a crucial part of their workforce required to address higher health needs and issues, crippling their healthcare systems. The reason for this potential for migration was the increasing shortages in the nursing workforces of developed countries. This would inhibit and undermine global health initiatives aimed at developing countries, and demonstrates an issue related to the systems, funding, status and conditions that nurses face in developing countries and questions over why developed countries are unable to produce or retain enough domestic nurses to supply their own health services. Prescott and Nichter (2014) argue that such transnational migration leads to serious global health issues and hinders progress towards health and development goals (which were highlighted at the beginning of this chapter).

As discussed earlier, the ageing population across the world is leading to a multitude of health issues that require serious attention and focus for professional healthcare providers. Aligned with this is the fact that the nursing workforce itself is ageing at a time when healthcare demands are increasing. Afentakis and Maier (2013) showed that the average age of a migrant nurse is 46 compared to 41 for domestic nurses, suggesting that migrant nurses actually increase the average age of the workforce and therefore add to this issue. According to Sherman et al. (2013), the WHO considers at least 57 countries to be in crisis in relation to their workforce. To address this 'greying' of the workforce, healthcare providers will need to consider generational diversity, how work is done, and pay closer attention to technologies that may assist an increasingly ageing workforce. Sherman et al. (2013) suggested there would be a potential shortage of 600,000 nurses across Europe alone by 2020, with more nurses expected to leave the workforce in developed countries in the next two decades. Bittner et al. (2017) highlight that the issue is compounded by the shortages of appropriately qualified nurse educators, which led to around 69,000 applicants to nursing courses in the USA being turned away due to lack of faculty capacity to accommodate the demand. Nardi and Gyurko (2013) suggested that the shortage of nurse educators arises from a number of similar factors that lead to the shortage of nurses globally, that is global migration, ageing nurse educators, a reduced pool of younger staff to recruit from, lack of funding and poor salaries. They found a number of recommendations including creating international cooperative programs, managing migration, and a change in the educational paradigm to incorporate high-tech delivery systems and non-traditional experiences.

—————————————————— ACTIVITY 10.3 ——————————————————

Think of the factors that might need to be in place in order for an ageing nursing workforce to be able to continue to provide quality healthcare to patients.
    What are the barriers that an ageing workforce might face?

So, it can be seen that there are issues and concerns related to the situation from a source country perspective, where there is a move 'away from' nursing within their own domestic environments, with some moving 'towards' nursing within the host country in differing cultural contexts. These are known as 'push-pull' factors. Nurses pushed by the conditions of their home (source) countries and pulled towards improved conditions and circumstances in the overseas (host) country. According to Li et al. (2014), job availability, personal and professional development, career advancement, attractive salaries, stable socio-political environments and retirement benefits are recognized as pull factors. Low wages, limited career and educational opportunities, lack of resources, unstable or dangerous working conditions and unstable political environments are recognized as push factors. The flow of nursing migration is normally from developing countries to more developed industrialized countries. The Philippines is currently the largest source of migrant nurses worldwide. Sasso et al. (2019) suggest some other factors within nursing work areas that lead to nurses leaving the profession or migrating. They identify push factors such as understaffing, emotional exhaustion, poor patient safety, performing non-nursing duties and being male (around 88 percent of the nursing workforce internationally is female). The pull factors identified were positive perception of quality and safety of care, and performing core nursing activities. This suggests that the actual roles of the nurses themselves can lead to dissatisfaction and therefore the motivation to migrate, as well as the status, economic prospects and quality of life issues that influence the desire for migration.

It was identified by de Vries et al. (2016) that nursing migration was linked to the factors of nurses tending to move to countries with language matches, near neighbours or to countries that hold former colonial relationships. They also found clear positive evidence that nursing migrant workers often received higher levels of pay than those that stayed in their source country. A final interesting finding was that they found that such migrants did not necessarily experience discrimination in relation to wages and level of occupational status. However, there are still some issues related to other stressors such as lower levels of life satisfaction in some migrant populations.

Delucas (2014) highlights the risks associated with the global migration of nurses. She states that migration might be seen as an advantageous exchange of nursing information and creates the potential for professional growth. However, the benefits to the host country will often outweigh the consequences to the source country which may be left with a diminished workforce, the potential for brain drain and a decrease in access to quality care (the very issues which cause the 'brain drain'). Jacobson (2015) suggests that countries such as the USA, which is a large draw for migrating nurses, should take some ethical responsibility in relation to their recruitment policies. This includes developing strategies to recruit more diverse students domestically rather than importing nurses.

Another issue highlighted by Eckenwiler (2014) is that of 'status drop'. Quite often qualified nurses that migrate take up positions for which they are over-qualified. This leads to de-skilling or down-skilling and the apparent loss of status. This may also occur if the qualifications gained in their source country are not recognized by the host countries. In such cases the migrating nurse may have to take further courses/qualifications before being eligible for roles. They may also have to take on lower positions than they left because of this. The roles may tend to be in services such as long-term care which are deemed less popular than other jobs. This can lead to high rates of job stress and low levels of satisfaction with their working conditions.

Marginson (2014) looked at adjustment of students that chose to undertake study abroad. It is suggested that there are issues involved in managing the identities, perceptions, values, actions, and a sense of what is important. The material conditions, social relationships, and the agency of the individual all contribute to how successful or detrimental this experience might be. If not managed well and combined with the above-mentioned factors of status drop, low job satisfaction and having to deal with the host country's language, culture, customs and expectations, this can affect the health of those nurses moving to other countries. Schilgen et al. (2017) explain that such poor health in migrants can be attributed to the 'exhausted migrant effect' or through 'acculturation stressors', often caused by separation from families, loss of support networks and social exclusion. However, their study was inconclusive, stating that the health of the migrating nurse may decrease or increase over time, amongst those nurses that demonstrate more resilience considering the stressors (remember the concept of resilience was also identified as an important factor in transition discussed in Chapter 2). There were three main factors that affected health: acculturation; discrimination in the workplace; and in the context of race and ethnic background. Nurses from India and the Philippines tended to be affected by the stressful factors mentioned above. Korean and Chinese immigrants tended to decline in health at the same rate as their hosts, probably to the exposure of westernized dietary and exercise habits which are currently known to be playing a part in an increase in morbidities amongst populations.

Nurses however, are also considered to be instrumental in promoting health and assisting in the needs of other migrants. Shaffer et al. (2019) suggest that nurses are able to empathize with migrants and refugees and are at the forefront of contributing to the UN 'Global Compacts' and the 'Sustainable Development Goals'. They have a pivotal role in advocating for vulnerable populations, and because they are 'migrants in demand' they can shift the toxic narratives currently being associated with migrant and refugee populations by acting as positive role models. A migrant or refugee nurse would be appropriately qualified and positioned to provide care and support for refugee and migrant populations, so have a key role to play in advancing health in a world where migration is rapidly increasing.

Therefore, it can be seen that migrating nurses are crucial in helping to achieve the health goals outlined in the sustainable development goals mainly in developing countries. They are also highly valued and instrumental in delivering high-quality care in developed countries where there are comparatively healthy numbers of nurses per head of population, yet there are still highlighted and forecasted nursing shortages. You can see how factors in transitioning to becoming a qualified nurse at the end of your pre-registration nurse education might be challenging. Imagine how much more challenging this would be if you also decided to migrate to another country to practise your nursing.

--------------------------------- ACTIVITY 10.4 ---------------------------------

Think of the countries you could consider migrating to (this can be hypothetical or realistic). What are the factors of that country, their populations and health service situations that might make you wish to migrate there to work for a period of time?

1   Identify which of these factors are 'pull' factors.
2   What factors in your current situation might be considered 'push' factors?

Should you decide to migrate to another country to practise your nursing, as well as the factors about the country itself and its lifestyle properties, you would also need to be aware of the standards and requirements needed in order to be eligible for entry onto nursing registers in the host country.

Registering as a nurse in other countries

Moving to live and work in another country, whilst exciting can also be daunting. There are obvious issues related to financial security, geographical, living and accommodation issues, language, family, culture and social experiences that would influence this decision. There are also political issues and the rules and laws of the country you intend to move to in order to start or experience living and working there. Aspects such as the type of visa you would require and the requirements for those would have to be checked. However, this section will not be focusing on these issues; rather it will focus on the requirements needed from a nursing registration perspective in some selected countries. This includes Canada, Australia, the USA and Singapore.

There are numerous factors associated with registering in other countries. For nurses educated overseas, they must demonstrate that they meet several requirements in the host country. For example, in the UK, for nurses outside of the European Economic Area (EEA) (although this may also change with the UK leaving the European Union in 2020) to register with the Nursing and Midwifery Council (NMC), the incoming nurse must meet the requirements for the specific field (adult, children's, mental health or learning disabilities nursing) and must demonstrate that they are suitable for the intended field of nursing practice. This includes 'part one', completing a computer-based test via Pearson VUE (a company that provide computer-based testing services to international organizations) to demonstrate this competency based on 120 multiple choice questions, and 'part two', an objective structured clinical observation (OSCE). The first can be taken at a recognized Pearson VUE test centre around the world and the second at a test centre in the UK (NMC, 2020). They also need to demonstrate proficiency in English.

Within the European Union (EU), there has been a sustained push for the mobility of nursing professionals across the member states (which may be subject to change depending on the outcomes of the negotiations, processes and deals as they develop following the UK leaving the EU). This requires professional recognition of an academic and practice nature for mobility of the qualifications across states.

Kortese (2016) points out that EU directive 2005/36/EC (amended by directive 2103/55/EU) is an instrument that provides the requirement to recognize the profession of nursing (amongst others) across the member states of the EU. The NMC (2018f: Article 31) highlight that programmes for nurses entering into general care (adult/child) must fulfil a number of criteria related to theoretical and practical experiences. If these criteria are met then as long as nurses demonstrate appropriate language proficiency in the country they migrate to then mobility is made easier due to this professional recognition and mutual standards.

Allan and Westwood (2016) highlight that the UK, Australia, Canada and the USA are major host countries for nurses migrating from overseas. They often include mandatory English language proficiency testing, mainly using the International English Language Testing System (IELTS) to demonstrate this. The NMC (2020), for example, state that the IELTS score must be a minimum of seven across the range of speaking, listening and reading, and a minimum of six point five in writing. Such a nurse must hold a nursing qualification (diploma or degree), the equivalent to a UK level one nurse (having completed a course with a minimum of three years of study). They will also need to demonstrate good health, so occupational health or other certified medical records might be required, plus demonstration of good character, usually confirmed by an official police record check. The following sections will look at some of the countries that are popular destinations for migrating nurses. These factors are open to change due to policy reviews and amendments in each location, so you must check with the relevant nursing regulatory systems in whichever country, state, territory or district you are interested in practising your nursing for the time-specific relevant requirements, and not make assumptions about them and your eligibility for entry.

Canada

Canada is a popular destination for nurses wishing to migrate. Giblin et al. (2016) highlighted that Canada has launched a recruitment campaign aimed at Internationally Educated Nurses (IENs). Canada is comprised of 11 provinces/territories which individually regulate nurses and their licensure/registration. The College and Association of Registered Nurses Alberta (CARNA) saw a ten-fold rise in such IEN applicants in the 2000s. This was halted slightly following the financial crisis in 2008/9. Nordstrom et al. (2018) state that, due to the slowdown in recruitment to nursing, efforts have focused on IENs and the number is growing again. They point out that international nurses wishing to enter Canadian nursing practice are normally assessed for proficiency by demonstrating completion of an approved course of nursing study and successful completion of a national practice examination similar to the one required in the UK accessed via Pearson VUE.

The Canadian Nurses Association (CNA, 2019) outline that although there is no national licensure body in Canada each of the 11 provinces/territories provides its own regulatory body. However, they chose the National Council of State Boards of Nursing (NCSBN) as the provider of the Canadian entry to practice exam. Internationally Educated Nurses must show that their nursing practice experience and proficiencies are equivalent to what domestic nursing graduates would have on entry to the Canadian nursing profession. This is attained via a 'Substantially Equivalent Competency' (SEC) assessment by an independent assessor to ascertain that appropriate knowledge, skills and attitudes are demonstrated by the nurse. Nordstrom et al. (2018) highlight that if this SEC highlights gaps between the applicant's experience and qualifications and the requirements for entering into the specific province's nursing board register/licensure then a bridging course may have to be taken to address this. Covell et al. (2018) suggest that these bridging programmes are useful in helping IENs to integrate into the nursing systems of another country. They suggest that immigrants from high-income countries' nursing systems tend to be educated in similar ways, so are perhaps more closely aligned to the requirements in countries that are similar. However, those from lower-income countries may have more requirements in order to be able to register due to the differences in the educational quality of their training, cultural contexts and standards of regulation.

The bridging programmes help to prepare them for the cultural context and standards required and to reduce the gaps in their experiences. Cruz et al. (2017) looked at such programmes across four popular destinations for IENs (Australia, New Zealand, United Kingdom and Canada) and found value in such programmes for acclimatising the participants into the differing expectations of the nursing systems and regulatory bodies, and increasing English fluency where it is a second language, and that they are helpful in personal and professional development. However, nurses from the USA, Canada and Australia when migrating to the UK found less value in such courses, due to similarities in systems, nursing status and language. The English proficiency requirements are very similar to the UK for those from non-English speaking backgrounds and educational systems, with applicants for registration in some territories requiring IELTS academic test scores as follows: 'Listening' seven point five; 'Writing' seven; 'Reading' six point five; and 'Speaking' seven. You may need to check the specific territory for their own requirements. There is also a recency of practice requirement of completing 1,125 hours in the previous five years.

Australia

Another very popular place for migrating nurses to travel to is Australia. It is a popular destination to those nurses educated in the Asia

Pacific area, and also popular for western nurses as it is a recognized high-income country based on English as the primary language. Health Professionals in Australia come under the umbrella auspices of the 'Australian Health Practitioner Regulation Agency' (AHPRA). AHPRA oversees the health professions regulatory aspects via 15 national boards that set standards and policies which health professionals must meet (AHPRA, 2019a). The Nursing and Midwifery Board of Australia (NMBA) governs the nursing and midwifery boards from each of the Australian states and territories (Müller, 2016). The NMBA roles and functions are in relation to registering nursing and midwifery practitioners and students, developing standards, codes and guidelines, assessing overseas trained practitioners who wish to practise in Australia and approving accreditation standards and accredited courses of study (NMBA, 2019a).

As with other countries highlighted above there are some very rigorous requirements and expectations that must be met in order to register in Australia. There are requirements related to criminal history checks. This includes providing information on any past or pending charges. Any offences punishable by imprisonment must be declared to the NMBA. English language requirements, if the student has not studied in English in their tertiary nursing course and if English is not their first language, is an IELTS pass with a mean of seven and a minimum score of seven across all factors (or equivalent tests) (NMBA, 2019b). You would need to demonstrate a recency of practice of 450 hours within the previous three years. If you are registering for the first time you must not have completed the course more than two years prior to application.

Philip et al. (2015) highlight that nurses trained in culturally different settings than Australia may find challenges in their transition even if they pass the English language test. They recognize that many overseas nurses require the completion of a bridging course before registering fully. They suggest that these should include much more emphasis on communication and acculturation skills to recognize the subtleties of language, culture, humour and acceptable approaches.

As with Canada these courses may help bridge the gaps between educational systems and levels of nursing courses from other countries. The NMBA (2019b) reduced the number of assessment criteria of the 'Internationally Qualified Nurses and Midwives' (IQNMs) from eight to three. This includes the following:

- The qualification is recognized by a statutory/licensing/registering body in the country where the nurse education took place. The level must be that of registered nurse.
- The qualification is based on standards recognized, accredited and quality assured by a regulatory body external to the education institution.
- The academic level of the course is equivalent to level seven (degree qualification) in the Australian Qualification framework.

(AHPRA, 2019b)

United States of America

As in Australia and Canada the United States is a large geographical area made up of states, territories and districts. Each of these has their own nursing board with responsibility for licensure, registration and legislature. These nursing boards are affiliated to the umbrella organization the National Council of State Boards for Nursing (NCSBN).

> NCSBN developed the uniform licensure requirements to provide boards of nursing (BONs) with a standardized set of criteria for making licensure decisions in order to assure that all nurses, whether educated domestically or abroad, are safe and qualified to practice. (NCSBN, 2015: 1)

According to the NCSBN (2019) all of the state boards require that candidates pass an examination to demonstrate competency to perform safely and effectively to ensure public protection. The examination used by all boards is the 'National Council Licensure Examination for Registered Nurses' (NCLEX-RN). Similar to Canada and the UK this examination can be accessed via the Pearson VUE company.

NCSBN (2015) highlight that for an IEN to gain licensure they need to:

- Provide verification of graduating from a nursing programme comparable to a nursing board approved programme.
- Successful completion of the NCLEX-RN.
- Self-disclosure and verification of licensure in the home country.
- Successful completion and verification of an English exam approved by a nursing board to demonstrate proficiency in English

speaking, listening, reading and writing (unless educated to the expected qualification level in English).

- Self-disclosure of any criminal records and assessment of any provided, judged on a case-by-case basis.
- Self-disclosure of any substance use disorder in the last five years.
- Self-disclosure of any professional actions taken against the individual.

Interestingly the IELTS expectation for English proficiency is six point five, with no factor lower than six, or equivalents.

The NCSBN (2015) highlights the importance of transition to practice programmes for IENs commencing their roles as practising registered nurses in order to acclimatize to the cultural, communication and technological aspects of nursing in new settings.

Maryniak (2019) points out that each state may have some slight differences in how they legislate, license and regulate nurses so it is pertinent to check in detail the requirements. She states that the American Nurses Association (ANA) is the largest professional organization that represents all nurses and provides a scope of practice and codes of conduct for nurses. The Nurse Practice Act (NPA) includes statutes and rules on nursing but these may also vary among states. Therefore, if you are considering nursing in the USA it is imperative not to apply a broad rule to the whole country, but to check the rules, regulations and legalities in the specific one you are interested in.

Singapore

Singapore is included here as it is recognized as one of the best healthcare systems in the world, once ranked number two in the world on the Bloomberg Health Efficiency Index (Miller and Lu, 2018). It is also included here as an interest of one of the authors who has experience of living and working in Singapore within the nurse education sector. As an Asian country, with many historical ties to western influence, it provides an appealing draw to migrating nurses from Asia and surrounding areas as well as from other countries all around the world.

Healthcare in Singapore is governed by the Ministry of Health (MOH) and nursing is regulated through the ministry via the Singapore

Nursing Board (SNB). The SNB (2019a) identify that the Nurses Act (Chapter 209) outlines its scope and functions in the regulation and registering of nurses in Singapore.

In order to register as a 'foreign trained nurse' you must already hold an offer of employment with a recognized healthcare organization within Singapore, and the organization has responsibility to enquire on their eligibility to employ foreign nurses before applying for registration on your behalf.

Similar to other countries mentioned above the SNB requires that you hold a current valid registration/license to practice from your home country or country of initial registration with evidence that the nursing programme undertaken is comparable to those eligible for registration in Singapore (SNB, 2019b). These must be verified, along with verification of no outstanding criminal offences or actions against you.

As an IEN you may be asked (on a case-by-case basis) to take a licensure examination in order to be able to enter the register. In some cases a competency examination may also be required. An application to practice may also be deemed as conditional by the SNB, who would clarify what the required conditions would be.

Within the region there is a body known as the Association of Southeast Asian Nations (ASEAN). This organization basically promotes the economic growth of the region and collaboration across the ten member nations (Brunei Darussalam, Cambodia, Indonesia, Lao PDR, Malaysia, Myanmar, Philippines, Singapore, Thailand and Vietnam). In a similar way to the EU, ASEAN's objectives also relate to nursing in promoting mobility and collaboration of nursing bodies. Within ASEAN, nursing falls under the auspices of the ASEAN Joint Coordinating Committee on Nursing (AJCCN). This committee set out domains and nursing core competencies relating to nursing practice, as well as a 'Mutual Recognition Arrangements' (MRA) agreement to:

> Facilitate the mobility of nursing services professionals within ASEAN, enhance exchange of information and expertise on standards and qualifications, promote adoption of best practices for professional nursing services and provide opportunities for capacity building and training of nurses. (Association of Southeast Asian Nations, 2019)

Although there is the MRA in place to facilitate mobility, the process for nurses within the region to register with the SNB are very similar to those highlighted above and are reviewed on a case-by-case basis.

Summary

This chapter has focused on a number of issues related to Global and international aspects of nursing. The concepts of changing global demographics including rapidly ageing populations, changes in the prevalence of non-communicable diseases and healthcare economics have been discussed.

The WHO/UN Sustainable Development Goals have highlighted how nurses across the globe will be instrumental in moving towards the targets and improving health and peoples' lives. Factors related to mobility and migration of nurses, increasing economic and technological advances and a need for collaboration demonstrate how nurses training in one country may now find it much easier to find themselves working in another in an increasingly smaller world.

Issues related to nursing migration, including the 'push-pull' factors that may influence such a decision, have been discussed. There are tensions between developed countries with large shortages in their nursing workforces needing to recruit internationally educated nurses to meet these demands. These obviously have effects on the source countries which, although they are most likely in greater need due to the healthcare issues facing their countries and the resources required to meet them, are losing their highly skilled nurses seeking better conditions for themselves and their families. There are obviously opportunities and benefits to moving for qualified nurses, not least developing wider collaborative networks and intercultural skills.

Finally, should you decide to migrate to practise nursing in another country, you will need to demonstrate that you meet the requirements for registering in the host country. Aspects covering some of this detail in certain countries have been discussed. However, policies, procedures and regulations do change regularly over time so it is imperative that you contact the specific nursing boards in whichever country you decide to move to, and check on any of the issues and approaches discussed to ensure you access the most up-to-date information and current requirements.

Working internationally is an exciting prospect, and as a registered nurse you will find that your skills are highly desired and provide you with excellent opportunities that should enhance your nursing career. Just as in the changes you will face or have faced in becoming a qualified nurse, you will also face similar transition issues should you decide to migrate to pursue your nursing career in another country.

11

CONCLUSION

Preparing for Transition: Putting it all Together

Graham Ormrod and Rob Burton

THE AIMS OF THIS CHAPTER ARE TO:

- Consolidate the topics discussed in Chapters 1–10 in order to enhance your understanding of the roles and responsibilities of a newly qualified nurse.
- Draw together the underpinning theories and explore how they are connected and related to each other by applying them to practice.
- Explore the common challenges experienced by the newly qualified nurse and give you guidance on how to manage them.

Introduction

As highlighted in the preceding chapters of this book, while the role of a newly qualified nurse is complex and challenging, it is also rewarding and fulfilling. Hopefully, you are now ready to start this new period of your career, in which the benefits of your hard work and your hopes, plans and aspirations will come to fruition. You are now, finally, about to become a registered nurse.

The preceding chapters will have helped you to clarify and confirm the roles and responsibilities of a registered nurse, such as:

- Recognizing the transition from student to registered nurse.
- Maintaining standards in the workplace.
- Making decisions (accountable, ethical and legal).
- Leading, managing and teamworking.
- Teaching and mentoring others.

You should have gained insight and awareness into your current level of preparedness and been able to recognize areas requiring further development. You will have also recognized where you might choose to invest your efforts and prioritize your time to ensure that you get the job that your commitment and hard work so richly deserves. There has also been scope to investigate the nature of your continuing personal and professional development.

This final chapter is an occasion to revisit some of the key learning opportunities that have been previously highlighted. We will look at how all of the complex and occasionally confusing aspects of professional practice can be brought together to ensure that you are appropriately confident and ready to take on the role of a qualified nurse. This should help to guarantee that you are fit for purpose as a nurse ready for registration. The aspects of a nurse's roles listed above may have been addressed as separate issues, however, in the real-world setting, everyday situations are not compartmentalized in such a way. You are not able to think 'I'll do the decision-making bit', then 'Now, I'll do the teamworking bit', followed by 'Now, I'll think about the leadership aspects'. All of these are inherent in each and every situation that you will face as a registered nurse. Therefore, it is essential to recognize the interplay and interconnected nature of the concepts involved in your nursing practice.

First of all, it is important to be aware that some nervousness and anxiety are inevitable at this point. Consideration of what the future might hold and your preparedness for this are understandable and to be expected. Anyone about to embark on their new career who says that they have no hint of uneasiness is either being a little untruthful or profoundly lacking in self-awareness. Such overconfidence should also probably worry any future employer, as the potential employee will be implying that they have little or nothing left to learn. It is almost a truism to say that no one applies for a position or role for which they are already totally competent, and in the ever-changing professional context, reflection, self-awareness and the grasping of the ethos of lifelong learning should be encouraged. This understandable nervousness is hopefully also coupled with a genuine enthusiasm and excitement at the career step that you are about to take.

What it means to be a front-line member of staff

According to the independent regulator the Nursing and Midwifery Council (NMC, 2020b) their role is to:

> ... make sure nurses, midwives and nursing associates have the skills they need to care for people safely, with integrity, expertise, respect and compassion, from the moment they step into their first job.

This and other NMC documents such as *The Code* (NMC, 2018a) and *Future Nurse: Standards of Proficiency for Registered Nurses* (NMC, 2018b) continually highlight the need for nurses to ensure delivery of high-quality care in changing situations and environments, and consistently place an emphasis on the development and leadership aspects of nursing. There is an importance placed on measuring outcomes and making sure that standards are met, as well as the innovation and promotion of nursing itself. The previous chapters in this book covered such aspects to raise your awareness of the complexities of each of these activities. Now, we will show you how these are brought together in everyday practice as we revisit some of the scenarios from earlier chapters and analyse them in relation to all of these activities.

Common issues faced by newly qualified nurses

As mentioned previously in Chapter 1, it was pointed out that the challenges faced by most newly qualified nurses did not necessarily always involve service user contact. Indeed, at this time, you may find yourself with more duties that relate to contacting and dealing with other professionals and services. Others may now expect you to provide the advice, guidance and answers in some very complex situations. We have already emphasized that you should have a **preceptor** on qualifying to aid you through these transitions; however, the literature suggests there are still likely to be difficulties in this transition process and that, on occasion, you may have to face and take responsibility for some challenging situations. As Suresh et al. (2012) point out, individual accountability, managerial responsibilities, delegating duties and managing clinical situations such as death and dying may be some of the things with which qualifying nurses have to deal.

Let's revisit the thoughts of a newly qualified learning disability nurse from Chapter 6:

When I qualified, I went to work in a group home (registered nursing) for seven adults with learning disabilities and complex needs. Once there, I was often the shift leader and found that most of the challenging issues that I faced were related to managing the shift team. As the only qualified nurse on shift, delegation of duties was to unqualified staff; many of whom had worked within the home and/or company for several years. I had to overcome a significant age difference in conjunction with my newly qualified status – 'proving my worth' was my most difficult task.

Sheena Hiller

This nurse identifies some of the leadership and management skills required of a nurse when they take charge as a shift leader. These skills, as suggested by Magnusson et al. (2017), include managing the team and delegating duties. Managing the care of seven individuals in any setting requires appropriate teamwork in order to make sure that all standards of care are met. There is a need to be aware of the relevant standards and policies and be accountable for their implementation. This requires decision-making based on the knowledge of legal, ethical and professional principles. Delegation needs firm leadership awareness, while also recognizing that the accountability

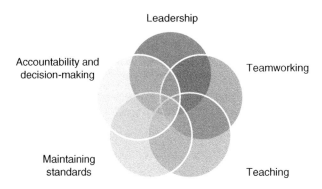

Figure 11.1   The overlapping concepts that newly qualified nurses face

still rests with those delegating. There may also be some practices or skills that need to be taught to the junior staff, as discussed in detail in the preceding chapters. Now, it is important to gain an overview of how all of these aspects contribute to successfully managing different situations. There is no line where leadership stops and management starts, or where accountability stops and maintaining standards starts, or where teamwork stops and teaching starts. These concepts overlap. Awareness of this in such situations gives you scope to draw on your knowledge and skills and find alternatives that can help you to develop the best solutions available to you, as seen in Figure 11.1.

Before going any further, it is appropriate to reflect on Rob's own experience of becoming a qualified nurse. Rob also provides an insight into the challenges he faced, and how he overcame them.

For me the period of transition was challenging. The safety net of having a supervisor no longer being there to confirm decisions can be a daunting experience. I found my self being challenged by staff more than patients, yet realizing that those issues with staff were all related to benefitting the patient experience. I found I had to make decisions and had to be strong in the light of pressure from staff that did not necessarily agree. I also found that mistakes could happen but with appropriate support could be addressed.

As I progressed into my academic and other leadership roles, I understood that these situations are an amalgam of many issues all happening at once. I would observe leaders and managers responding to situations of an emergency nature or dealing with longer-term strategic planning and realized this was a multifaceted approach. It involved responding to and making decisions based on a number of factors, and in taking action, employing a number of approaches. I realized that it is not until you analyse a situation that you can recognize these factors. By identifying the factors, aspects can be learned about them. Using evidence-based practice and research (as well as learning from experience) can actually help you to improve and learn these approaches.

So, in any given situation, there are issues related to governance and policy, locally, nationally and globally that may have an impact. Therefore, there is a need to understand and be aware of these. There is a need to lead and manage whilst at the same time recognizing ethical and legal implications. Understanding the theories and evidence behind these approaches and employing them can help you develop.

In nursing there is the need for teamwork, and you may find you are teaching others almost on a daily basis, and you may be assessing students. In order to do this, you also need to develop yourself personally and professionally. In my 35+ years within the profession I have been involved in formal study (mostly part-time since qualifying) for around 19 years, not including smaller short-term courses, and general updating. This professional development has been vital in my roles at all levels and has been a major factor in me being able to draw on lots of differing disciplines to 'put it all together' and perform in my various jobs.

ACTIVITY 11.1

Responding to a medication error

Consider the scenario in Activity 6.9 (Chapter 6):

> A nurse has just completed a consecutive run of five night shifts. Arriving on duty, the shift leader finds that the nurse has made a medication error, which fortunately has not resulted in any harm to a patient.

From the brief information that you have in the above scenario:

1   What do you consider to be the leadership priorities?
2   What issues are there in relation to accountability?
3   What elements might be considered important for teamworking?
4   What actions do you need to take in relation to maintaining standards?
5   What teaching might need to occur?

A medication error demonstrates an alarming and worrying, but all too common, occurrence that can happen in differing kinds of health-care services. As we have discussed, the leadership issues in the scenario can be related to the leadership styles required in dealing with the situation (Marquis and Huston, 2012). Some authoritarian steps may need to be taken in dealing with the immediate issue of ensuring that the patient is safe. There are transactional leadership or trans-formational leadership considerations (Wong and Giallonardo, 2015) to be made in how to approach the member of staff. Should you use sanctions or suggestions? Although you will not be directly involved in the human resource aspects of the care environment, you will still need to alert your senior colleagues to the situation, identifying any human resource factors that may have contributed to it. It is likely that you will be closest to the patient, and this will mean that both junior and senior colleagues will view you as the prime information-holder.

Clearly, there are also significant aspects of quality and clinical governance. As highlighted in Chapter 3, the complex aspects of risk management are the responsibility of all involved in the care of the patient (Aiken and Sloane, 2020). This relates to your responsibilities in the processes of maintaining standards, including passing on and recording information accurately, and the subsequent steps taken. King et al. (2017) emphasize that teams need collaboration, coordination and communication with regards to issues of skill mix and accountability. A nurse having completed five nights might not be a good reflection of a positive team approach. The solving of this problem may need a team meeting of all staff to resolve it, as there may be fundamental issues that are beyond the scope of one qualified nurse to change on their own. The nurse in question and even the rest of the team may need to be involved in further training or instruction on the safe ways of medicine management in the workplace. Here, your skills of teaching may be put to the test, along with your understanding of learning styles and teaching approaches that are best suited to the learners, the topic and the environment (Hughes and Quinn, 2013).

Delivering an evidence-based nursing teaching session

To continue on the notion of teaching and learning, once you are qualified, there will be an expectation that you not only contribute to the teaching of patients and their families, but also the development of junior nurses and the supervision and development of student nurses. Clearly, you will be expected to utilize evidence-based practice in such instances. Providing instruction, demonstrations and education is a recognized part of your role (NMC, 2018e). Although most of this will take place informally, there may be occasions when you are asked to do this in a more formal setting.

────────────────── **ACTIVITY 11.2** ──────────────────

Your charge nurse has set up a series of lunchtime seminars for the multidiscipli-nary team in your care area and you have been asked to fill one of the slots in two weeks' time as someone has backed out. You are given freedom to choose whatever relevant topic you want.

How would you approach this to make it relevant and beneficial for the whole interprofessional team?

──

The most important factor involved in this is the need to plan thoroughly (Hughes and Quinn, 2013). This may include canvassing the staff team to find out what relevant topics they might be interested in. Getting to know what is on the rest of the programme is also important to avoid duplication or repetition. It would be good practice to attend similar seminars if possible, to get a 'feel' for the environment, the topics and the approaches taken. Muijs and Reynolds (2018) suggest that understanding the 'climate' of a learning environment is important. This relates to the general relationship dynamics in the setting. For example, how formal would it be? Is it likely to be a didactic session in which you are required to 'lecture' and provide information, or is it more likely to be an interactive environment in which you can act as a facilitator and create discussion? It is also essential to confirm what resources will be available, and as Race (2015) suggests, carefully check that all equipment needed is present, available and in working order.

In the session itself, you will need to present up-to-date, evidence-based information. Stevens and Duffy (2017) highlight that part of the essential contribution you make to good nursing care is to ensure that you are knowledgeable and skilled and possess up-to-date knowledge in order to teach others. This ensures that standards for good practice can be identified and met. It also confirms your accountability to the NMC (2018a) that you must deliver care based on the best and current available evidence and practice. Such sessions can help to develop collaborative teamworking approaches to care. Handy (1993) suggests that teamworking approaches can help to develop motivation and joint working towards an organization's goals, and that being provided with such opportunities lends itself to more positive group cohesion, raised staff morale and improved working relationships.

Professional behaviour

The maintenance of professional behaviour in the workplace is something with which you may have to deal with on a regular basis. In order to qualify as a nurse, there is a requirement to have a statement of good character provided at the end of your course. The NMC (2018a) suggests that good character is based on a person's conduct, behaviour, and attitude. Treating people as individuals with respect and integrity and upholding the reputation of your profession is paramount. Obviously, more extreme examples, such as violence, criminal activity and dishonesty, may be more easily identified, and may be managed in a relatively straightforward way due to clearly defined policies and laws. Similarly, there are sometimes situations in which professional behaviours are absent, demonstrated in behaviours such as rudeness to clients or colleagues, or staff with persistent inappropriate attitudes or behaviour, such as poor communication skills and failure to accept and follow advice. However, it is also important to realize that, as a qualified nurse, you have a responsibility to manage situations and behaviours that are not always so explicit, with aspects that can be difficult to define or demonstrate.

ACTIVITY 11.3

You are working with a third-year student while visiting a group of clients in a community nursing caseload. While conducting an assessment of a client, you notice that the student is distracted and disengaged. You note that she is using her mobile phone to send texts.

1   What professional issues are raised in this scenario?
2   How would you deal with this situation?

Activity 11.3 clearly shows an example of inappropriate behaviour, and you might need to employ several strategies in order to fully address it. For example, it would appear to be appropriate to quietly and politely advise the student to put away the phone and to refocus on the client. In doing so, the student should be reminded that the client is their first concern, demonstrating dignity and respect. This would again be an example of adopting an authoritarian leadership style. It would also be important to remind the student that the NMC (2018b) emphasizes that all students conduct themselves professionally at all times in order to justify the trust that the public places in the nursing profession. Such discussions should take place away from the immediate care environment to ensure confidentiality and fairness. This also relates to both your and their accountability.

You might conduct a tutorial with the student at a specified time during which you facilitate their understanding of the NMC (2019e) guidance on conduct for student nurses and the NMC *Code* (NMC, 2018a). Setting objectives with an action plan related to the standards of proficiency in their portfolio could be undertaken as a formative assessment. This particularly relates to the ethical and professional practice domain. The incident would also need to be reported to their mentor, including the actions taken and the student's response to the situation. Passing on information in such a circumstance helps to promote teamwork as it ensures that all involved are apprised of the situation. However, working in community services might mean taking on more of a lone role, in which case you need to communicate with the student's mentor and teachers if further action is needed.

Creating a staff rota

─────────────────── **ACTIVITY 11.4** ───────────────────

Let us revisit the scenario from Chapter 6.

You arrive on duty on a Monday morning. The charge nurse has phoned in sick, leaving you in charge of the area. You receive a phone call from the unit manager asking about the next monthly rota that they were expecting to be ready. You search the office to find that the charge nurse had started but not completed it. The unit manager requests that you provide them with the rota by the end of the day.

What do you need to do now that the responsibility to complete this task has fallen on you?

───

Although this scenario is very likely to raise anxiety and might be described as fundamentally unfair, it does indicate the need for all staff to recognize how the various aspects of an organization link together and how the management of an individual unit inevitably impacts in some way on the wider needs of the organization. This highlights the complexity and variety of the teams within which nurses work and confirms that healthcare systems require significant and varied resources to ensure that patients receive appropriate services and high-quality care.

Similarly, it highlights the need for robust managerial leadership and clear recognition and understanding of accountability in relation to quality, patient safety, and risk management. You will need to demonstrate some action in response to this situation to enable those you work with to establish some trust in your abilities.

Clinical governance is fundamentally concerned with the culture of an organization and it would be legitimate to investigate whether such a situation had occurred previously. While the formulation of duty rotas might well be an appropriate development opportunity in the context of lifelong learning and professional development for a junior member of staff, it requires appropriate planning and supportive facilitation rather than simply having to deliver in such a pressured and acute situation, even if there is technology available to support such a task.

Such a situation will give you an opportunity to recognize the skills and insights that you have gained from your experience on the unit. As always, the safety of patients is paramount, and it would be appropriate to negotiate time to complete this task if necessary. However, you will have gained awareness of the needs and requirements of those for whom you are caring, and you may be very well placed to complete the rota, recognizing both the client dependency and the requisite skill mix. This will also offer you the opportunity to call on the support and experience of colleagues, both to ensure the safe running of the unit and to contribute ideas and thoughts to complete the rota.

Summary

This chapter has focused on bringing together the principles and examples described throughout the previous chapters of the book.

It is undoubtedly true that the transition to becoming a qualified nurse is a very challenging and complex one. It incorporates the application of a variety of diverse, multifaceted, principle-based concepts within a multiplicity of dynamic environments. Crucially, the diversity of experience and the vital support and input from patients, service users and carers and the entire interdisciplinary team provides a uniquely rewarding, fulfilling and ever-changing journey.

A note on the scenarios

The scenarios above provide a glimpse into some of the complex situations that you may face as a qualified nurse. The underpinning theories discussed throughout this book apply to them all. By raising your awareness of the theories, concepts, models, strategies and approaches, you should be able to gain further understanding of the various aspects of nursing practice that you need to consider in solving such problems.

The above examples have not been field-specific, as they relate to principles that nurses in all settings and disciplines will recognize as familiar. Neither have we attempted to investigate all of the situations that you may face or provided answers to such. Rather, we have given you a flavour of the kinds of situation in which you may find yourself and with which you may have to deal with as a qualified nurse. Do remember that once you are a qualified nurse, you will gain experience in such situations; you will have someone to turn to for help, or at least you will be able to find some reference within this book or others that may provide you with insight into solving problems you may encounter.

Conclusion: Putting it all together

We have covered with differing approaches the professional skills of improving safety and quality of care, making ethical and legal decisions, being accountable, teamworking, teaching others, and being in charge. All of these are aspects of the role that you will undertake as a qualified nurse. It is necessary to reiterate for a final time that there is a certain amount of overlap in these concepts and you may be taking decisions and actions in day-to-day practice that are influenced by the concepts discussed.

This book has explored the 'quality agenda', the expectations of the public, and the changing responsibilities and expectations of nurses in maintaining standards and ensuring quality of care. Healthcare is seen as a partnership between health professionals and patients, and nurses, already accountable, will be scrutinized more closely in relation to various clinical outcomes – nurses may well be judged against measures such as nursing metrics. We have emphasized that nurses have a key role as advocates for patients and in their lead role within the multidisciplinary team. This may mean being involved in certain ethical dilemmas from time to time.

The use of an ethical framework can assist you in engaging in 'principled discussion' and subsequent actions; being aware of the principles of autonomy, beneficence, non-maleficence and justice may help you to formulate solutions and inform your decision-making in relation to such challenging dilemmas. As discussed in scenarios within this chapter and elsewhere in this book, respect for individuals is the underpinning moral and ethical principle that informs current healthcare practice and the law. The essential concept of informed consent and capacity are reinforced throughout the book – once you qualify, it is imperative that you stay up to date with developments in relevant laws, initiatives and policies and their implications for your practice. We have discussed the differences in the accountability of students and registered nurses in practice – and don't forget, soon you will be the nurse and students will ask you: 'Can I do this?'

You may soon find yourself in charge after qualifying. The major leadership theories, such as trait, style, situational, transactional and transformational, have been discussed earlier in the book. In addition, some of the scenarios in this chapter have highlighted the fact that you need to be aware of these so that you can be flexible in your response to the workplace situations in which you find yourself. Leadership is related to your people skills and your ability to observe the situation, identify problems and create solutions. You need to be seen to be taking action, leading by example, evidence and commitment, and being involved and participating in the tasks that you would expect others to do. The concept of being a manager may seem to be some distance away for you in your career when you first become a qualified nurse. However, we have emphasized that awareness of theories of management can assist you by describing how organizational goals are aligned and your part in the strategies that are put in place to realize them. Management is about formal mechanisms in the day-to-day running of services and following the policies and procedures set in place by your employing organization and profession. You may find yourself formally dealing with colleagues at all levels of an organization and have responsibility for reporting situations from the ground or 'coalface' level of service provision.

The importance of teamwork in healthcare has been highlighted, including what teamwork is and what the ingredients of an effective team are. We have emphasized that, during their career, nurses can work in a huge range of different types of team, so they will always need teamworking skills, as well as the skills required to overcome the potential problems of teamworking!

The concepts of teaching and mentoring will be an important aspect of your role as a qualified nurse, and we have explored the NMC standards (NMC, 2018e) about the nature of teaching, learning and assessment in practice. Recognizing the individual learning needs and styles of students and junior staff provides a basis to develop appropriate strategies to meet their educational needs, including assessing and giving feedback.

Within the book, we have also provided some advice for you to consider once qualified, so don't give this book away just yet! Chapter 8 includes ways in which to develop an effective CV and strategies for performing well in interview to get the jobs that you want, for the career that you want. Over the coming years, continuing professional development will be very important to you, and we have provided some advice on how you can meet these requirements in Chapter 9.

Chapter 10 introduced the concept of global migration. You never know you may one day decide to practise your nursing overseas, so it is important to understand some of the major health issues and agendas being faced worldwide and in specific countries. You need to understand the requirements of any nursing board/council to whom you may be applying to register with in order to practise in various countries to which you might migrate to.

A final note

Although there are many overlapping complexities in the theories and scenarios presented in this book and in the various issues that you may face as a qualified nurse, essentially nursing is an engaging and fulfilling profession. It is often stated that no two days are the same, and that the wide variety of people and situations that you encounter is rewarding.

You may reflect on your reasons for entering the nursing profession and remember what made you take those first steps. It may have been a necessity that led you to nursing, or a vocational drive. Whatever the reason, you can be assured that although a career in nursing is challenging, and at times stressful, you will find that it is a wonderful privilege to care for people in a variety of dynamic and exciting environments, in a professional field that is constantly changing and developing, yet highly publicly valued.

Remember that policies, procedures and regulations do change regularly over time, so be aware to check up on any of the issues and approaches discussed within this book to ensure you access the most up-to-date information to help you in your nursing career.

We know that you will be glad of the efforts you put in when you attain your goals. We wish you the very best for your future as a qualified nurse.

Rob and Graham

REFERENCES

Abbott, M.R.B. and Shaw, P. (2018) Multiple modalities for APA instruction: Addressing diverse learning styles. *Teaching and Learning in Nursing*, 13(1): 63–65.

Adair, J. (2010) *Effective Leadership* (electronic edn). London: Pan Books.

Adams, J.E. and Gillman, L. (2016) Developing an evidence-based transition program for graduate nurses. *Contemporary Nurse: A Journal for the Australian Nursing Profession*, 52(5): 511–521.

Adults with Incapacity (Scotland) Act (2000) London: HMSO. Available at: www.legislation.gov.uk/asp/2000/4/contents

Afentakis, A. and Maier, T. (2013) Can nursing staff from abroad meet the growing demand for care? Analysis of labor migration in nursing professions in 2010. *Bundesgesundheitsblatt-Gesundheitsforschung-Gesundheitsschutz*, 56(8): 1072–1080.

Age of Legal Capacity (Scotland) Act (1991). Available at: www.legislation.gov.uk/ukpga/1991/50/contents

Ahmad, S.Z. and Buchanan, F.R. (2016) Choices of destination for transnational higher education: 'Pull' factors in an Asia Pacific market. *Education Studies*, 42(2): 163–180.

Aiken, L.H. and Sloane, D. (2020) Nurses matter: More evidence. *BMJ Quality and Safety*, 29(1): 1–3.

Aiken, L.H., Buchan, J., Sochalski, J., Nichols, B. and Powell, M. (2004) Trends in international nurse migration: The world's wealthy countries must be aware of how the 'pull' of nurses from developing countries affects global health. *Health Affairs*, 23(3): 69–77.

Aiken, L.H., Sermeus, W., Van den Heede, K., Sloane, D.M., Busse, R., McKee, M., Bruyneel, L., Rafferty, A., Griffiths, P., Moreno-Casbas, T., Tishelman, C., Scott, A., Brzostek, T., Kinnunen, J., Schwendimann, R., Heinen, M., Zikos, D., Smith, H. and Kutney-Lee, A. (2012) Patient safety, satisfaction, and quality of hospital care: Cross sectional surveys of nurses and patients in 12 countries in Europe and United States. *BMJ*, 344: 1–14.

Aiken, L.H., Sloane, D.M., Bruyneel, L., Van den Heede, K., Griffiths, P., Busse, R., Diomidous, M., Kinnunen, J., Kozka, M., Lesaffre, E., McHugh, M., Moreno-Casbas, M., Rafferty, A., Schwendimann, R., Schwendimann, R., Scott, A. and Tishelman, C. (2014) Nurse staffing and education and hospital mortality in nine European countries: A retrospective observational study. *The Lancet*, 383: 1824–1830.

Ailey, S., Lamb, K., Friese, T. and Christopher, B. (2015) Educating nursing students in clinical leadership. *Nursing Management*, 21(9): 23–28.

Alder, H. (2017) Handbook of NLP: A Manual for Professional Communicators. London: Routledge.

Alexander, C. and Lopez, R.P. (2018) A thematic analysis of self-described authentic leadership behaviors among experienced nurse executives. *JONA: The Journal of Nursing Administration*, 48(1): 38–43.

All Party Parliamentary Group (2016) Triple Impact: How Developing Nursing Will Improve Health, Promote Gender Equality and Support Economic Growth (APPG Report on Global Health). London: APPG.

Allan, H.T. and Westwood, S. (2016) English language skills requirements for internationally educated nurses working in the care industry: Barriers to UK registration or institutionalized discrimination? *International Journal of Nursing Studies*, 54: 1–4.

Allan, H.T., Magnusson, C., Horton, K., Evans, K., Ball, E., Curtis, K. and Johnson, M. (2015) People, liminal spaces and experience: Understanding recontextualisation of knowledge for newly qualified nurses. *Nurse Education Today*, 35(2): e78–e83.

Ankers, M.D., Barton, C.A. and Parry, Y.K. (2018) A phenomenological exploration of graduate nurse transition to professional practice within a transition to practice program. *Collegian*, 25(3): 319–325.

Appleby, J. and Harrison, A. (2006) *Spending on Health: How Much is Enough?* London: King's Fund.

Arnold, E.C. and Underman Boggs, K. (2016) *Interpersonal Relationships: Professional Communication Skills for Nurses* (7th edn). St Louis, MO: Elsevier.

Arrowsmith, V., Lau-Walker, M., Norman, I. and Maben, J. (2016) Nurses' perceptions and experiences of work role transitions: A mixed methods systematic review of the literature. *Journal of Advanced Nursing*, 72(8): 1735–1750.

Arunasalam, N.D. and Burton, R. (2018) Investigating Malaysian nurses' perspectives of intercultural teaching in transnational higher education learning environments. *Nurse Education Today*, 69: 165–171.

Association of Southeast Asian Nations (2019) Nursing Services (AJCCN). (https://asean.org/asean-economic-community/sectoral-bodies-under-the-purview-of-aem/services/healthcare-services/nursing-services-ajccn/)

Aubrey, K. and Riley, A. (2016) *Understanding and Using Educational Theories*. London: Sage.

Australian Health Practitioner Regulation Agency (2019a) About AHPRA: Who We Are. (www.ahpra.gov.au/About-AHPRA/Who-We-Are.aspx)

Australian Health Practitioner Regulation Agency (2019b) Registration Standards. (www.ahpra.gov.au/Registration/Registration-Standards.aspx)

Ausubel, D.P., Novak, J.D. and Hanesian, H. (1978) *Educational Psychology: A Cognitive View* (2nd edn). New York: Holt, Rinehart and Winston.

Avery, G. (2016) Law and Ethics in Nursing and Healthcare: An Introduction (2nd edn). London: Sage.

Baggott, R. (2015) *Understanding health policy* (2nd edn). London: Policy Press.

Baggott, R. (2016) Health policy and the coalition government. In Bochel, H. and Powell, M. (eds), *The Coalition Government and Social Policy: Restructuring the Welfare State.* London: Policy Press.

Bagley, K., Hoppe, L., Brenner, G.H., Crawford, M. and Weir, M. (2018) Transition to nursing faculty: Exploring the barriers. *Teaching and Learning in Nursing,* 13(4): 263–267.

Baillie, L. (2017) An exploration of the 6Cs as a set of values for nursing practice. *British Journal of Nursing,* 26(10): 558–563.

Baldwin, K.M., Black, D.L., Normand, L.K., Bonds, P. and Townley, M. (2016) Integrating retired registered nurses into a new graduate orientation program. *Clinical Nurse Specialist,* 30(5): 277–283.

Bamford, M., Wong, C.A. and Laschinger, H. (2013) The influence of authentic leadership and areas of worklife on work engagement of registered nurses. *Journal of Nursing Management,* 21(3): 529–540.

Barr, J. and Dowding, L. (2016) *Leadership in Health Care* (3rd edn). London: Sage.

Barron, K. and Sloan, G. (2015) Clinical coaching for early clinical careers fellows: Promoting compassionate care values. *British Journal of Mental Health Nursing,* 4(3): 140–145.

Bates, B. (2016) Learning Theories Simplified … and How to Apply Them to Teaching: 100+ Theories and Models from Great Thinkers. London: Sage.

Baumann, A., Hunsberger, M., Crea-Arsenio, M. and Akhtar-Dunesh, N. (2018) Policy to practice: Investment in transitioning new graduate nurses to the workplace. *Journal of Nursing Management,* 26(4): 373–381.

Beauchamp, T.L. and Childress, J.F. (2019) *Principles of Biomedical Ethics* (5th edn). Oxford: Oxford University Press.

Benner, P.E. (1984) From Novice to Expert: Excellence and Power in Clinical Nursing Practice. Menlo Park, CA: Addison Wesley.

Benton, D., and Shaffer, F. (2016) How the nursing profession can contribute to sustainable development goals. *Nursing Management,* 23(7): 29–34.

Bichel-Findlay, J. and Doran, C. (2015) Leadership in health informatics: A pathway to twenty-first century patient care. In Daly, J., Speedy, S. and Jackson, D. (eds), *Leadership and Nursing: Contemporary Perspectives* (2nd edn). Sydney: Churchill Livingstone/Elsevier.

Billings, D.M. and Halstead, J.A. (2020) (eds) *Teaching In Nursing: A Guide For Faculty* (6th edn; ebook). St Louis, MO: Elsevier.

Bing-Jonsson, P.C., Bjork, I.T., Hofoss, D., Kirkevold, M. and Foss, C. (2015) Competence in older people nursing: Development of nursing older people – competence evaluation tool. *International Journal of Older People Nursing*, 10(1): 59–72.

Bittner, N.P. and Bechtel, C.F. (2017) Identifying and describing nurse faculty workload issues: A looming faculty shortage. *Nursing Education Perspectives*, 38(4): 171–176.

Blackman, I., Henderson, J., Willis, E., Hamilton, P., Toffoli, L., Verrall, C., Abery, E. and Harvey, C. (2014) Factors influencing why nursing care is missed. *Journal of Clinical Nursing*, 24(1–2): 47–56.

Blanchard, K.H. and Ken Blanchard Companies. (2010) *Leading at a Higher Level: Blanchard on Leadership and Creating High Performing Organizations* (revised and expanded edn). Upper Saddle River, NJ: FT Press.

Blevins, S. (2018) From nursing student to registered nurse: The challenge of transition. *MEDSURG Nursing*, 27(3): 199–200.

Bloom, S.B. (1956) Taxonomy of educational objectives: The classification of educational goals. New York: Longmans, Green.

Bochel, H. and Powell, M. (2016) The Coalition Government and Social Policy: Restructuring the Welfare State. London: Policy Press.

Bolam v Friern Hospital Management Committee (1957) 2 All ER 118–128.

Bonello, M., Morris, J. and Azzopardi Muscat, N. (2018) The role of national culture in shaping health workforce collaboration: Lessons learned from a case study on attitudes to interprofessional education in Malta. *Health Policy*, 122(10): 1063–1069.

Bostridge, M. (2008) Florence Nightingale: The Woman and Her Legend. London: Viking.

Boychuk Duchscher, J.B. and Windey, M. (2018) Stages of transition and transition shock. *Journal for Nurses in Professional Development*, 34(4): 228–232.

Bradbury-Jones, C. and Clark, M. (2017) Globalisation and global health: Issues for nursing. *Nursing Standard*, 31(39): 54.

Bradshaw, P. and Bradshaw, G. (2004) *Health Policy for Health Care Professionals*. London: Sage.

Brazier, M. and Cave, E. (2016) *Medicine, Patients and the Law*. Manchester: Manchester University Press.

Brennan, G. and McSherry, R. (2009) Exploring the transition and professional socialisation from health care assistant to student nurse. In Meleis, A.I. (ed.), *Transitions Theory: Middle-Range and Situation-Specific Theories in Nursing Research and Practice*. New York: Springer.

Broad, P., Walker, J., Boden, R. and Barnes, A. (2011) Developing a 'model of transition' prior to preceptorship. *British Journal of Nursing*, 20(20): 1298–1301.

Bruner, J. (1960) *Acts of Meaning*. Cambridge, MA: Harvard University Press.

Buckner, E.B., Anderson, D.J., Garzon, N., Hafsteinsdóttir, T.B., Lai, C.K.Y. and Roshan, R. (2014) Perspectives on global nursing leadership:

International experiences from the field. *International Nursing Review,* 61(4): 463–471.

Burnard, P. and Chapman, C. (2005) *Professional and Ethical Issues in Nursing* (3rd edn). London: Bailliere Tindall.

Buscemi, C.P. (2011) Acculturation: State of the Science in Nursing. *Journal of Cultural Diversity,* 18(2): 39–42.

Canadian Nurses Association (2019) Regulation of RNs. (www.cna-aiic.ca/en/nursing-practice/the-practice-of-nursing/regulation-of-rns)

Candela, L. (2020) Theoretical foundations of teaching and learning. In Billings, D.M. and Halstead, J.A. (eds), *Teaching In Nursing: A Guide For Faculty* (6th edn; ebook). St Louis, MO: Elsevier.

Care Quality Commission (2015) *The State of Health Care and Adult Social Care in England.* London: Care Quality Commission.

Care Quality Commission (2018) Adult inpatient survey. (www.cqc.org.uk/publications/surveys/adult-inpatient-survey-2018)

Care Quality Commission (2019a) The independent regulator of health and social care in England. (www.cqc.org.uk/what-we-do)

Care Quality Commission (2019b) Cygnet Whorlton Hall Quality Report. (www.cqc.org.uk/sites/default/files/new_reports/AAAJ5381.pdf)

Cassidy-Rice, J. (2014) NLP promotes personal development and professional success: Process gives the edge to both companies and individuals. *Human Resource Management International Digest,* 22(3): 38–41.

Caulfield, H. (2005) *Accountability.* Oxford: Blackwell Publishing.

Cave, E. and Reinach, N. (2019) Patient rights to participate in treatment decisions: Choice, consultation and knowledge. *Journal of Medical Law and Ethics,* 7(2): 157–176.

Chang, E. and Daly, J. (2016) *Transitions in Nursing: Preparing for Professional Practice* (4th edn; ebook). Chatswood, NSW: Elsevier Australia.

Chantrell, G. (2004) *Oxford Dictionary of Word Histories.* Oxford: Oxford University Press.

Chávez, E.C. and Yoder, L.H. (2015) Staff nurse clinical leadership: A concept analysis. *Nursing Forum,* 50(2): 90–100.

Church, M. and Watts, S. (2007) Assessment of mental capacity: A flow chart guide. *Psychiatrist,* 31: 304–307. (http://citeseerx.ist.psu.edu/viewdoc/download?doi=10.1.1.855.4196andrep=rep1andtype=pdf)

Clancy, C. (2014) The importance of emotional intelligence: Cheri Clancy explains how self-awareness can be used to benefit staff morale and patient experience. *Nursing Management,* 21(8): 15.

Coffield, F., Moseley, D., Hall, E. and Ecclestone, K. (2004) *Learning Styles and Pedagogy in Post 16 Learning: A Systematic and Critical Review.* London: Learning and Skills Research Centre.

Collins Dictionary (2014) *Collins English Dictionary* (12th edn; Kindle edn). Glasgow: Harper Collins.

Concilio, C., Lockhart, J., Oermann, M., Kronk, R. and Schreiber, J. (2019) Newly licensed nurse resiliency and interventions to promote resiliency in the first year of hire: An integrative review. *Journal of Continuing Education in Nursing*, 50(4): 153–161.

Cooper, J. (2013) Building good leadership through personal development. *Australian Nursing and Midwifery Journal*, 21(5): 28.

Cope, V. and Murray, M. (2017) Leadership styles in nursing. *Nursing Standard*, 31(43): 61–70.

Coster, S., Watkins, M. and Norman, I.J. (2018) What is the impact of professional nursing on patients' outcomes globally? An overview of research evidence. *International Journal of Nursing Studies*, 78: 76–83.

Courtney, M., Nash, R., Thornton, R. and Potgeiter, I. (2015) Leading and managing in nursing practice: Concepts, processes and challenges. In Daly, J., Speedy, S. and Jackson, D. (eds), *Leadership and Nursing: Contemporary Perspectives* (2nd edn). Sydney: Churchill Livingstone/ Elsevier.

Covell, C.L., Primeau, M.D. and St-Pierre, I. (2018) Internationally educated nurses in Canada: Perceived benefits of bridging programme participation. *International Nursing Review*, 65(3): 400–407.

Coventry, T.H., Maslin-Prothero, S.E. and Smith, G. (2015) Organizational impact of nurse supply and workload on nurses continuing professional development opportunities: An integrative review. *Journal of Advanced Nursing*, 71(12): 2715–2727.

Covey, S. (2013) The 7 Habits of Highly Effective People: Powerful Lessons in Personal Change (25th anniversary electronic edn). LLC: Rosetta Books.

Crinson, I. (2009) Health Policy: A Critical Perspective. London: Sage.

Crisp, N.L. (2016) Triple Impact: How developing nursing will improve health, promote gender equality and support economic growth: A Report by the All-Party Parliamentary Group on Global Health. London: AAPG.

Crisp, N.L. and Watkins, M. (2018) The triple impact of nursing. *International Journal of Nursing Studies*, 78: A3–A4.

Crown Prosecution Service (CPS) (2014) Suicide: Policy for Prosecutors in Respect of Cases of Encouraging or Assisting Suicide. (www.cps.gov.uk/ legal-guidance/suicide-policy-prosecutors-respect-cases-encouraging- or-assisting-suicide)

Croy, S.R. (2018) Development of a group work assessment pedagogy using constructive alignment theory. *Nurse Education Today*, 61: 49–53.

Cruz, E.V., Felicilda-Reynaldo, R.F. and Mazzotta, C.P. (2017) Return to nursing: A meta-synthesis of academic bridging programs' effect on internationally educated nurses. *Qualitative Report*, 22(4): 1092–1111.

Currie, I. and Watts, C. (2012) *Preceptorship and Pre-Registration Nurse Education*. London: Department of Health.

Currie, L. Morrell, C. and Scrivner, R. (2003) *Clinical Governance: An RCN Resource Guide*. London: Royal College of Nursing.

Curry, L. (1983) *Learning Styles in Continuing Medical Education*. Ottawa, ON: Canadian Medical Association.

Cutler, A. and Steptoe-Warren, G. (2014) *Leadership Psychology: How the Best Leaders Inspire their People* (1st edn). London: Kogan Page.

Dalpezzo, N.K. (2000) Nursing care: A concept analysis. *Nursing Forum*, 44(4): 256–264.

Daly, J., Hill, M.N. and Jackson, D. (2015) Leadership and healthcare change management. In Daly, J., Speedy, S. and Jackson, D. (eds), *Leadership and Nursing: Contemporary Perspectives* (2nd edn). Sydney: Churchill Livingstone/Elsevier.

Darvill, A. (2013) A qualitative study into the experiences of newly qualified children's nurses during their transition into children's community nursing teams. Unpublished PhD thesis, University of Salford.

Darvill, A. and Croughan, C. (2018) Managing the transition from student to registered nurse. In Darvill, A., Stephens, M. and Leigh, J. (eds), *Transition to Nursing Practice: From Student to Registered Nurse*. London: Sage.

Darvill, A., Fallon, D. and Livesley, J. (2014) A different world? The transition experiences of newly qualified children's nurses taking up first destination posts within children's community nursing teams in England. *Issues in Comprehensive Pediatric Nursing*, 37(1): 6–24.

Darvill, A., Stephens, M. and Leigh, J. (eds) (2018) *Transition to Nursing Practice: From Student to Registered Nurse*. London: Sage.

Davenport, M., Castle, R., Brady, M., Smith, P. and Keen, M. (2015) Choosing the right field of nursing. In Elcock, K. (ed.), *Getting into Nursing* (2nd edn). London: Sage.

David, F.R. and David, F.R. (2015) *Strategic Management Concepts and Cases: A Strategic Management Approach* (15th edn; global edn). Harlow: Pearson Education.

Davis, A., Tschudin, V. and De Raeve, L. (eds) (2006) *Essentials of Teaching and Learning in Nursing Ethics: Perspectives and Methods*. Edinburgh: Churchill Livingstone.

Davis, J., Lister, J. and Wrigley, D. (2015) *NHS for Sale: Myths Lies and Deception*. London: The Merlin Press.

de Vries, D.H., Steinmetz, S. and Tijdens, K.G. (2016) Does migration 'pay off' for foreign-born migrant health workers? An exploratory analysis using the global WageIndicator dataset. *Human Resources for Health*, 14(1): 40.

Delucas, A.C. (2014) Foreign nurse recruitment: Global risk. *Nursing Ethics*, 21(1): 76–85.

Department of Health (1992) *The Patient's Charter and You: A Charter for England*. London: Department of Health.

Department of Health (1997) *The New NHS: Modern and Dependable*. London: Department of Health.

Department of Health (1998) *A First Class Service: Quality in the New NHS*. London: Department of Health.

Department of Health (1999) Making a Difference: Strengthening the Nursing, Midwifery and Health Visiting Contribution to Health and Health Care. London: HMSO.

Department of Health (2000) *The NHS Plan*. London: Department of Health.

Department of Health (2006) *Modernising Nursing Careers: Setting the Direction*. London: Department of Health.

Department of Health (2007a) *Chief Nursing Officer Report on Privacy and Dignity: Mixed Sex Accommodation in Hospitals*. London: Department of Health. (www.nhs.uk/nhsengland/aboutnhsservices/nhshospitals/documents/privacy%20and%20dignity.pdf)

Department of Health (2007b) Trust, Assurance and Safety: The Regulation of Health Professionals in the 21st Century. London: Department of Health.

Department of Health (2008a) *High Quality Care for All: NHS Next Stage Review*. London: Department of Health.

Department of Health (2008b) *A High Quality Workforce: NHS Next Stage Review*. London: Department of Health.

Department of Health (2008c) Principles for Revalidation: Report of the Working Group for Non-Medical Revalidation; Professional Regulation and Safety Programme. London: Department of Health.

Department of Health (2010) Preceptorship Framework for Newly Registered Nurses, Midwives and Allied Health Professionals. London: Department of Health.

Department of Health (2012) Compassion in Practice: Nursing, Midwifery and Care Staff, Our Vision and Strategy. London: Department of Health.

Department of Health (2013a) A Promise to Learn – A Commitment to Act: Improving the Safety of Patients in England, National Advisory Group on the Safety of Patients in England. London: Department of Health.

Department of Health (2013b) *Compassion in Practice: One Year On*. London: Department of Health.

Department of Health (2015) *NHS Constitution*. London: Department of Health.

Department of Health (2019) *Handbook to the NHS Constitution for England*. London: Department of Health.

Dewar, B. and MacBride, T. (2017) Developing caring conversations in care homes: An appreciative inquiry. *Health and Social Care in the Community*, 25(4): 1375–1386.

Deyo, P., Swartwout, E. and Drenkard, K. (2017) Nurse manager competencies supporting patient engagement. *The Journal of Nursing Administration*, 46(3; Supplement): S19–S26.

Dimond, B. (2015) *Legal Aspects of Nursing* (7th edn). Harlow: Pearson Longman.

Dimond, B. (2016) Legal Aspects of Mental Capacity: A Practical Guide for Health and Social Care Professionals. Oxford: Wiley-Blackwell Publishing.

Dirik, H.F. and Seren Intepeler, S. (2017) The influence of authentic leadership on safety climate in nursing. *Journal of Nursing Management*, 25(5): 392–401.

Dommett, K. and Pearce, W. (2019) What do we know about public attitudes towards experts? Reviewing survey data in the United Kingdom and European Union. *Public Understanding of Science*, 28(6): 669–678.

Donaldson, S.I. and Dollwet, M. (2013) Taming the waves and wild horses of positive organizational psychology. *Advances in Positive Organizational Psychology*, 1: 1–21.

Donnelly, G.F. (2017) Normative and cataclysmic career transitions a nurse's memoir. *Nursing Administration Quarterly*, 41(3): 223–232.

Donoghue v Stevenson (1932) AC 562. In Griffith, R. and Dowie, I. (eds), *Dimond's Legal Aspects of Nursing* (8th edn). Harlow: Pearson.

Doody, O., Tuohy, D. and Deasy, C. (2011) Final-year student nurses' perceptions of role transition. *British Journal of Nursing*, 21(11): 684–688.

Doria, H. (2015) Successful transition from staff nurse to nurse manager. *Nurse Leader*, 13(1): 78–81.

DuBois, C.A. and Zedreck Gonzalez, J.F. (2018) Implementing a resilience-promoting education program for new nursing graduates. *Journal for Nurses in Professional Development*, 34(5): 263–269.

Duff, L. (1995) Standards of care, quality assurance and accountability. In Watson, R. (ed.), *Accountability in Nursing Practice*. London: Chapman and Hall.

Eckenwiler, L. (2014) Care worker migration, global health equity, and ethical place-making. *Women's Studies International Forum*, 47: 213–222.

Edwards, D., Hawker, C., Carrier, J. and Rees, C. (2015) A systematic review of the effectiveness of strategies and interventions to improve the transition from student to newly qualified nurse. *International Journal of Nursing Studies*, 52(7): 1254–1268.

Egan, G. (2014) The Skilled Helper: A Problem-Management and Opportunity-Development Approach to Helping (10th edn). Belmont, CA: Brooks/Cole, Cengage Learning.

Ekström, L. and Idvall, E. (2015) Being a team leader: Newly registered nurses relate their experiences. *Journal of Nursing Management*, 23(1): 75–86.

Ellis, P. (2017) *Understanding Ethics for Nursing Students* (2nd edn). Exeter: Learning Matters.

Fallatah, F. and Laschinger, H.K. (2016) The influence of authentic leadership and supportive professional practice environments on new graduate nurses' job satisfaction. *Journal of Research in Nursing*, 21(2): 125–136.

Family Law Reform Act 1969. London: HMSO. Available at: www.legislation.gov.uk/ukpga/1969/46

Family Law (Scotland) Act (2006). London: HMSO. Available at: www.legislation.gov.uk/asp/2006/2/contents

Fealy, G., McNamara, M. and Casey, M. (2015) Leading contemporary approaches to nursing practice. In Daly, J., Speedy, S. and Jackson, D. (eds), *Leadership and Nursing: Contemporary Perspectives* (2nd edn). Sydney: Churchill Livingstone/Elsevier.

Fearon, D., Hughes, S. and Brearley, S. (2018) A philosophical critique of the UK's National Institute for Health and Care Excellence guideline 'Palliative care for adults: Strong opioids for pain relief'. *British Journal of Pain*, 12(3): 183–188.

Feltrin, C., Newton, J.M. and Willetts, G. (2019) How graduate nurses adapt to individual ward culture: A grounded theory study. *Journal of Advanced Nursing*, 75(3): 616–627.

Fleming, N. (2014) The nature of preference. https://vark-learn.com/wp-content/uploads/2014/08/THE-NATURE-OF-PREFERENCE.pdf. Accessed 14.04.2020.

Francis, R. (2013) The Mid Staffordshire NHS Foundation Trust, Final Report of Public Inquiry. London: The Stationery Office.

Freeth, P. (2016) *The NLP Master Practitioner Manual* (3rd edn). Birmingham: CGW Publishing.

Fry, S.T. and Johnstone, M. (2008) *Ethics in Nursing Practice: A Guide to Ethical Decision Making* (3rd edn). Oxford: Wiley-Blackwell Publishing.

Fuller, B.L. and Mott-Smith, J.A. (2017) Issues influencing success: Comparing the perspectives of nurse educators and diverse nursing students. *Journal of Nursing Education*, 56(7): 389–396.

Gage, W. (2016) Role of the nurse in managing complaints in their clinical area. *Nursing Standard*, 30(32): 51–60.

Gallagher, A. (2010) Whistleblowing: What influences nurses' decisions on whether to report poor practice? *Nursing Times*, 106: 4.

Gallo, K. (2007) The new nurse manager: A leadership development program paves the road to success. *Nurse Leader*, 5(4): 28–32.

Gardner, H.E. (1993) Frames of mind: The theory of multiple intelligences. New York: BasicBooks.

General Pharmaceutical Council (2018) *Revalidation for pharmacists and pharmacy technicians*. London: GPhC.

George, B., Sims, P., McLean, A.N. and Mayer, D. (2018) Discovering your authentic leadership: Why self-awareness is so critical. In George, B., Ibarra, H., Goffee, R. and Jones, G. (eds), *Authentic Leadership* (HBR Emotional Intelligence Series). Boston, MA: Harvard Business Review Press.

Giblin, C., Lemermeyer, G., Cummings, G., Wang, M. and Kwan, J.A. (2016) Learning from experience: Improving the process of internationally educated nurses' application for registration – A study protocol. *Journal of Advanced Nursing*, 72(3): 650–657.

Goleman, D., Boyatzis, R. and McKee, A. (2002) The New Leaders: Transforming the Art of Leadership into the Science of Results. London: Time Warner.

Goodrich, J. and Cornwell, J. (2008) *Seeing the person in the patient*. King's Fund. London.

Gopee, N. (2018) Supervision and Mentoring in Healthcare (4th edn). London: Sage.

Gottwald, M. and Lansdown, G. (2014) Clinical Governance: Improving the Quality of Healthcare for Patients and Service Users. New York: McGraw-Hill Education.

Grant, A.M., Cavanagh, M.J., Kleitman, S., Spence, G., Lakota, M. and Yu, N. (2012) Development and validation of the solution-focused inventory. *The Journal of Positive Psychology*, 7(4): 334–348.

Grant, L. and Kinman, G. (2013) The Importance Of Emotional Resilience for Staff and Students in the 'Helping' Professions: Developing an Emotional Curriculum. *York, Higher Education Academy Research Briefing*. (www.heacademy.ac.uk/sites/default/files/emotional_resilience_louise_grant_march_2014_0.pdf)

Greer, S., Jarman, H. and Azorky, A. (2014) *A Reorganisation You Can See from Space: The Architecture of Power in the New NHS*. London: Centre for Health and the Public Interest.

Griffiths, P. (2019) Nursing, midwifery, and the sustainable development goals: An editorial series leading up to the World Health Organization's 'Year of the Nurse and Midwife', *International Journal of Nursing Studies*, 94: A1–A2.

Griffith, R. and Dowie, I. (2019) *Dimond's Legal Aspects of Nursing* (8th edn). Harlow: Pearson.

Grossman, S. and Valiga, T. (2016) *The New Leadership Challenge: Creating the Future of Nursing* (5th edn). Pennsylvania, PA: F.A. Davis Company.

Halpin, Y., Terry, L.M. and Curzio, J. (2017) A longitudinal, mixed methods investigation of newly qualified nurses' workplace stressors and stress experience during transition. *Journal of Advanced Nursing*, 73(11): 2577–2586.

Ham, C. (2017) Next steps on the NHS five year forward view. *BMJ*, 357: 1678.

Handy, C. (1993) *Understanding Organizations* (4th edn). London: Penguin.

Harkess, L. and Kaddoura, M. (2015) Culture and cultural competence in nursing education and practice: The state of the art. *Nursing Forum*, 51(3): 211–222.

Harrison, S.R. and McDonald, E.R. (2008) *The Politics of Healthcare in Britain*. London: Sage.

Hayter, M. (2013) The UK Francis Report: The key messages for nursing. *Journal of Advanced Nursing*, 69(8): 1–3.

Health and Care Professions Council (2019) *Standards for Continuing Professional Development*. London: HCPC.

Health and Social Care Act 2012. London: Department of Health.

Health Education England (2015) Raising the Bar: Shape of Caring – A Review of the Future Education and Training of Registered Nurses and Care Assistants. London: Health Education England.

Health Education England (2017) *Preceptorship and Return to Practice for Nursing*. London: Health Education England.

Health Education England (2020) How to Become a Nurse. (www.healthcareers.nhs.uk/explore-roles/nursing/studying-nursing)

Healthwatch (2019) Care Quality Commission (CQC) London. (www.healthwatch.co.uk/)

Heizer, J. and Render, B. (2014) *Operations Management* (11th edn; global edn). Harlow: Pearson Education.

Henwood, S. and Lister, J. (2009) *NLP and Coaching for Healthcare Professionals*. Chichester: John Wiley and Sons.

Herring, J. (2018) *Medical Law and Ethics* (7th edn). Oxford: Oxford University Press.

Hodge (2018) The transition to registered nurse. In Hodge, A., Varndell, W. and West, R. (eds), *Professional Transitions in Nursing: A Guide to Practice in the Australian Healthcare System*. Sydney: Allen and Unwin.

Hofstede, G., Hofstede, G.J. and Minkov, M. (2010) Cultures and Organizations: Software of the Mind: Intercultural Cooperation and its Importance for Survival. New York: McGraw-Hill.

Holmgren, J. (2017) Global nursing: Educating future nurses for tomorrow's nursing care needs. *Nordic Journal of Nursing Research*, 37(3): 172–174.

Holmgren, J., Eriksson, H., Tegnestedt, C., Röda Korsets Högskola, and Hälsovetenskapliga institutionen. (2018) Global nursing as visualised on the internet: An ethnographic analysis of the emerging global paradigm in nursing. *Contemporary Nurse*, 54(4–5): 443–455.

Honey, P. and Mumford, A. (1992) *The Manual of Learning Styles* (3rd edn). Maidenhead: Peter Honey.

Hood, L.J. (2017) *Leddy and Pepper's Professional Nursing* (9th edn). Philadelphia, PA: Lippincott, Williams and Wilkins.

Howard, S. (2009) How to make your teaching effective. In Hinchliff, S.M. (ed.), *The Practitioner as Teacher* (4th edn). Philadelphia, PA: Elsevier.

Hughes, S.J. and Quinn, F.M. (2013) *Quinn's Principles and Practice of Nurse Education* (6th edn). Andover: Cengage Learning EMEA.

Human Rights Act 1998. London: HMSO.

Ibarra, H. (2018) The authenticity paradox. In George, B., Ibarra, H., Goffee, R. and Jones, G. (eds), *Authentic Leadership* (HBR Emotional Intelligence Series). Boston, MA: Harvard Business Review Press.

Ignatavicius, D. (2018) Teaching and Learning in a Concept-Based Nursing Curriculum: A How-To Best Approach. Burlington: Jones and Bartlett Learning.

Iheduru-Anderson, K.C. and Wahi, M.M. (2018) Experiences of Nigerian internationally educated nurses transitioning to United States health care settings. *Journal of Transcultural Nursing*, 29(6): 603–610.

Illeris, K. (2018) A comprehensive understanding of human learning. In Illeris, K. (ed.), *Contemporary Theories of Learning: Learning Theorists… In Their Own Words* (2nd edn). London and New York: Routledge.

International Council of Nurses (2012) The ICN Code of Ethics for Nurses. Geneva, Switzerland. (www.icn.ch/sites/default/files/inline-files/2012_ICN_Codeofethicsfornurses_%20eng.pdf)

International Council of Nurses (2013) Position Statement: Cultural and Linguistic Competence. (www.icn.ch/sites/default/files/inline-files/B03_Cultural_Linguistic_Competence.pdf)

International Council of Nurses (2014) *ICN Strategic Plan 2014–2018*. Geneva: International Council of Nurses.

International Council of Nurses (2019) *ICN Mission, Vision and Strategic Plan*. (www.icn.ch/who-we-are/icn-mission-vision-and-strategic-plan)

Irwin, C., Bliss, J. and Poole, K. (2018) Does preceptorship improve confidence and competence in newly qualified nurses: A systematic literature review. *Nurse Education Today*, 60: 35–46.

Isaac, M. and Carson, K. (2012) A Guide to Belbin Team Roles: How to Increase Personal and Team Effectiveness. Humberside: Bridge Publications.

Jacobs, K. (2004) Accountability and clinical governance in nursing: A critical overview of the topic. In Tilley, S. and Watson, R. (eds), *Accountability in Nursing and Midwifery* (2nd edn). Oxford: Blackwell Publishing.

Jacobson, J. (2015) The complexities of nurse migration. *American Journal of Nursing*, 115(12): 22–23.

Jakeman, R.C., Henderson, M.M. and Howard, L.C. (2017) Reflective pedagogy: The integration of methodology and subject-matter content in a graduate-level course. *Teaching in Higher Education*, 22(2): 207–221.

Jensen, E. (2008) *Brain-Based Learning: The New Paradigm of Teaching* (2nd edn). Thousand Oaks, CA: Corwin Press.

Johnson, T.C. and Johnson, T. (2015) Missionary nursing life among an Indonesian tribe. In Harlan, C.A. (ed.), *Global Health Nursing: Narratives from the Field*. New York: Springer Publishing Company.

Jones, C.B. and Sherwood, G. (2014) The globalization of the nursing workforce: Pulling the pieces together. *Nursing Outlook*, 62(1): 59–63.

Jones, S. and Jenkins, R. (2004) *The Law and the Midwife* (2nd edn). Oxford: Blackwell Publishing.

Kaihlanen, A., Haavisto, E., Strandell-Laine, C. and Salminen, L. (2018) Facilitating the transition from a nursing student to a registered nurse in the final clinical practicum: A scoping literature review. *Scandinavian Journal of Caring Sciences*, 32(2): 466–477.

Keeling, J. and Major, D. (2018) Self-assessment of knowledge, skills and attitudinal values through critical reflection. In Darvill, A., Stephens, M. and Leigh, J. (eds), *Transition to Nursing Practice: From Student to Registered Nurse*. London: Sage.

Kemp, S. and Baker, M. (2013) Continuing professional development: Reflections from nursing and education. *Nurse Education in Practice*, 13(6): 541–545.

Keogh, B. (2013) Review into the Quality of Care and Treatment Provided by 14 Hospital Trusts in England: Overview Report. London: NHS.

King, N., Bravington, A., Brooks, J., Melvin, J. and Wilde, D. (2017) 'Go make your face known': Collaborative working through the lens of personal relationships. *International Journal of Integrated Care*, 17(4): 3.

King's Fund (2014) A New Settlement for Health and Social Care: Final Report. London: The King's Fund.

King's Fund (2019a) The Politics of Health: What do the Public Think About the NHS? (www.kingsfund.org.uk/publications/public-think-about-nhs)

King's Fund (2019b) Workforce Implementation Plan: Five Key Issues to Look Out For. (www.kingsfund.org.uk/blog/2019/05/workforce-implementation-plan)

King's Fund (2019c) The King's Fund Responds to the Interim NHS People Plan. (www.kingsfund.org.uk/press/press-releases/interim-nhs-people-plan)

Knowles, M. (1980) The Modern Practice of Adult Education: From Pedagogy to Andragogy. Englewood Cliffs, NJ: Cambridge.

Kolb, D. (1984) Experiential Learning: Experience as the Source of Learning and Development. London: Prentice-Hall.

Kortese, L. (2016) Exploring professional recognition in the EU: A legal perspective. *Journal of International Mobility*, 1(4): 43–58.

Kramer, M. (1974) *Reality Shock: Why Nurses Leave Nursing*. St Louis, MO: Mosby.

Kramer, M. and Crespy, D.A. (2011) Communicating collaborative leadership. *The Leadership Quarterly*, 22: 1024–1037.

Kramer, M., Maguire, P., Halfer, D., Brewer, B. and Schmalenberg, C. (2013) Impact of residency programs on professional socialization of newly licensed registered nurses. *Western Journal of Nursing Research*, 35(4): 459–496.

Kulka, J.M., De Gagne, J.C., Mullen, C. and Robeano, K. (2016) Mindfulness-based stress reduction for newly graduated registered nurses. *Creative Nursing*, 24(4): 243–250.

Kumaran, S. and Carney, M. (2014) Role transition from student nurse to staff nurse: Facilitating the transition period. *Nurse Education in Practice*, 14(6): 605–611.

Labrague, L.J. and McEnroe-Petitte, D.M. (2018) Job stress in new nurses during the transition period: An integrative review. *International Nursing Review*, 65(4): 491–504.

Laschinger, H., Duffield, C. and Read, E. (2015) Leadership and empowerment in nursing. In Daly, J., Speedy, S. and Jackson, D. (2015) *Leadership and Nursing: Contemporary Perspectives* (2nd edn). Sydney: Churchill Livingstone/Elsevier.

Law, H. (2013) *Coaching Psychology: A Practitioners Guide* (1st edn). Malden, MA: Wiley.

Lawrence, P. (2017) Managerial coaching: A literature review. *International Journal of Evidence Based Coaching and Mentoring*, 15(2): 43.

Lazarus, J. (2015) NLP: The Essential Handbook for Business – Communication Techniques to Build Relationships, Influence Others, and Achieve your Goals. Pompton Plains, NJ: Career Press.

Leadership Alliance for the Care of Dying People (LACDP) (2014) One Chance to Get it Right. (https://assets.publishing.service.gov.uk/government/uploads/system/uploads/attachment_data/file/323188/One_chance_to_get_it_right.pdf)

Lekan, D.A., Ward, T.D. and Elliott, A.A. (2018) Resilience in baccalaureate nursing students: An exploration. *Journal of Psychosocial Nursing and Mental Health Services*, 56(7): 46–55.

Lewis, S. and McGowan, B. (2015) Newly qualified nurses' experiences of preceptorship. *British Journal of Nursing*, 24(1): 41–43.

Li, J., Li, H. and Nie, W. (2014) The benefits and caveats of international nurse migration. *International Journal of Nursing Sciences*, 1(3): 314–317.

Lidster, J. and Wakefield, S. (2019) Student Practice Supervision and Assessment: A Guide for NMC Nurses and Midwives. Exeter: Learning Matters.

Lin, H. (2016) Impact of nurses' cross-cultural competence on nursing intellectual capital from a social cognitive theory perspective. *Journal of Advanced Nursing*, 72(5): 1144–1154.

Lindh, I., Barbosa da Silva, A., Berg, A. and Severinsson, E. (2010) Courage and nursing practice: A theoretical analysis. *Nursing Ethics*, 17(5): 551–565.

Loftus, I. (2019) Not so NICE guidelines for patients with aortic aneurysms. *CVIR Endovascular* 2:38.

Maben, J. and Griffiths, P. (2008) *Nurses in Society: Starting the Debate.* London: National Nursing Research Unit, King's College.

Magnusson, C., Allan, H., Horton, K., Johnson, M., Evans, K. and Ball, E. (2017) An analysis of delegation styles among newly qualified nurses. *Nursing Standard*, 31(25): 46–53.

Mannix, J., Wilkes, L. and Daly, J. (2013) Attributes of clinical leadership in contemporary nursing: An integrative review. *Contemporary Nurse*, 45(1): 10–21.

Marć, M., Bartosiewicz, A., Burzyńska, J., Chmiel, Z. and Januszewicz, P. (2019) A nursing shortage: A prospect of global and local policies. *International Nursing Review*, 66(1): 9–16.

Marginson, S. (2014) Student self-formation in international education. *Journal of Studies in International Education*, 18(1): 6–22.

Marquis, B.L. and Huston, C.J. (2012) *Leadership and Management Tools for the New Nurse: A Case Study Approach*. Philadelphia, PA: Lippincott, Williams and Wilkins.

Marton, F. and Saljo, R. (1976) On qualitative differences in learning: I – outcome and process. *British Journal of Educational Psychology*, 46: 4–11.

Marx, M. (2014) Examining the structural challenges to communication as experienced by nurse managers in two US hospital settings. *Journal of Nursing Management*, 22(8): 964–973.

Maryniak, K. (2019) *Professional Nursing Practice in the United States: An overview for international nurses, and those along the continuum from new graduates to experienced nurses*. [Kindle edition]. Copyright @ Kim Maryniak.

Maslow, A. (1943) A theory of human motivation. *Psychological Review*, 50(40): 370–396.

Maslow, A. (1954) *Motivation and Personality*. New York: Harper and Row.

Mason, T. and Whitehead, E. (2003) *Thinking Nursing*. Maidenhead: Open University Press.

McAllister, M. and Lowe, J. (eds) (2011) *The Resilient Nurse: Empowering Your Practice*. New York: Springer Publishing.

McDonald, G., Jackson, D., Vickers, M.H. and Wilkes, L. (2016) Surviving workplace adversity: A qualitative study of nurses and midwives and their strategies to increase personal resilience. *Journal of Nursing Management*, 24(1): 123–131.

McHugh, M.D., Kutney-Lee, A., Cimiotti, J.P., Sloane, D.M. and Aiken, L.H. (2011) Nurses' widespread job dissatisfaction, burnout, and frustration with health benefits signal problems for patient care. *Health Affairs*, 30(2): 202–210.

McKenna, L., Copnell, B., Butler, A.E. and Lau, R. (2018) Learning style preferences of Australian accelerated postgraduate pre-registration nursing students: A cross-sectional survey. *Nurse Education in Practice*, 28: 280–284.

McMahon, A. and White, M. (2017) Compassion in practice: Connected, contested, conflicted, conflated and complex. *Journal of Research in Nursing*, 22(1–2): 3–6.

Meleis, A.I. (2009) Transitions Theory: Middle-Range and Situation-Specific Theories in Nursing Research and Practice. New York: Springer.

Melia, K. (2013) Ethics for Nursing and Healthcare Practice. London: Sage.

Mental Health Act (1983). London: HMSO. Available at: www.legislation.gov.uk/ukpga/1983/20/contents

Mental Capacity Act (2005). London: HMSO.

Mental Health Act (2007). London: HMSO. Available at: www.legislation.gov.uk/ukpga/2007/12/contents

Mental Health (Care and Treatment) (Scotland) Act (2015). Edinburgh: Scottish Executive.

Merriam, S.B. and Bierema, L.L. (2013) *Adult Learning: Linking Theory and Practice*. San Francisco, CA: Jossey-Bass.

Merriam, S.B. (2018) Adult learning theory: evolution and future directions. In Illeris, K. (ed.), *Contemporary Theories of Learning: Learning Theorists ... In Their Own Words* (2nd edn). London and New York: Routledge.

Meyer, E. (2015) The Culture Map: Decoding How People Think, Lead, and Get Things Done Across Cultures. New York: Public Affairs.

Meyer, G. and Shatto, B. (2018) Resilience and transition to practice in direct entry nursing graduates. *Nurse Education in Practice*, 28: 276–279.

Mezirow, J. (2018) Transformative learning theory. In Illeris, K. (ed.), *Contemporary Theories of Learning: Learning Theorists ... In Their Own Words* (2nd edn). London and New York: Routledge.

Miller, L.J. and Lu, W. (2018) *These Are the Economies with the Most (and Least) Efficient Health Care*. (www.bloomberg.com/news/articles/2018-09-19/u-s-near-bottom-of-health-index-hong-kong-and-singapore-at-top)

Mitchell, C., Del Fabbro, L. and Shaw, J. (2017) The acculturation, language and learning experiences of international nursing students: Implications for nursing education. *Nurse Education Today*, 56: 16–22.

Moore, L.W., Sublett, C. and Leahy, C. (2017) Nurse managers speak out about disruptive nurse-to-nurse relationships. *The Journal of Nursing Administration*, 47(1): 24–29.

Morgan, S. (2010) Nursin' USA: Why do UK nurses consider restraints unacceptable? *Nursing Times*. (www.nursingtimes.net/roles/older-people-nurses/nursin-usa-why-do-uk-nurses-consider-restraints-unacceptable/5016114.article)

Morrell, N. and Ridgway, V. (2014) Are we preparing student nurses for their final placement? *British Journal of Nursing*, 23(10): 518–523.

Mühlberger, M.D. and Traut-Mattausch, E. (2015) Leading to effectiveness: Comparing dyadic coaching and group coaching. *The Journal of Applied Behavioral Science*, 51(2): 198–230.

Muijs, D. and Reynolds, D. (2018) *Effective Teaching: Evidence and Practice* (4th edn). London: Sage.

Müller, A. (2016) Language proficiency and nursing registration. *International Journal of Nursing Studies*, 54, 132–140.

Mullins, L.J. and Christy, G. (2016) *Management and Organisational Behaviour* (11th edn). Harlow: Pearson Education Limited.

Murray, E. (2017) Nursing Leadership and Management for Patient Safety and Quality Care. Philadelphia, PA: F.A. Davis.

Naidoo, V. and Sibiya, M.N. (2019) Graduate experiences with transnational nursing education: A qualitative enquiry. *International Journal of Health Care Quality Assurance*, 32(3): 562–573.

Narayanasamy, A. and Penney, V. (2014) Coaching to promote professional development in nursing practice. *British Journal of Nursing*, 23(11): 568–573.

Nardi, D.A. and Gyurko, C.C. (2013) The global nursing faculty shortage: Status and solutions for change. *Journal of Nursing Scholarship*, 45(3): 317–326.

National Council of State Boards for Nursing (2015) *U.S. Nursing Licensure for Foreign-Educated Nurses – Resource Manual*. Chicago, IL: NCSBN.

National Council of State Boards for Nursing (2019) *Nursing Regulation*. (www.ncsbn.org/boards.htm)

National Quality Board (2011) Quality Governance in the NHS: A Guide for Provider Boards. London: NQB.

NHS Employers (2018) Preceptorships for Newly Qualified Staff. London: NHSE.

NHS England (2014) *Five Year Forward View*. London: NHS.

NHS England (2016) Compassion in Practice: Evidencing the Impact. London: NHS.

NHS England (2017a) Leading Change, Adding Value: A Framework for Nursing, Midwifery and Care Staff. London: NHS England.

NHS England (2017b) Next Steps on the NHS Five Year Forward View. London: NHS.

NHS England (2019a) *The NHS Long Term Plan*. London: NHS.

NHS England (2019b) *Interim NHS People Plan*. London: NHS.

Nicholas, P.K. and Breakey, S. (2015) Global health and global nursing. In Breakey, S., Corless, I.B., Meedzan, N., Nicholas, P.K. and ProQuest Ebooks (eds), *Global Health Nursing in the 21st Century*. New York: Springer.

Nordstrom, P.M., Kwan, J.A., Wang, M., Qiu, Z, Cummings, G.G. and Giblin, C. (2018) Internationally educated nurses' competency assessment and registration outcomes. *International Journal of Migration, Health and Social Care*, 14(3): 332–346.

Northouse, P.G. (2016) *Leadership: Theory and Practice* (7th edn). London: Sage.

Nursing and Midwifery Board of Australia (2019a) About. (www.nursingmidwiferyboard.gov.au/About.aspx)

Nursing and Midwifery Board of Australia (2019b) Registration Standards. (www.nursingmidwiferyboard.gov.au/Registration-Standards.aspx)

Nursing and Midwifery Council (2006) *Preceptorship Guidelines* (NMC Circular 21/200: 3 October). London: NMC.

Nursing and Midwifery Council (2008a) Focus Group Consultation Report on Have Your Say on Equality and Diversity. London: NMC.

Nursing and Midwifery Council (2008b) Standards to Support Learning and Assessment in Practice. London: NMC.

Nursing and Midwifery Council (2016a) Revalidation: Your Step-By-Step Guide through the Process. London: NMC.

Nursing and Midwifery Council (2016b) Revalidation: How to Revalidate with the NMC, Requirements for Renewing Your Registration. London: NMC.

Nursing and Midwifery Council (2016c) Advice and Information for Employers of Nurses and Midwives. London: NMC.

Nursing and Midwifery Council (2018a) The Code: Professional Standards of Practice and Behaviour for Nurses, Midwives and Nursing Associates. London: NMC.

Nursing and Midwifery Council (2018b) Future Nurse: Standards of Proficiency for Registered Nurses. London: NMC.

Nursing and Midwifery Council (2018c) Delegation and Accountability: Supplementary Information to the NMC Code. London: NMC.

Nursing and Midwifery Council (2018d) Realising Professionalism: Standards for Education and Training. *Part 1: Standards Framework for Nursing and Midwifery Education.* London: NMC.

Nursing and Midwifery Council (2018e) Realising Professionalism: Standards for Education and Training. *Part 2: Standards for Student Supervision and Assessment.* London: NMC.

Nursing and Midwifery Council (2018f) *Standards for Pre-Registration Nursing Programmes.* London: NMC.

Nursing and Midwifery Council (2018g) Realising Professionalism: Part 3 Standards for Pre-Registration Nursing Programmes. London: NMC.

Nursing and Midwifery Council (2019a) Raising Concerns: Guidance for Nurses, Midwives and Nursing Associates. London: NMC.

Nursing and Midwifery Council (2019b) Revalidation: How to revalidate with the NMC, requirements for renewing your registration. London: NMC.

Nursing and Midwifery Council (2019c) *Guidance on using social media responsibly.* London: NMC.

Nursing and Midwifery Council (2019d) *Standards for Prescribers.* London: NMC.

Nursing and Midwifery Council (2019e) *Guidance on health and character.* London: NMC.

Nursing and Midwifery Council (2020a) Registering as a Nurse or Midwife in the UK: Information for Applicants Trained Outside the European Union (EU) or European Economic Area (EEA). London: NMC.

Nursing and Midwifery Council (2020b) Who we are. London: NMC. Available at: www.nmc.org.uk/about-us/careers/who-we-are/

Nursing and Midwifery Council and General Medical Council (2014) *Openness and Honesty When Things Go Wrong: The Professional Duty of Candour.* London: NMC.

Nursing Now (2018) Our Aims for 2020. (www.nursingnow.org/our-aims/)

Nystrom, S., Dahlberg, J., Hult, H. and Dahlgren, M. (2016) Enacting simulation: A sociomaterial perspective on students' interprofessional collaboration. *Journal of Interprofessional Care,* 30(4): 441–447.

O'Driscoll, M., Allan, H., Liu, L., Corbett, K.S. and Errant, L. (2018) Compassion in practice: Evaluating the awareness, involvement and perceived impact of a national nursing and midwifery strategy amongst healthcare professionals in NHS trusts in England. *Journal of Clinical Nursing*, 27(5–6): e1097–e1109.

OECD (2017) Health at a Glance 2017: OECD Indicators. Paris: OECD Publishing.

Ohr, S.O., Holm, D. and Brazil, S. (2016) The transition of overseas qualified nurses and midwives into the Australian healthcare workforce. *Australian Journal of Advanced Nursing*, 34(2): 27–36.

Ong, G.L. (2013) Using final placements to prepare student nurses. *Nursing Times*, 109(3): 12–14.

Ortega, J., Mitchell, E.M. and Peragallo, N. (2016) Beyond borders: Global nursing education for the future. *Nursing Education Perspectives*, 37(4): 227–229.

Ortiga, Y.Y. and Rivero, J.A. (2019) Bodies of work: Skilling at the bottom of the global nursing care chain. *Globalizations*, 16(7): 1–14.

Orupabo, J. (2018) Cultural stereotypes and professional self-socialisation in the transition from education to work. *Journal of Education and Work*, 31(3): 234–246.

Oxtoby, K. (2015) Making the most of complaints. *Nursing Standard*, 29(47): 64.

Pendleton, D. and Furnham, A.F. (2016) *Leadership: All You Need to Know* (2nd edn). London: Springer Nature.

Pepin, J., Dubois, S., Girard, F., Tardif, J. and Ha, L. (2011) A cognitive learning model of clinical nursing leadership. *Nurse Education Today*, 31(3): 268–273.

Philip, S., Manias, E. and Woodward-Kron, R. (2015) Nursing educator perspectives of overseas qualified nurses' intercultural clinical communication: Barriers, enablers and engagement strategies. *Journal of Clinical Nursing*, 24(17–18): 2628–2637.

Phillips, C., Esterman, A. and Kenny, A. (2015) The theory of organisational socialisation and its potential for improving transition experiences for new graduate nurses. *Nurse Education Today*, 35(1): 118–124.

Phillips, J.M. (2020) Strategies to promote student engagement and active learning. In Billings, D.M. and Halstead, J.A. (eds), *Teaching In Nursing: A Guide For Faculty* (6th edn; ebook). St Louis, MO: Elsevier.

Pidgeon, K. (2017) The keys for success: Leadership core competencies. *Journal of Trauma Nursing*, 24(6): 338–341.

Pishghadam, R. and Shayesteh, S. (2014) Neuro-linguistic programming (NLP) for language teachers: Revalidation of an NLP scale. *Theory and Practice in Language Studies*, 4(10): 2096–2104.

Presado, M., Colaco, S., Rafael, H., Baixinho, C., Felix, I., Saraiva, C. and Rebelo, I. (2018) Learning with high fidelity simulation. *Ciencia and Saude Coletiva*, 23(1): 51–59.

Prescott, M. and Nichter, M. (2014) Transnational nurse migration: Future directions for medical anthropological research. *Social Science and Medicine*, 107: 113–123.

Prime Minister's Commission (2010) Front Line Care: The Future of Nursing and Midwifery in England – Report of the Prime Minister's Commission on the Future of Nursing and Midwifery in England 2010. London: HMSO.

Pugh, W.T.G. (1944) *Practical Nursing Including Hygiene and Dietetics* (4th edn). London: Blackwood and Sons.

Quality Assurance Agency for Higher Education (2008) The Framework for Higher Education Qualifications for England, Wales and Northern Ireland. Gloucester: QAA.

Race, P. (2015) The Lecturer's Toolkit: A Practical Guide to Assessment, Learning and Teaching (4th edn). London: Routledge.

Rao, M.S. (2013) Soft leadership: A new direction to leadership. *Industrial and Commercial Training*, 45(3): 143–149.

Regulation and Quality Improvement Authority, Mental Health and Learning Disability Directorate (2014) *Awareness and Use of Restrictive Practices in Mental Health and Learning Disability Hospitals*. Belfast: RQIA.

Richards, S. and Mughal, A.F. (2006) *Working with the Mental Capacity Act 2005*. North Waltham: Matrix Training Associates.

Roberts, M. (2016) A critical analysis of the failure of nurses to raise concerns about poor patient care. *Nursing Philosophy*, 18: 3.

Rogers, A., Kennedy, A., Nelson, E. and Robinson, A. (2005) Uncovering the limits of patient-centeredess: Implementing a self-management trial for chronic illness. *Qualitative Health Research*, 15(2): 224–239.

Rogers, C.R. and Freiberg, H.J. (1994) *Freedom to Learn* (3rd edn). New York, Toronto: Merrill.

Rosa, W. (2017) Public health nursing and transnational agendas: Local to global health advocacy. *Public Health Nursing*, 34(3): 197–199.

Rossler, K.L., Hardin, K., Hernandez-Leveille, M. and Wright, K. (2018) Newly licensed nurses' perceptions on transitioning into hospital practice with simulation-based education. *Nurse Education in Practice*, 33: 154–158.

Royal College of Nursing (2004) *The Future Nurse: The RCN Vision*. London: RCN.

Royal College of Nursing (2016) RCN Factsheet: Continuing Professional Development (CPD) for Nurses Working in the United Kingdom (UK). London: RCN.

Royal College of Nursing (2017a) *Safe and Effective Staffing: The Real Picture* (UK Policy Report). London: RCN.

Royal College of Nursing (2017b) *Raising Concerns*. London: RCN.

Royal College of Nursing (2017c) Three Steps to Positive Practice: A Rights-Based Approach when Considering and Reviewing the Use of Restrictive Interventions. London: RCN.

Royal College of Nursing (2018) Principles of Nursing Practice: Eight Principles that Apply to all Nursing Staff and Nursing Students in any Care Setting. (www.rcn.org.uk/professional-development/principles-of-nursing-practice)

Royal College of Nursing (2020) Guidance for members: Refusal to treat due to lack of adequate PPE during the pandemic (www.rcn.org.uk/-/media/royal-college-of-nursing/documents/publications/2020/april/009-231.pdf?la=en)

Royal Pharmaceutical Society (2019) Professional Guidance on the Administration of Medicines in Healthcare Settings. (www.rpharms.com/recognition/setting-professional-standards/safe-and-secure-handling-of-medicines/professional-guidance-on-the-safe-and-secure-handling-of-medicines)

Sasso, L., Bagnasco, A., Catania, G., Zanini, M., Aleo, G. and Watson, R. (2019) Push and pull factors of nurses' intention to leave. *Journal of Nursing Management*, 27(5): 946–954.

Savage, J. and Moore, L. (2004) *Interpreting Accountability*. Oxford: Royal College of Nursing Institute.

Scheckel, M. (2020) Designing courses and learning experiences. In Billings, D.M. and Halstead, J.A. (eds), *Teaching in Nursing: A Guide for Faculty* (6th edn; ebook). St Louis, MO: Elsevier.

Schilgen, B., Nienhaus, A., Handtke, O., Schulz, H. and Moèsko, M. (2017) Health situation of migrant and minority nurses: A systematic review. *Plos One*, 12(6): e0179183.

Schroyer, C.C., Zellers, R. and Abraham, S. (2016) Increasing registered nurse retention using mentors in critical care services. *Health Care Manager*, 35(3): 251–265.

Scully, N. (2015) Leadership in nursing: The importance of recognising inherent values and attributes to secure a positive future for the profession. *Collegian*, 22(4): 439–444.

Shaffer, F., Bakhshi, M., Farrell, N. and Álvarez, T. (2019) The role of nurses in advancing the objectives of the global compacts for migration and on refugees. *Nursing Administration Quarterly*, 43(1): 10–18.

Sherman, R.O., Chiang-Hanisko, L. and Koszalinski, R. (2013) The ageing nursing workforce: A global challenge. *Journal of Nursing Management*, 21(7): 899–902.

Silvestre, J., Ulrich, B., Johnson, T., Spector, N. and Blegen, M. (2017) A multisite study on a new graduate registered nurse transition to practice program: Return on investment. *Nursing Economics*, 35(3): 110–118.

Sinclair, A. (1995) The chameleon of accountability: Forms and discourses. *Accounting, Organisations and Society*, 20(2–3): 219–237.

Sinclair, P.M., Levett-Jones, T., Morris, A., Carter, B., Bennett, P.N. and Kable, A. (2017) High engagement, high quality: A guiding framework for developing empirically informed asynchronous e-learning programs for health professional educators. *Nursing and Health Sciences*, 19(1): 126–137.

Singapore Nursing Board (2019a) SNB Functions. (www.health professionals.gov.sg/snb/about-snb/snb-functions)

Singapore Nursing Board (2019b) Foreign Trained Nurses/Midwives. (www.healthprofessionals.gov.sg/snb/registration-enrolment/application-for-registration-enrolment/foreign-trained-nurses-midwives)

Slate, K.A., Stavarski, D.H., Romig, B.J. and Thacker, K.S. (2018) Longitudinal study: Transformed onboarding nurse graduates. *Journal for Nurses in Professional Development*, 34(2): 92–98.

Smith, C. (2001) Trust and confidence: Possibilities for social work in 'high modernity'. *British Journal of Social Work*, 31: 287–305.

Speakman, E. (2020) Interprofessional education and collaborative practice. In Billings, D.M. and Halstead, J.A. (eds), *Teaching in Nursing: A Guide For Faculty* (6th edn; ebook). St Louis, MO: Elsevier.

Speedy, S. (2015) Psychological influences in leadership style. In Daly, J., Speedy, S. and Jackson, D. (2015) *Leadership and Nursing: Contemporary Perspectives* (2nd edn). Sydney: Churchill Livingstone/Elsevier.

Stein-Parbury, J. (2018) *Patient and Person: Interpersonal Skills in Nursing* (6th edn). Chatswood, NSW: Elsevier.

Stephens, T.M. (2013) Nursing student resilience: A concept clarification. *Nursing Forum*, 48(2): 125–133.

Stevens, K. and Duffy, E.A. (2017) A toolkit for nursing clinical instructors. *Teaching and Learning in Nursing*, 12(2): 170–172.

Stevens, K., Engh, E.P., Tubbs-Cooley, H., Conley, D.M., Cupit, T., D'Errico, E. and Withycombe, J.S. (2017) Operational failures detected by frontline acute care nurses: Operational failures in frontline nursing. *Research in Nursing and Health*, 40(3): 197–205.

Stirling, B.V. (2017) Results of a study assessing teaching methods of faculty after measuring student learning style preference. *Nurse Education Today*, 55: 107–111.

Sullivan, D.T. (2020) An introduction to curriculum development. In Billings, D.M. and Halstead, J.A. (eds), *Teaching In Nursing: A Guide For Faculty* (6th edn; ebook). St Louis, MO: Elsevier.

Suresh, P., Matthews, A. and Coyne, I. (2012) Stress and stressors in the clinical environment: A comparative study of fourth-year student nurses and newly qualified nurses in Ireland. *Journal of Clinical Nursing*, 22: 770–779.

Talbot-Smith, A. and Pollock, A. (2006) *The New NHS: A Guide*. Oxford: Routledge.

Taylor, G. and Hawley, H. (2010) *Key Debates in Health Care*. Maidenhead: Open University Press.

The Patients' Association (2009) NHS Constitution. (www.patients-association.org.uk/News/254)

Thompson, G. and Glasø, L. (2015) Situational leadership theory: A test from three perspectives. *Leadership and Organization Development Journal*, 36(5): 527–544.

Tingle, J. and Cribb, A. (2013) *Nursing Law and Ethics* (4th edn). Oxford: Blackwell.

Townsend, K., Wilkinson, A. and Kellner, A. (2015) Opening the black box in nursing work and management practice: The role of ward managers. *Journal of Nursing Management*, 23(2): 211–220.

Transforming Care and Commissioning Steering Group (2014) Winterbourne View – Time for a Change: Transforming the Commissioning of Services for People with Learning Disabilities and/or Autism. (www.england.nhs.uk/wp-content/uploads/2014/11/transforming-commissioning-services.pdf)

Truss, C., Mankin, D. and Kelliher, C. (2012) *Strategic Human Resource Management*. Oxford: Oxford University Press.

Tyndall, D.E., Firnhaber, G.C. and Scott, E.S. (2018) The impact of new graduate nurse transition programs on competency development and patient safety. *Advances in Nursing Science*, 41(4): e26–e52.

United Kingdom Central Council for Nursing, Midwifery and Health Visiting (1986) *Project 2000: A New Preparation for Practice*. London: UKCC.

United Nations (2015) Sustainable Development Goals. (www.un.org/sustainabledevelopment/sustainable-development-goals/)

Unsworth, J., Melling, A., Tuffnell, C. and Allan, J. (2016) Improving performance amongst nursing students through the discovery of discrepancies during simulation. *Nurse Education in Practice*, 16(1): 47–53.

van Camp, J. and Chappy, S. (2017) The effectiveness of nurse residency programs on retention: A systematic review. *AORN Journal*, 106(2): 128–144.

van den Broek, D. and Groutsis, D. (2017) Global nursing and the lived experience of migration intermediaries. *Work, Employment and Society*, 31(5): 851–860.

van Rooyen, D.R., Jordan, P.J., ten Ham-Baloyi, W. and Caka, E.M. (2018) A comprehensive literature review of guidelines facilitating transition of newly graduated nurses to professional nurses. *Nurse Education in Practice*, 30: 35–41.

Vardaman, S.A. and Mastel-Smith, B. (2016) The transitions of international nursing students. *Teaching and Learning in Nursing*, 11(2): 34–43.

Verret, G. and Lin, V. (2016) Easing the transition: An innovative generational approach to peer mentoring for new graduate nurses. *Journal of Pediatric Nursing*, 31(6): 745–756.

Waite, M. (ed.) (2012) *Concise Oxford English Dictionary* (7th edn). Oxford: Oxford University Press.

Watson, J. (2019) Nursing's global covenant with humanity: Unitary caring science as sacred activism. *Journal of Advanced Nursing*, 76(2): 699–704.

Watson, R. (1992) Justifying your practice. *Nursing*, 5(3): 11–13.

Weiss, S.A. and Tappen, R.M. (2015) *Essentials of Nursing Leadership and Management* (6th edn). Philadelphia, PA: F.A. Davis Company.

Welch, E. (2018) *The NHS at 70: A Living History.* Barnsley: Pen and Sword Books.

West, D. (2014) Patient choice is not key to improving performance says Hunt. *Health Service Journal*, 26 November. (www.hsj.co.uk/acute-care/exclusive-patient-choice-is-not-key-to-improving-performance-says-hunt/5077051.article)

Whitehead, B., Owen, P., Holmes, D., Beddingham, E., Simmons, M., Henshaw, L. and Walker, C. (2013) Supporting newly qualified nurses in the UK: A systematic literature review. *Nurse Education Today*, 33(4): 370–377.

Wilkes, Z., Joyce, L. and Edmond, L. (2013) *Nursing and Mentorship: Survival Guide.* New York: Routledge.

Williams, F.S., Scott, E.S., Tyndall, D.E. and Swanson, M. (2018) New nurse graduate residency mentoring: A retrospective cross-sectional research study of nurse residency programs. *Nursing Economics*, 36(3): 121.

Williamson, G., Jenkinson, T. and Proctor-Childs, T. (2008) *Nursing in Contemporary Healthcare Practice.* Exeter: Learning Matters.

Willmott, A. (2010) Consent and confidentiality. In Redsell, S. and Hastings, A. (eds), *Listening to Children and Young People in Healthcare Consultations.* Oxford: Radcliffe Publishing

Wilson, L., Mendes, I.A.C., Klopper, H., Catrambone, C., Al-Maaitah, R., Norton, M.E. and Hill, M. (2016) 'Global health' and 'global nursing': Proposed definitions from the global advisory panel on the future of nursing. *Journal of Advanced Nursing*, 72(7): 1529–1540.

Wilson, T., Weathers, N. and Forneris, L. (2018) Evaluation of outcomes from an online nurse residency program. *Journal of Nursing Administration*, 48(10): 495–501.

Wiseman, A. and Horton, K. (2011) Developing clinical scenarios from a European perspective: Successes and challenges. *Nurse Education Today*, 31(7): 677–681.

Wlodkowski, R.J. and Ginsberg, M.B. (2017) *Enhancing Adult Motivation to Learn: A Comprehensive Guide for Teaching all Adults* (4th edn). San Francisco, CA: Jossey-Bass.

Wong, C. and Giallonardo, L. (2015) Leadership and its influence on patient outcomes. In Daly, J., Speedy, S. and Jackson, D. (eds), *Leadership and Nursing: Contemporary Perspectives* (2nd edn). Sydney: Churchill Livingstone/Elsevier.

Wong, C.A., Cummings, G.G. and Ducharme, L. (2013) The relationship between nursing leadership and patient outcomes: A systematic review update. *Journal of Nursing Management*, 21(5): 709–724.

Wong, F.K.Y., Liu, H., Wang, H., Anderson, D., Seib, C. and Molasiotis, A. (2015) Global nursing issues and development: Analysis of world health organization documents. *Journal of Nursing Scholarship*, 47(6): 574–583.

Wood, J., Weisner, R., Morrison, R., Zeffane, R., Fromholtz, M., Factor, A., McKeown, T., Schermerhorn, J., Hunt, J. and Osborn, R. (2016) *Organisational Behaviour: Core Concepts and Applications* (4th Australasian edn). Milton, QLD: Wiley.

World Health Organisation (2016) Global Strategic Directions for Strengthening Nursing and Midwifery 2016–2020. Geneva: WHO.

Young, L.E. and Maxwell, B. (2007) Student-centred teaching in nursing: From rote to active learning. In Young, L.E. and Patterson, B.L. (eds), *Teaching Nursing: Developing a Student-Centered Learning Environment.* Philadelphia, PA: Lippincott, Williams and Wilkins.

INDEX

NOTE: Page numbers in *italic* type refer to figures and tables.